Fremantle Hospital

A SOCIAL HISTORY TO 1987

'. . . an institution belonging to the people and for the people . . .'
Evening Mail, 21 August 1909

'It is perhaps not out of place to state that the Fremantle Hospital occupies a very important position in the Community, and its name and objects have become familiar to everyone in the District.'
Fremantle Hospital
Annual Report for Year Ended 30 June 1942

'The Fremantle Hospital continues to enjoy the respect of the Community it serves . . .'
Fremantle Hospital
Annual Report for Year Ended 30 June 1983

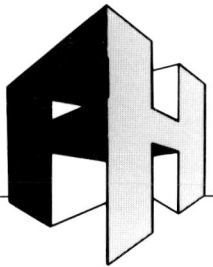

Fremantle Hospital

A SOCIAL HISTORY TO 1987

Phyl Garrick and Chris Jeffery

PUBLISHED BY FREMANTLE HOSPITAL, WESTERN AUSTRALIA, 1987

First published in 1987
by Fremantle Hospital
Alma Street, Fremantle, Western Australia 6160

All enquiries should be directed to above address.

National Library of Australia
Cataloguing-in-Publication data

Garrick, Phyl, 1943- .
    Fremantle Hospital.

    Bibliography.
    Includes index.
    ISBN 0 7316 1196 9.
    ISBN 0 7316 1212 4 (pbk.).

    1. Fremantle Hospital—History. 2. Hospitals—
    Western Australia—Fremantle—History.
    I. Jeffery, Chris, 1926- . II. Fremantle
    Hospital.   III. Title.

362.1'1'099411

Photoset by University of Western Australia Press, Nedlands, W.A.
Printed by Frank Daniels Pty Ltd, Perth, Western Australia.
Bound by Printers Trade Services, Belmont, Western Australia.

Contents

List of Figures and Plates

FIGURES

PLATES

CONVERSION TABLE

Imperial	Metric
one ounce (oz.)	28.35 grams (g)
one pound (lb.)	0.454 kilograms (kg)
one ton	1.016 tonnes (t)
one gallon	4.546 litres (l)
one pint	0.568 litres (l)
one inch	2.54 centimetres (cm)
one foot (feet or ft)	0.305 metre (m)
one yard	0.914 metre (m)
one mile	1.609 kilometres (km)
one acre	0.405 hectare (ha)

Monetary

one pound (£1)	two dollars ($2)
ten shillings (10s)	one dollar ($1)
one penny	one cent (1c)
one guinea (£1 1s 0d)	$2.10

Acknowledgements

It is true, as Jenny Carter points out in *Bassendean: A Social History 1829–1979*, that 'the totality of the past cannot be recreated', but like Lucy Snowe in Charlotte Bronte's *Villette,*

> ... I got books, read up the facts, laboriously constructed a skeleton out of the dry bones of the real, and then clothed them, and tried to breathe into them life, and in this last aim I had pleasure ... it was a difficult and anxious time till my facts were found, selected, and properly jointed ...

Many people have contributed to the clothing of the dry bones of this history. Without the laboriously hand-written records and reports of early secretaries and matrons of the hospital, in huge leather-bound volumes that are now musty with age, there would be little understanding of the hospital's past. The enthusiasm of Olga Hedemann, Roy Marshall and Peter Smith until his retirement, as Director of Nursing, Administrator and Medical Superintendent, respectively, have been infectious and their support and that of the Board, unstinting. The staffs at Fremantle Hospital Library and the Battye Library, especially Cheryl Hamill and Teresa Ives at the former and Tom Reynolds and Robin South at the latter have been unfailingly helpful, and no request for information at the Fremantle City Library was ever too much trouble for Larraine Stevens. The warmth and co-operation of Fremantle Hospital staff, past and present, will always be remembered—that of Pat Pettit, Kay Bolton, Yvonne Gowegati, Lindy Pratt and the staff on Level 6, in particular. For Judith Lancaster's research assistance and her support, despite routine nursing administration duties and her responsibility for the production of a historical pageant to mark the final graduation of nurses from Fremantle Hospital, we are deeply appreciative. For use of material, we are indebted to the Health Department of Western Australia, the Building Management Authority, the Master of the Supreme Court of Western Australia and staff at the Dixon Gallery at the Mitchell Library, Sydney. For the excellent mapwork illustrations by David Peake of Centagraph in Fremantle; Vic Greaves, Susannah Crowe, Ray Firkin and other production staff at the University of Western Australia Press who have generously and gently shared their wisdom and experience; until her recent resignation, Noelle McGlew, who typed most of the manuscript, and Daphne Pyke and Carolyn Burdge who completed it—to all these people, sincere thanks are due. For Tom Stannage's valued encouragement and support and his reading of the manuscript, we are especially grateful. We were two of many students at the University of Western Australia who, through his teaching, became aware of the richness of Western Australia's past.

Perhaps the most exciting historical aspect of Fremantle Hospital's 90th anniversary celebrations is the bank of oral history interviews being compiled which flesh the dry bones of statistics and routine reports as few other historical sources can. When completed, Chris Jeffery's interviews of a cross-section of people connected with the hospital—from doctors to domestics, an orderly, an engineer, a seamstress, patients, pharmacists, a plumber, teacher, carpenter, nurses, administrators and board members—will be an invaluable record of Fremantle Hospital's past. There will be fifty interviews, recorded on 150 tapes. The tapes and transcripts, will be lodged at the hospital's library, and at the Battye Library. Transcripts will also be available at Fremantle City Council Library. These will be a source of enjoyment and knowledge for people in decades and perhaps centuries to come. In conception and execution it is a brilliant project, unequalled by any individual institution anywhere in Australia. We thank the many who have willingly shared their recollections.

We are grateful to Kath Grimshaw and Fremantle-trained nurses for information, photographs and enthusiasm which so many have shared. Some even took time to complete detailed questionnaires. It was a privilege to attend two of the Fremantle Hospital Ex-trainee Nurses' Association annual dinners, and from the conversation there, came a real appreciation of Fremantle Hospital as it was in the past.

Special appreciation for their encouragement is also extended to the Tangs, the Skidmores, to Tom Garrick, the Rays and the Stewarts. Nor would this list be complete without Shanon, Tom, Kailie, sons-in-law Richard and Kevin, and especially Debbie and Sheri, who have understood, co-operated and endured.

Preface

When, in 1856, Captain Henderson, as Comptroller-General of the Convict Establishment in Western Australia, erected his two-storeyed home in Fremantle, little did he realise that it would develop into Fremantle Hospital. Captain Henderson called his home 'The Knowle', which he occupied until his return to England in 1863.

In addition to Captain Henderson, 'The Knowle' also became a residence for the Comptroller of Customs, Mr Clifton, until 1892 when it became a branch of the Fremantle Lunatic Asylum, now the Fremantle Museum, Finnerty Street, Fremantle.

With a grant of £1,500 from the Colonial Secretary, alterations were commenced in 1895 to convert 'The Knowle' into a Cottage Hospital and the Knowle/Fremantle Hospital was 'born' and opened with 52 beds in January, 1897.

Over the past 90 years there have been many changes to Fremantle Hospital although, through foresight, the original 'Knowle' building is largely the same today as it was when constructed in 1856.

In the 90 years of its existence as a hospital many persons have shaped its destiny. It is mainly the contribution of these persons that has been captured and placed on record for future generations by Phyllis Garrick and Chris Jeffery in this publication.

H. W. OLNEY
Chairman
Board of Management Fremantle Hospital

Foreword

This is the shortest foreword I have prepared. It is so out of respect to the Hospital's administrators, staff and patients, past and present; and from an unwillingness to impinge on their story so brilliantly told. A place, and a people of consequence indeed.

Fremantle Hospital is an institution which belongs to the community of Fremantle and which works for the people of Fremantle, and for visitors, often maritime, to the town. The history of Fremantle Hospital is a mirror to the commercial and social history of Western Australia. So how should its 'history' be written? Vibrantly, insightfully, sensitively, and based on wide reading and listening and deep research. It should be written as Phyllis Garrick and Chris Jeffery have written it in *Fremantle Hospital: A Social History to 1987*.

TOM STANNAGE
Associate Professor
Department of History
The University of Western Australia

ABBREVIATIONS

ANUP	Australian National Universtiy Press
ATNA	Australian Trained Nurses Association
BC	Building Committee
BL	Battye Library (State Reference Library of Western Australia)
BM	Board of Management, Fremantle Hospital
BMA	British Medical Association
CSD	Central Sterilising Department
CSO	Colonial Secretary's Office Records
FACP	Fremantle Arts Centre Press
FH	Fremantle Hospital
FLBH	Fremantle Local Board of Health
FMC	Fremantle Municipal Council
FCL	Fremantle City Library
HC	House Committee
MUP	Melbourne University Press
OUP	Oxford University Press
PHD	Public Health Department
PWD	Public Works Department
RMO	Resident Medical Officer
RPH	Royal Perth Hospital
RWAHS	*Early Days, Journal of the Royal Western Australian Historical Society*
SRMO	Senior Resident Medical Officer
UQP	University of Queensland Press
UWAP	University of Western Australia Press
VD	Venereal Disease
WAIG	*Western Australian Industrial Gazette*
WAPD	*Western Australian Parliamentary Debates*
WAVP	*Votes and Proceedings of the Western Australian Parliament*

Introduction

In 1973, Athol Thomas in the *West Australian* attempted to define the distinct identity of Fremantle, and not surprisingly, found the task difficult. 'The Fremantle feeling', he perceptively wrote, 'must be a synthesis of the whole—the shape of the city, its blues and greens and tawny yellows, the textures of its walls and its people, its history, its sounds and smells.' Fremantle Hospital, with its own very strong sense of identity, is an integral part of the town's history, and the 'Fremantle feeling' permeates the history of the hospital. The story of a hospital is a record of building and progress, but it is also a focus through which many aspects of a society may be explored. Community attitudes to poverty, to women, and to work can be isolated; the influence of technology, the effect of public health conditions and the changes they generate, medical discoveries and their application—all are aspects of a hospital's past. Social distinctions can be revealed, the medical hierachy observed, and the politics of power both at the level of the hospital and in relation to state and federal medical services, can be examined. Although a hospital may 'start' at a particular time, its foundations are firmly grounded in early medical services, and the forces which have brought about the establishment of the institution. Because it is a general hospital history, the focus on particular areas can only be brief and often frustratingly cursory. Each decade, each area, could be a study in its own right.

Perth is fortunate. The histories of most of its major public hospitals have been considered important enough to be written. That of Royal Perth Hospital by Geoffrey Bolton and Prue Joske was published in 1982. Prue Joske proceeded to write the history of King Edward Memorial Hospital (yet to be published) and Carolyn Polizzotto has been commissioned to compile a short history of Sir Charles Gairdner Hospital. Only the history of Princess Margaret Hospital for Children remains unwritten. When laid side by side, these studies will cast more light on Perth's medical and social history.

Until recent years, those who tended patients in Fremantle Hospital, lived in homes provided on or near the hospital site, ate in hospital dining rooms, talked about hospital affairs, and often took their recreation together, albeit usually in different work-related groups. In effect, the hospital became a close, supportive, loyal community within the local community. Because it was a comparatively small hospital and everyone knew each other; because many of the staff in all areas tended to stay—often for decades or even for a life work-span—because some patients

1

came, and brought their children and were followed by their grandchildren, a strong loyalty to the hospital developed. At best, the history of Fremantle Hospital is a history of people—those who came as patients, those who administered it, and those who worked within its precincts.

This is their story.

Chapter I

'... but for the natural ills which flesh is heir to,
there would seem no apparent provision.'
West Australian, 19 May 1886.

When Captain Charles Fremantle, under instruction to take possession of the 'Western Coast of New Holland', first set out to examine the Swan River on 2 May 1829, Aborigines on both sides of the river gathered in concern and '... halloo'd ... very loud ... "Warra Warra"'. Perhaps they sensed the ill that would come with these strange, pale invaders. The gestures and the menace in the cries effectively bridged a gaping cultural difference centuries of experience wide, and Fremantle had little doubt that the message was to 'go away'.[1]

For 40,000 years Aborigines had lived in harmony with the land, learning their place in relation to it and each other and becoming aware of the secrets of its ability to heal. Although Captain Fremantle noted that some Aborigines were 'affected with bad eyes',[2] it had become common tribal knowledge that medicines and applications could be prepared from plants and used with effect in both sickness and injury. In time, members of different Aboriginal tribes became recognized as doctors to their communities and their specialised abilities were passed on from generation to generation through male lines. These unique skills extended beyond the tangible elements of the land to realms of the spirit. The patient was nursed in a known, familiar environment close to kin and friends, and treatment was based on a shared faith between patient and doctor.[3]

This treatment seemed strange to the new settlers. Thomas Dodds wrote from Cobham, near Toodyay, to a friend in England in 1839, of a sick Aboriginal woman for whom 'the doctor or charmer' was sent:

> He commenced by placing one foot on the body of the woman, pressing very hard, in order to dislodge the snake which they suppose to have entered the body of the afflicted ... After using a variety of incantations, which he concluded by biting the part affected, making the patient believe that he has succeeded in drawing the snake out ... he goes round the company to find two persons willing to receive the said snake between them, which he pretends he is carrying in his mouth ...[4]

[1] Lord Cottesloe (ed.), *Diary and Letters of Admiral Sir C. H. Fremantle, G.C.B.*, 1979, pp. 37, 41.
[2] *Ibid.*, p. 54.
[3] See D. Gray, 'Traditional Medicine on the Carnarvon Aboriginal Reserve', in R. and C. Berndt (eds), *Aborigines of the West. Their Past and Their Present*, 1979, pp. 169–83. Includes useful list of related literature. See also J. Hagger, *Australian Colonial Medicine*, 1979, pp. 15–30.
[4] E. D. Cowan, 'Letters of Early Settlers', RWAHS, Vol. 1, Part 1, 1927, p. 57.

At the place which became known as Fremantle, where river and sea merged in sheets of spray across a bar of sand, Aborigines spent their springs and summers foraging and feasting.[5] Here as elsewhere, a native healer treated his people.

While their knowledge was often effective for wounds of the body and soul, a greater power than that held by either European or Aboriginal healers would have been needed to reverse the effects of diseases introduced by the encroachers. In the first decades of white settlement, whooping cough, venereal diseases, cholera, tuberculosis, influenza, and later measles, culled the Aboriginal population and no medicine could stay the carnage. It seemed, as one old survivor explained, 'Meenya Janga bomungur—the smell of the white man kills us'.[6]

The white men arrived ill-equipped for either settlement or the practice of medicine. One of the tents that mushroomed on the beach at Garden Island following Captain James Stirling's ignominious landing on a sandbank at Cockburn Sound on 1 June 1829, belonged to the young colonial surgeon, Dr Charles Simmons. The frail canvas membrane that protected the doctor from the directness of the elements served as hospital, surgery and home for the four months until September, when the colonial surgeon moved to the new capital of Perth. There another temporary hospital was pegged, which opened as it was needed, until a more sturdy room was rented in a hut in the wet winter of 1830. For over 20 years, stop gap measures were taken to provide hospital accommodation at Perth (including the conversion of stables into a sick ward), until a building specifically designed for the purpose was erected on a site between Goderich and Wellington Streets in mid-1855. In this new two-storey brick and shingle building, Dr John Ferguson, as the colonial surgeon, treated the indigent sick of mind and body alongside accident victims.[7] Citizens of means, however, usually avoided the stigma of hospital treatment which had been provided for the needy, and were treated by a doctor and nursed in their own homes.

In the three years following proclamation in 1829, over 1,500 men, women and their children arrived in Swan River Colony and many were allocated farmland abutting rivers, or town lots which had to be speedily surveyed. Some of these settlers were farmers, generally arriving unprepared to cultivate in conditions very different to those in England; some were their servants, and others administrators. Ten who arrived and stayed were doctors—all men with medical experience of some kind. Charles Garrett M.D., as the surgeon of the *Lotus* on her long journey to the new colony, had served as a shop-boy for a chemist and druggist and knew as little about bleeding or operating as the seafarers he was called on to treat.[8] The others had been apprenticed to doctors and received training in British hospitals and universities.

Two of the ten men treating colonists in Western Australia with Garrett between 1829 and 1832 were a private practitioner named Thomas Harrison, and William

[5] S. O'Connor and R. Thomson, 'Report into the Aboriginal Heritage of the Arthur Head Area, Fremantle City Council', June 1984.

[6] Monnop, last of the Victoria district men to Daisy Bates, cited in N. Green, 'Aborigines and White Settlers in Nineteenth Century', in C. T. Stannage (ed.), *A New History of Western Australia*, 1981, p. 119. See also pp. 118–21.

[7] See P. Joske, 'Health and Hospital: A Study of Community Welfare in Western Australia 1829–55', MA thesis, UWA, 1973; G. C.Bolton and P. Joske, *History of Royal Perth Hospital*, 1982, pp. 3–17.

[8] I. Berryman (ed.), *A Colony Detailed. The First Census of Western Australia 1832*, 1979, p. 165.

Milligan, a last-minute replacement for Dr Tully Daly, who had drowned at Cape Town on the voyage out. Drs J. Lyttleton and Nicholas Langley arrived with Peel's disastrous expedition[9] to South Rockingham in 1829, while John Whatley combined medicine and farming at Bayswater. Charles Simmons was the first colonial surgeon, for which he received 15 shillings a day. There was also Alexander Collie, who would succeed Simmons in his appointment and who shared a deep friendship with the Aborigine, Mokare, before both men died—one from 'a kind of influenza', the other from tuberculosis. Alfred Green went to Augusta before his appointment as the assistant surgeon to the Colonial Hospital in 1830, the year that George Cowcher, describing himself as 'Apothecary and Agriculturalist', arrived in the colony. Dr Davidson, an assistant surgeon who accompanied the 21st Fusiliers, also practised in the colony for a while in 1833.[10]

Despite the fact that there were few providing medical care in the far-settled colony, three of the 157 buried in the 'new' land in the first three years were doctors. The portly 42-year-old Garrett was discovered standing upright just under the surface of the Swan at Perth, after he failed to ford the river which effectively cut the new settlement in two.[11] His death in 1829 was one of the first recorded in the colony and a reminder that mortality was just as much a part of the human condition in this supposed Arcadia as anywhere else. A year later, John Whatley kissed his wife Ann goodbye before he set out down-river for Fremantle to buy a cow to supplement the small array of stock on their 1,000-acre grant. Although he was used to travelling by both foot and boat to treat the patients requiring his services, the doctor chose to travel by the faster means to get the cow home. It was an unfortunate decision and the colonist Joseph Hardey sadly recorded in his diary that September night:

> Dr. Whatley and Capt. Jones was drowned in crossing the Ferry at Fremantle, they foolishly put a beast into the Boat, and it brought it over and it is supposed they were both disabled . . .[12]

At that time, when a semblance of English propriety, order and prosperity was being wrested from the alien conditions of Swan River Colony, the loss of a precious cow could be a blow, the death of a husband a tragedy, but the loss of a man versed in healing was also disastrous. The deprivation was increased in 1831, when Charles Simmons died suddenly at the age of only 28 years.[13]

As settlement thrust outwards from the centre of administration in Perth to areas such as the Leschenault district, King George Sound, Augusta and the fertile Avon Valley, access to doctors by many colonists was increasingly reduced.[14] The problem

9   C. T. Stannage, *The People of Perth: A Social History of Western Australia's Capital City*, 1979, pp. 20–2; A. Hasluck, *Thomas Peel of Swan River*, 1965.
10 See B. C. Cohen, *A History of Medicine in Western Australia*, 1965. See also Bolton and Joske, *History of Royal Perth Hospital*; *Dictionary of Western Australians 1829–1914*, Vol. 1.
11 Berryman, *A Colony Detailed*, p. 165.
12 Diary of Joseph Hardey, 21 January 1830–16 November 1839. (Battye Library Acc. No. 466.)
13 Bolton and Joske, *History of Royal Perth Hospital*, p. 6.
14 This was different from Victoria where by the 1850s, before the discovery of gold, so many doctors had arrived that the profession was glutted. See K. S. Inglis, *Hospital and Community: A History of the Royal Melbourne Hospital*, 1958, p. 30.

continued into the twentieth century, as new regions such as the goldfields, the pastoral districts of the north and the wheatbelt to the east were settled. It was different at Fremantle. Situated at the mouth of the Swan River, which connected Perth with the ships that brought settlers, vital stores and mail on the four-month journey from England, Fremantle was settled quickly and its inhabitants benefited by the attendance of a trained doctor from 1829 onward.

Of the passengers on the third ship to arrive at Swan River Colony by the end of August 1829, one was listed as Dr Thomas Harrison. Like other excited immigrants on the *Marquis of Anglesea* who watched the welcome smudge of land take the shape of sand hills and clumps of trees, his excitement soon turned to dismay. Passengers and their possessions, stock, cargo—all had to be loaded from the sailing ship into small rowing boats able to skim the treacherous shoals. They landed anywhere on the coast between Arthur Head at Fremantle, and Cottesloe to the north. New arrivals pitched tents on beaches, built makeshift huts, which in some cases looked little different from humpies, and dragged furniture and stores into windbreaks to shelter from the winter rain and winds that howled in from the sea. Unsecured canvas flapped and cracked in storms that sometimes beached ships. Fine Fremantle sand was hurled into eyes and ears and penetrated food and bedding and crevices wherever they occurred.[15]

Although most settlers were waiting for farming land to be plotted and allocated to them, John Septimus Roe was ordered by Captain James Stirling to first survey the towns of Perth and Fremantle. By 18 September 1829, the contours of the Port of Fremantle had been shaped across and around the promontory jutting west into the Indian Ocean. As Cliff Street linked the ocean landing site at South Bay with the northern river jetty from which boats and barges sailed up to Perth, it was the route which all new colonists had to trudge with their possessions, and the town grew quickly across narrow Arthur Head.[16] After the port had been surveyed, 26-year-old Dr Thomas Harrison was one of the first to purchase land at Fremantle. Lot 30 on the corner of High and Mouat Streets[17] was central and well placed for a doctor's residence in the town.

By April 1830, vessels had anchored off Fremantle 36 times to land passengers with their property and provisions to await land grants. Women slept in carts if they were lucky, or like the men and boys, had to hollow beds out of sand in the circle of their heaped possessions. Eliza Shaw recorded that her family lived 'up to our ankles in sand' and to one visitor it seemed as though the town might be 'run through an hour glass in a day'.[18] At the end of December 1830, Fremantle was still

> ... a bare, barren-looking district of sandy coast; the shrubs cut down for fire-wood, the herbage trodden bare, a few wooden houses, many ragged-looking tents and con-

[15] See R. T. Appleyard and T. Manford, *The Beginning: European Discovery and Early Settlement of Swan River Western Australia*, 1979, pp. 148–55. See also J. Nairn, *Walter Padbury—His Life and Times*, 1985, pp. 37–54; K. Spillman, *Identity Prized: A History of Subiaco*, 1985, pp. 25–6.

[16] J. L. Burton Jackson, *Not an Idle Man. A Biography of John Septimus Roe. Western Australia's First Surveyor-General 1797–1878*, 1982, pp. 64–6. See map of Fremantle.

[17] J. K. Ewers, *The Western Gateway: A History of Fremantle*, 1971, p. 6. Harrison later decided not to build on this lot.

[18] Eliza Shaw to *Leicester Journal*, 24.9.1830, cited in Appleyard and Manford, *The Beginning*, p. 150, and J. L. Burton Jackson, *Not an Idle Man*, p. 66.

trivances for habitations,—our hotel, a poor public-house into which everyone crowded,—our colony, a few cheerless dissatisfied people with gloomy looks, plodding their way through the sand from hut to hut to drink grog, and grumble out their discontents to each other.[19]

A skeletal framework of familiar British organisation was soon provided with the opening of a bakery, some stores and four public houses to supplement the 'good number' of grog tents which were well patronised.[20] Constables and justices of the peace were appointed to ensure that law and order prevailed and it seemed logical to use the storm-wrecked hulk of the *Marquis of Anglesea* for a prison as had been done 'at home'. This improvised gaol was soon replaced by the most substantial stone building in Fremantle. Situated high on the promontory and comprising eight stone cells, the Round House, sheltering the colony's recalcitrant, was capable of being seen far out to sea and served as a tangible proclamation of the colony's priorities. Although by 1832 the port was still barren from sharp salt winds that shifted the white sand at will, and bare from settlers who scrounged vegetation to fuel their fires and feed their stock, there was:

> . . . a town laid out in regular streets of stone houses with low walls, and in some places palisades in front; two or three large well kept inns or hotels, in which you could get clean beds and good private rooms.[21]

With so many inhabitants ill-housed and crowded into a small area with minimal sanitary precautions, it was not long before Thomas Harrison's professional services were required. The number of private patients varied with the town's population as immigrants arrived from ships and then left on the allocation of their land, often many months later. Sometimes patients did not survive their primitive living conditions. Far from the rest of his family in England, a young lad, Walter Padbury, watched in distress as his father wheezed out his life in a crude shelter on Fremantle Beach.[22] The dead man was not the only hopeful colonist whose sole land grant in the colony proved to be a plot in the Alma Street cemetery.

Due to the difficulties of travel between Perth and the port, and Simmon's pressure of duty as colonial surgeon for the state, it was not long before Thomas Harrison was attending coronial enquiries and inquests, performing quarantine inspections and taking on duty at the Fremantle prison in an official capacity for the Medical Department. Not only were there ill prisoners, the soldiers, civil officers and their families to attend to—all of whom received free medical treatment through the government—but Harrison was required to be present at floggings conducted outside the gaol. In a community in which an eight-year-old boy could be im-

[19] G. F. Moore, *Diary of Ten Years Eventful Life of an Early Settler in Western Australia*, 1884, Facsimile edition, 1978, p. 150.

[20] J. Munro McDermott, 'The Turners of Augusta', *RWAHS*, i, pt viii, 1930, p. 42, cited in Ewers, *The Western Gateway*, p. 10.

[21] Moore, *Diary*, p. 150.

[22] Nairn, *Walter Padbury*, p. 53. Walter Padbury would become a wealthy and respected philanthropist and on his death in 1907, Fremantle Hospital was just one of the public hospitals to benefit by his bequest.

prisoned for two years for stealing silver teaspoons,[23] painful sentences for larceny were frequent and six dozen lashes were considered a good, round, admonitory number. While the doctor was generally called immediately in the case of serious accident, many of the sick who were of few means endured pain and illness until their condition deteriorated before consulting Harrison. 'Surgeons charge very high and drugs are not to be bought at present,'[24] observed one colonist. Paupers could obtain treatment at no cost but to their self-respect.

If all who endured pain and illness at Fremantle in its first years had consulted the doctor, he would have been busy indeed. 'Everyone in the colony is suffering from sore legs occasioned by the want of green vegetables,' despaired an early settler, seeing the swollen legs and limping gait of those around her suffering from scurvy. Sores 'like boils fresh broken' lasting on the legs from one week to a year were also common. Few escaped the agony akin to 'scalding water poured on the eyeballs' and the temporary blindness that accompanied ophthalmia.[25] Dysentery lasting from three days to three weeks was also a familiar affliction.

Being a man of admirable order and observation, Harrison collated the particulars of his Fremantle patients between the year of settlement and 1833 for a report requested by William Barrett Marshall. The large number suffering from pneumonia was unknown however, and the total of those with ophthalmia was 'not to be obtained, every man in the colony being said to have experienced the disease once at least'. The cause was usually attributed to the glistening white, fine sand blown over land and sea. Six of the 101 suffering from acute dysentery who called the doctor could not be saved, and the six with empyema, like the three marasmus patients, also died. Forty received treatment for scurvy, but the illness 'proved fatal in numerous instances'. Intemperance originating in the grog tents also added a 'multitude of victims to the sick list'. Harrison's report strongly suggested the role of sailors, soldiers and new arrivals such as the Lascars from India, in introducing sickness to the colony, and foreshadowed a greater need for the enforcement of quarantine regulations.[26]

Although Harrison's medical treatments—including blood-letting, the use of antiphlogistics, emetics, purgatives, the application of refrigerant lotions to the head and dietetics—were sought after, so too, were his skills in treating accident victims. Like other medical practitioners of his period, a set of amputation instruments and others for post-mortem work and teeth extraction were part of his basic equipment.[27] Many he was called to visit suffered burns, or had been party to inevitable

---

23 Supreme Court Case File No. 120, April 1835.
24 P. Statham (Comp. and Researcher), *The Tanner Letters: A Pioneer Saga of Swan River and Tasmania 1831-1845*, 1981, p. 5. William Tanner to his mother, 11 April 1831: 'Bring a good supply of medicine for use on board as well as here . . .', he urges.
25 From the diary of Mrs Whatley, cited in Cohen, *A History of Medicine*, p. 47. See also report of Dr W. P. Dineley at Fremantle, in *Perth Gazette*, 7 October 1843. Ophthalmia and mild dysentery were mentioned as 'most prevalent'; P. Statham, *The Tanner Letters*, p. 12.
26 'Nosological Report, for the Town of Fremantle, in the Colony of Western Australia, from the Commencement of the Colony in 1828, to December 1833', in *Medico-Chirurgical Review and Journal of Practical Medicine*, n. 5, v. 28, 1838. See appendix 1. This reference was first used by Joske in 'Health and Hospital'. See also CSO, Vol. 142, Fol. 171-3.
27 CSO, Vol. 142, Fol. 190, 1845.

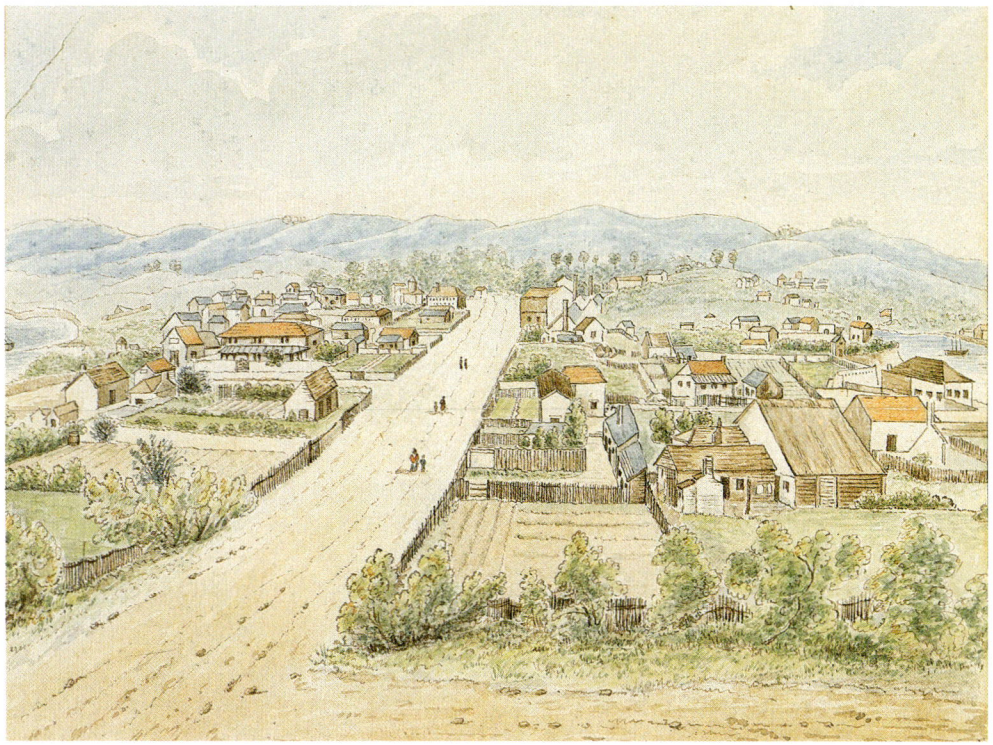

Watercolour by C. D. Wittenoom   Photograph courtesy Dixon Galleries, Sydney

Plate 1. View of High Street in 1838, looking inland from the Round House. In 1829 Dr Thomas Harrison was the original purchaser of Lot 30 on the corner of Mouatt and High Streets on which the first house on the left-hand side of the painting can be seen. Most dwellings were constructed from wood or local limestone.

fights, when drink and frustrations among servants and workers flowed equally freely. Occasionally there was an attempted suicide, as a dream of arcadia turned to private purgatory. Near drownings were very common.[28]

On 17 August 1832, Thomas Harrison witnessed a duel. Although any brush with eternity was a source of lively interest in the colony, the excitement of a duel between two of Fremantle's most respected citizens was the topic of reminiscence for decades. Unable to agree over a business matter, solicitor William Nairne Clark and merchant George French Johnson agreed to an 'indisputable and permanent settlement with pistols'. It was arranged that Dr Harrison should be present at a designated paddock outside the town when the protagonists met at sunrise on the appointed day. Both duelists fired. Clark survived unscathed and walked back to Fremantle, greatly agitated, but no nineteenth century medical knowledge and

---

[28] Of 155 deaths recorded in the colony between June 1829 and June 1832, 25 were specified as due to drowning. Calculated from figures in Berryman, *A Colony Detailed*, pp. 159–64.

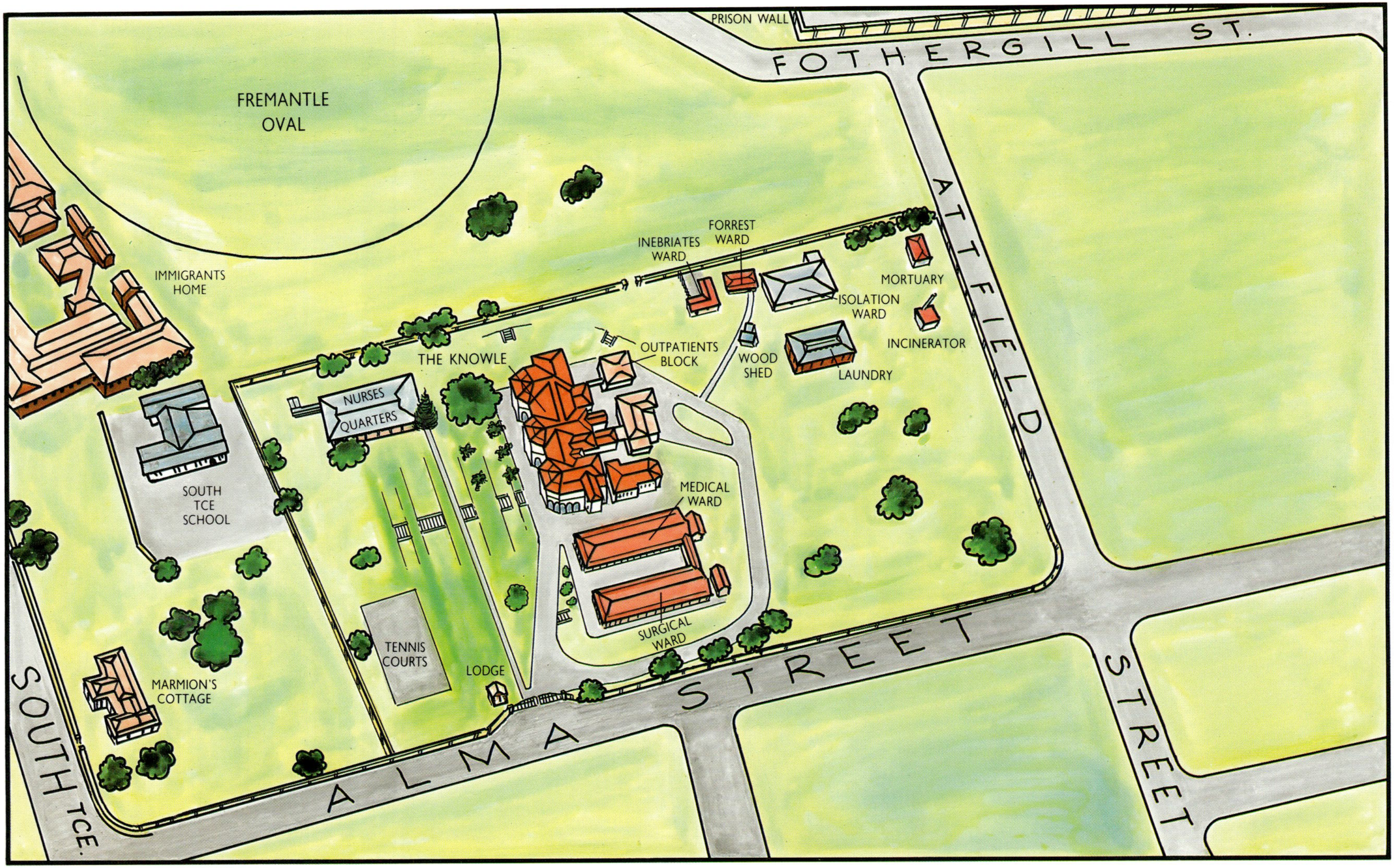

Fig. 1. Fremantle Hospital, 1915.

Mapwork illustration by David Peake, Centagraph, Fremantle, Western Australia

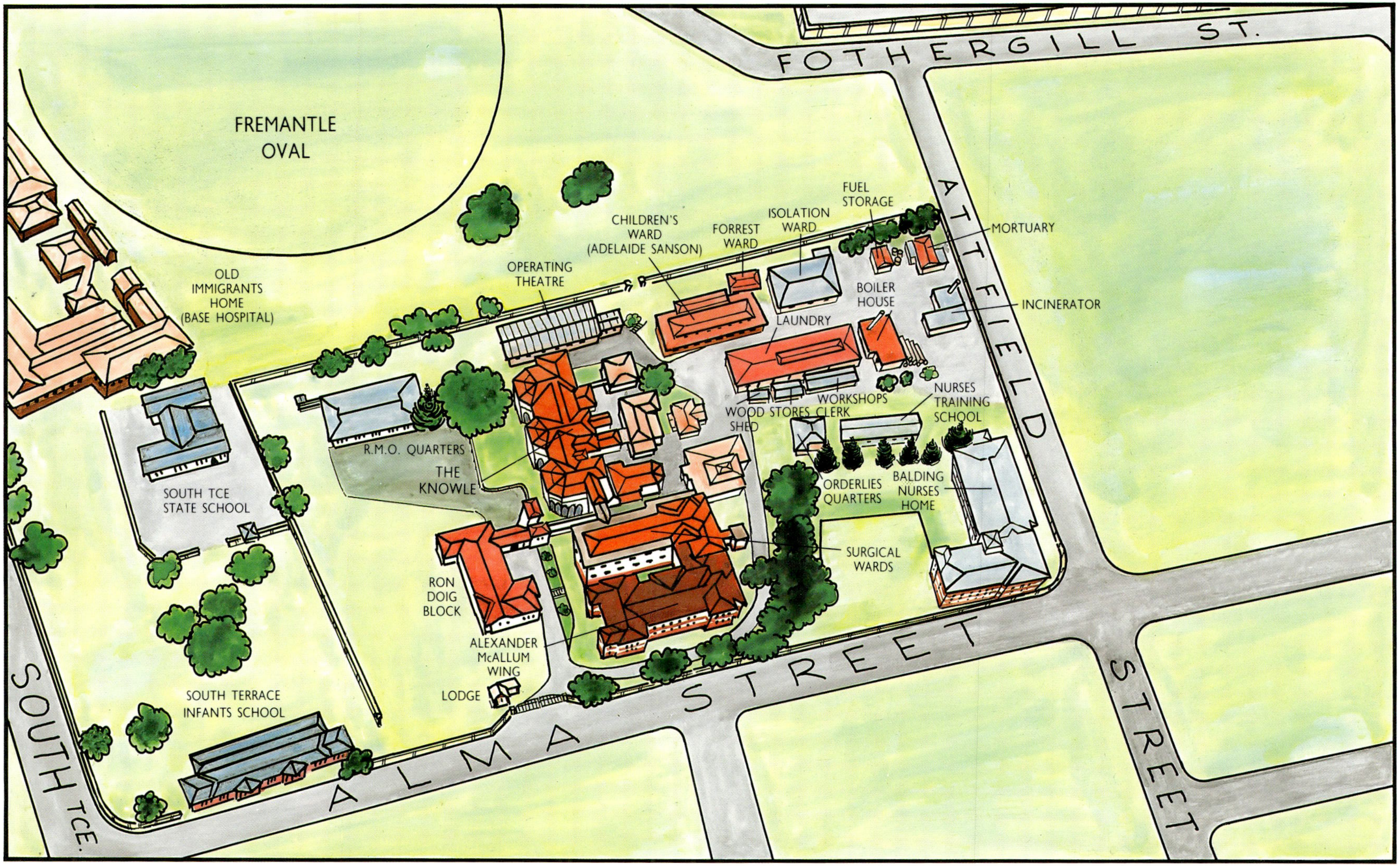

Fig. 2. Fremantle Hospital, 1951.

FREMANTLE OVAL

OLD IMMIGRANTS HOME (BASE HOSPITAL)

FOTHERGILL ST.

ATTFIELD STREET

ALMA STREET

SOUTH TCE.

MORTUARY

INCINERATOR

FUEL STORAGE

BOILER HOUSE

NURSES TRAINING SCHOOL

ISOLATION WARD

FORREST WARD

LAUNDRY

WORKSHOPS

WOOD STORES SHED

STORES CLERK

ORDERLIES QUARTERS

BALDING NURSES HOME

SURGICAL WARDS

CHILDREN'S WARD (ADELAIDE SANSON)

OPERATING THEATRE

R.M.O. QUARTERS

THE KNOWLE

RON DOIG BLOCK

ALEXANDER McALLUM WING

LODGE

SOUTH TCE STATE SCHOOL

SOUTH TERRACE INFANTS SCHOOL

Mapwork illustration by David Peake, Cenagraph, Fremantle, Western Australia

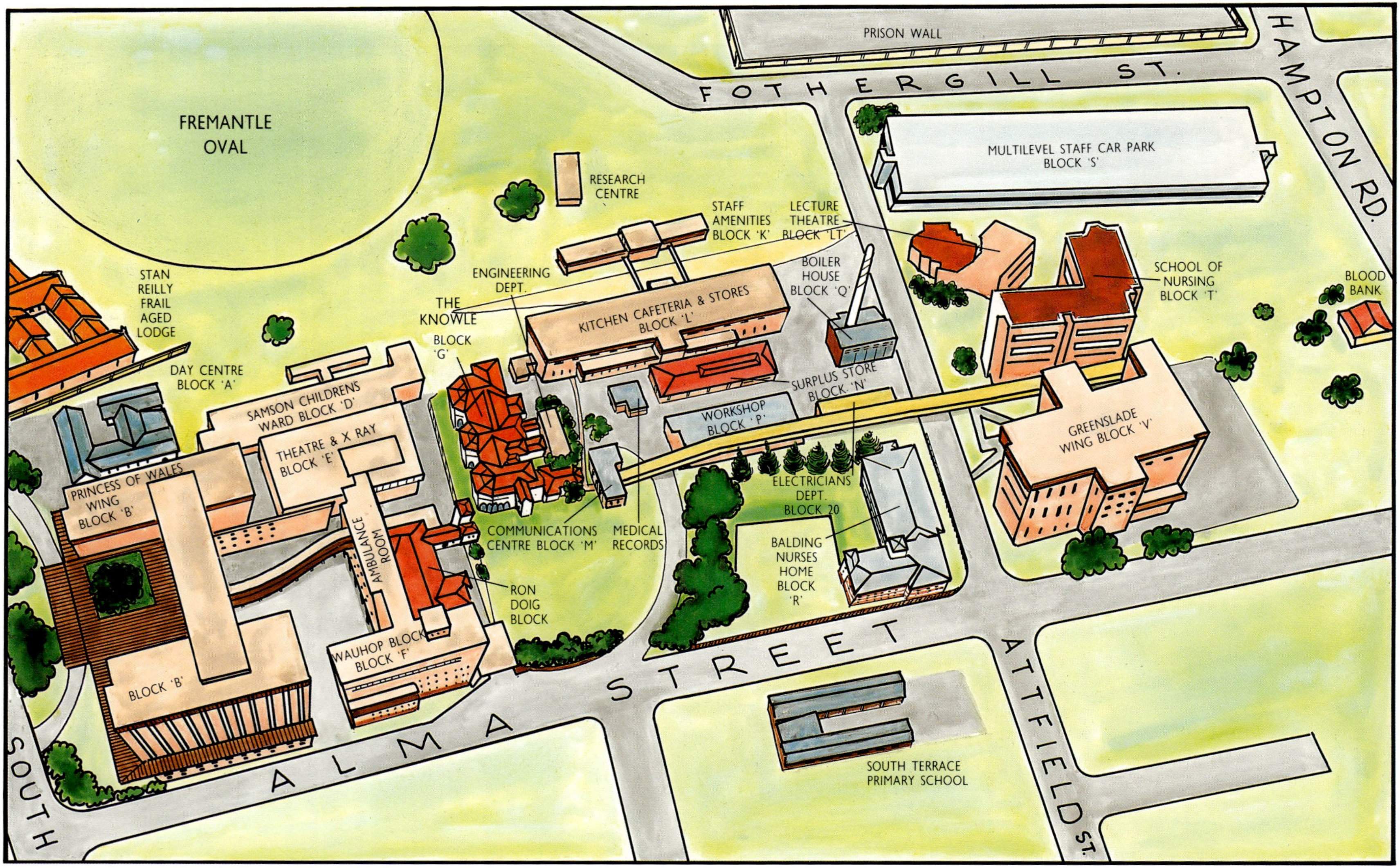

Fig. 3. Fremantle Hospital, 1987.

Mapwork illustration by David Peake, Centagraph, Fremantle, Western Australia

Labels on map:

HAMPTON RD.

FOTHERGILL ST.

ATTFIELD ST.

ALMA STREET

SOUTH

BLOOD BANK

PRISON WALL

MULTILEVEL STAFF CAR PARK BLOCK 'S'

SCHOOL OF NURSING BLOCK 'T'

GREENSLADE WING BLOCK 'V'

SOUTH TERRACE PRIMARY SCHOOL

LECTURE THEATRE BLOCK 'T'

BOILER HOUSE BLOCK 'Q'

SURPLUS STORE BLOCK 'N'

ELECTRICIANS DEPT BLOCK 20

BALDING NURSES HOME BLOCK 'R'

STAFF AMENITIES BLOCK 'K'

WORKSHOP BLOCK 'P'

RESEARCH CENTRE

KITCHEN CAFETERIA & STORES BLOCK 'L'

MEDICAL RECORDS

ENGINEERING DEPT

THE KNOWLE BLOCK 'G'

COMMUNICATIONS CENTRE BLOCK 'M'

RON DOIG BLOCK

FREMANTLE OVAL

SAMSON CHILDRENS WARD BLOCK 'D'

THEATRE & X RAY BLOCK 'E'

AMBULANCE ROOM

WAUHOP BLOCK BLOCK 'F'

STAN REILLY FRAIL AGED LODGE

DAY CENTRE BLOCK 'A'

PRINCESS OF WALES WING BLOCK 'B'

BLOCK 'B'

expertise could save Johnson from the fatal effects of the bullet that ripped deeply into his hip.[29]

Like the tides that constantly licked or lashed the town's western perimeter, the movement of doctors into and out from Fremantle became a regular occurrence during the remainder of the century. As it was the landing point, new arrivals with medical training sometimes chose to settle on the coast while making more permanent arrangements. The life plans of Fremantle's doctors were not always predictable. One of the first to follow Harrison in settling at Fremantle was George Cowcher with his family, household goods and husbandry implements, who practised in Fremantle in 1830 before taking up an allotment of land at Guildford. Despite a supplementary income gained from running a ferry across the river, luck frowned on the family with eight children, who soon returned to Fremantle, where the doctor practised until 1840, the year of his death.[30]

Dr Nicholas Langley boosted the available medical service at the port in 1832. He had arrived to join Peel's ill-fated company in 1830 and suffered mental instability soon after. On his recovery, he conferred with Thomas Harrison on the treatment of the severely wounded duelist Johnson, and worked as a doctor until his death from a stroke at the age of 34 in 1835.[31] In this year Thomas Harrison was the same age, and like Langley, a single man, so perhaps the death of his medical contemporary prompted Fremantle's first doctor to fulfill a private dream of becoming landed medical gentry. He went to King George Sound, where five or six years later he lost nearly three-quarters of the 800 sheep he imported on the *Cormandel*. Thomas Harrison's pride at being appointed Magistrate of Albany in November 1846, was short lived, as he died later that month from the dysentery that had afflicted so many of his patients in the colony.[32]

Following Harrison's departure from Fremantle, James Crichton, as the colonial surgeon, had to hire a horse in Perth, pay for its fodder and the ferry fee to cross the river, and ride 'ploughing through the heavy sand under the burning rays of a hot sun' to perform the necessary medical duties at the Fremantle prison.[33] With relief, he handed the task to Dr John Wight in April, 1837, but this gentleman remained in charge at Fremantle for only two years before leaving for the Murray District, where he had property. Crichton again had to endure the travel on a hired horse, from October 1839 until he resigned the Fremantle appointment at the end of a hot Western Australian summer in March, 1840. In this month, a year later, Dr John Shipton landed at Fremantle, planning to purchase land. He was persuaded instead to work as assistant colonial surgeon at Fremantle, to help Crichton who was 'the only medical man in Perth and its environs'.[34]

[29] See Ewers, *The Western Gateway*, pp. 15–16; Cohen, *History of Medicine*, pp. 44–5; *Dictionary of Western Australians 1829–1850*, Vol. 1, entries for Clark and Johnson; A. S. Ellis, *Eloquent Testimony: The Story of the Mental Health Services in Western Australia 1830–1975*, 1984, p. 7; P. E. C. de Mouncey, 'The Historic Duel at Fremantle between George French Johnson, a Merchant, and William Nairne Clark, a Solicitor, in the Year 1832', *RWAHS*, Vol. 1, Part V, 1929, pp. 1–15.

[30] Cohen, *A History of Medicine*, pp. 57–8; *Dictionary of Western Australians 1829–1914*, Vol. 1, entry for Cowcher.

[31] Cohen, *A History of Medicine*, pp. 41, 45–6; Ellis, *Eloquent Testimony*, pp. 2–10.

[32] *Dictionary of Western Australians 1829–1914*, Vol. 1, entry for Harrison.

[33] Joske, 'Health and Hospital', p. 102. Crichton to Colonial Secretary, 7 March 1840.

[34] CSO, Vol. 617, Fol. 246, 1841.

Until July, 1843, Shipton filled in at Fremantle. William Dineley then accepted the position as district medical officer and surgeon to the Fremantle prison. Perhaps it was no coincidence that when, after eight years with only an occasional day off, the task of quarantine officer was added to his duties in 1848, Dineley requested 18 months' leave to visit England and did not return. In the emergency, Shipton was again requested by the Governor to take office at Fremantle. While convicts were assigned to labour for the landed settlers Shipton had wished to emulate, they only increased the doctor's responsibilities when he was appointed for two years as the first surgeon to the Convict Establishment at Fremantle. For nearly 20 years, however, between January 1849 and December 1868, Shipton worked at Fremantle without any lengthened leave of absence until from 'age and bodily infirmity' he felt unable to continue and took a well-earned voyage to England.[35]

With the introduction of almost 1,000 convicts in 1850—who had been appealed for by the landed and opposed by free labourers[36]—and with their construction of the daunting, stone convict depot at Fremantle by 1858, to house themselves and those who continued to be sent, the demand for medical attendants for the convicts increased. In 1853, Charles Elliott relieved the overworked John Shipton, as the surgeon of the Fremantle Convict Establishment, until the following year, when he in turn was replaced by David Rennie, who retained the post for five years. George Galbraith was appointed medical officer of convict services in Western Australia in 1850 and attended at Fremantle until 1858. George Attfield was the imperial surgeon at the depot between 1857 and 1879 with charge of the lunatic asylum as well. These two establishments were worlds apart from the community that lived just outside their respective confining walls. For the two years from 1878 to 1880, Dr Alexander Milne-Robertson also doctored at the prison.[37]

All the Convict Establishment doctors were British trained, but in 1866, Henry Dickey, a graduate from Pennsylvania, arrived in the colony and temporarily replaced Shipton as assistant colonial surgeon, while also helping Attfield at the gaol and asylum. He took leave in 1872 and Henry Calvert Barnett arrived from the York district to accept the appointment of colonial surgeon at Fremantle and responsibility for colonial lunatics—a task which he shouldered for over twenty years.[38] Other doctors who served at Fremantle at different short periods included William L. Oliver, who practised in Fremantle before 1868, William Mayhew, William Sholl and Samuel Viveash. Their work in Fremantle was only part of a medical umbrella which was thinly stretched in an attempt to cover the whole state. While the colonial surgeon constantly battled to manage the colony's health concerns, the doctors under his close direction fought to minister to their patients with a minimal supply of drugs and a keenly-felt, small-sized salary. 'The stipend being so small, puts me to serious inconvenience to keep up the necessary appearances of the situation I hold,' Shipton pointed out in 1850.[39]

[35] CSO, Vol. 617, Fol. 246; *Dictionary of Western Australians 1829–1914*, entry for Shipton.
[36] C. T. Stannage, *The People of Perth*, pp. 79–83.
[37] See appropriate biographical references for doctors in Cohen, *A History of Medicine*; and *Dictionary of Western Australians 1829–1914*, various volumes. For Attfield, see also Ellis, *Eloquent Testimony*, pp. 18–22.
[38] See Ellis, *Eloquent Testimony*, pp. 26–7.
[39] CSO Recl 45, Vol. 207, 26 June 1850, p. 151.

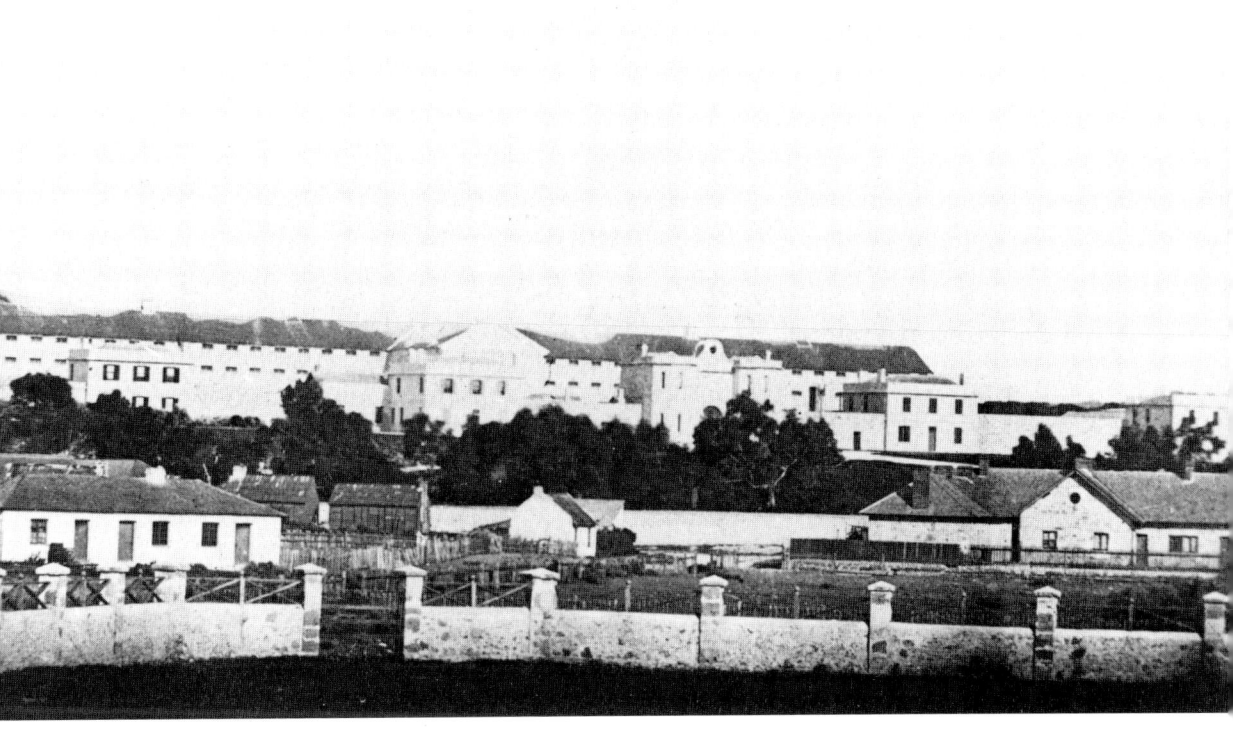

Photograph courtesy Battye Library

Plate 2. Convict establishment and houses of the convict officers, Fremantle, *c.* 1870s–1880s.

The duties of many Fremantle doctors increased with the growth of the colony, with its expanding areas of administration and with the needs of the community. Although he settled and planned only a private practice, from 1829 onwards Harrison was soon visiting gaol prisoners and treating sick Aborigines, paupers, soldiers and the civil officers stationed at Fremantle plus their families, as well as carrying out quarantine duties. When Dineley and Shipton in turn accepted the position of 'medical attendant at Fremantle' they inherited a similar list of responsibilities and medical dependents. Shipton looked around the town which had grown by the 1840s and wondered just who his 'civil officers' were.[40] The colonial surgeon listed the resident magistrate; the harbour master; the postmaster; the government clerk; the jailer; the government storekeeper; the Rottnest Island Establishment, including the pilot; all government officers visiting Fremantle and the families and servants of

---

[40] CSO, Vol. 190/4, 16 January 1849. The population of Fremantle in 1843 totalled 387. See J. K. Hitchcock, *The History of Fremantle: The Front Gate of Australia 1829–1929*, 1929, p. 29.

these employees. The schoolmaster was later included. The Fremantle doctors were appalled. 'I think the Government are rather hard to saddle one with all these families,' protested Shipton. In twelve months he made no more than £20, 'as allmost [sic] everyone in Fremantle is on the government list ...'[41] Dineley, too, wondered if there would be any private patients left in the town, and in 1845 he weighed up the duties and income from his government and private practices and announced through the *Inquirer* that:

> ... I shall for the future relinquish private practice in Fremantle, and merely attend to my Government duties; not finding the remuneration equivalent to the anxiety and trouble. Consequently, wishing to avoid the disagreeable task of refusing, I hope I shall not be called upon.[42]

Some of his patients felt 'grievously insulted' and Dineley was moved to elaborate:

> The literal meaning was simply this ... taking the whole of the inhabitants as a body, in the aggregate it was not sufficiently remunerative—at the best, it is an unthankful office ...[43]

His return to private practice was prompted less by altruism than as a result of swift, effective, colonial arm-twisting. The only doctor in the town was informed that if he declined to practise, his government allowance would be transferred to someone else '... as it is to encourage a Medicine Man such as himself at Fremantle for the benefit of the community there that this allowance is granted'.[44]

With the decision in the late 1830s to make Rottnest Island a prison for Aboriginal offenders,[45] the duties of Fremantle's doctor increased. As the first medical officer to undertake the responsibility of its inmates, Dineley was appalled to find:

> ... it particularly amazing not having a medicine chest over there and I can only say if Government cares anything about the unfortunate creatures—one must be granted—and moreover, it is my humble opinion that it is highly necessary if common justice was done—that a medical man should be stationed on the Island—for I thoroughly believe that if proper remedies had been used immediately—the native now dead—would in all probability be living.[46]

Dineley's words fell on an unresponsive official desk and were subsequently filed away. Three months later there was still no sign of a medicine chest, let alone a resident doctor. When medical aid was required at the island, a signal fire was lit, and the Rottnest pilot would sail across to the mainland to take the doctor to his patient.

[41] CSO, Vol. 207, Fol. 130–1, 7 February 1850.
[42] *Inquirer*, 4 June 1845.
[43] *Ibid.*, 11 June 1845.
[44] CSO, Vol. 139, Fol. 239, 6 June 1845. Dineley decided to continue serving in both private and government capacities. See also CSO, Vol. 139, Fol. 254, 31 July 1845.
[45] J. E. Thomas and A. Stewart, *Imprisonment in Western Australia: Evolution, Theory and Practice*, 1978, p. 125. See also CSO, Vol. 62, Fol. 229. The island commenced as a prison for Aborigines on 17 August 1838.
[46] CSO, Vol. 139, Fol. 196, 15 February 1845.

Sometimes rough seas meant a delay of days before a sick Aborigine could be seen, by which time, instead of diagnosis and treatment, there might be a post-mortem.[47]

White prisoners at the convict depot suffered dysentery, chest complaints (though not as frequently as the captives across the water), and all the diseases of a prison community. Their medical attendants also had the responsibility of patching up after fights between the convicts, of restoring a flogged offender so that he could morally benefit from his reformatory treatment and determining the point at which a man was unable to further survive a diet of bread and water in a dark, solitary, refractory cell.[48] They also treated the enrolled pensioners brought out with their families to police Western Australia's convicts, and who appear to have been viewed with some reserve by the Fremantle community.[49]

While the fortunes of landed settlers could rise and fall with market forces and seasonal influences, nineteenth century Fremantle doctors, dependent on their professional skills in private practice and employed by a tight-fisted colonial government, were reasonably sure that theirs was not a profession from which to shape a colonial empire. Prior to 1834, William Barrett Marshall spoke of medical practitioners engaged in agriculture 'to which they have been obliged to turn for that daily bread which the practice of medicine failed to secure to them' in the colony.[50] In 1841, Shipton came with 'ample means and with the full intention to purchase land'. When he agreed to undertake the health care of the port for £50 a year, however, he 'entailed considerable loss!' and complained '. . . had I not had some private means and used the greatest economy almost to penuriousness I could not have managed to live'.[51] For his two years of service at the Convict Establishment, Shipton received 'no remuneration or gratuity' and as district registrar he averaged 'a little in advance of £10' each year. As health officer for Fremantle, Dickey received only £75 a year and in 1860 Henry Wakefield, the Governor's private secretary, thought that it would not have been unreasonable to have offered a government position to Attfield who had attended the colonial lunatics 'without any remuneration whatever'.[52]

Nor did the climate appear to encourage a generous income. Despite a natural increase in the number of patients with the growth of population, many of whom remembered long, bitterly cold British winters and health problems accompanying the concentration of people in towns following industrialisation, colonial doctors eulogised the healthy climate of the colony. The temperature might drop 20 degrees in a day but Dr Joseph Harris, the colonial surgeon, still concluded that nothing had occurred to shake his confidence in the 'salubrity of the climate. The country is free from Malaria, the air generally being dry and fine, [and] peculiarly favourable to those suffering "chest affectations".'[53] When he was the sub-registrar for Fre-

---

[47] Dickey advised the Colonial Surgeon that in winter, 'sometimes for a week at a time it is impossible except at considerable risk, to cross in a Boat to the Island', CSO, Vol. 638, Fol. 128-9.

[48] See M. Brown, 'Probationary Prisoner 270: Thomas Bushell', in C. T. Stannage (ed.), *Studies in Western Australian History*, Vol. IV, December 1981, p. 53.

[49] For background on Pensioner guards, see G. C. Bolton, 'Who Were the Pensioners?', in C. T. Stannage (ed.), *Studies in Western Australian History*, Vol. IV, December 1981.

[50] 'Nosological Report', in *Medico-Chirurgical Review*, p. 212. See appendix 1.

[51] CSO, Vol. 617, Fol. 246; CSO, Vol. 207, Fol. 130-1, 7 February 1850.

[52] CSO, Vol. 617, Fol. 317, 31 December 1860.

[53] CSO, Vol. 142, Fol. 171-3, 24 February 1845.

mantle, William Dineley shared similar observations in enthusiastic terms and thought that apart from

> ... the common accidents which all occasionally are subject to—not forgetting the free patronage given to the Alcohol—the profession would do well to close the scene, and retire into the bush, to plough, to toil, and to reap ... under almost a cloudless sky, a clear dry atmosphere, and in a climate unsurpassed by any in the world.[54]

Many new colonists who became ill in this unsurpassed climate did not seek professional medical attention. George Fletcher Moore recorded on 29 May 1840: 'A blade of a pen-knife ran into my hand to-day, up to the handle. I bled like a stuck pig; still I stopped the cut with my thumb, and then bandaged it, without anything further.'[55] In outlying areas there might be no doctor to consult; some patients could not afford the medical fees anyway and other colonists shared a different medical learning gained from either personal experience, or family and community tradition. 'Diet cures more than the lancet' was a proverb common in the eighteenth century[56] and one Fremantle doctor wrote disparagingly of:

> ... the generality of invalids [who] think it needless to make application to the profession, until a certain routine, varying according to the patients own ideas of the matter, has been had recourse to, which invariably proves beneficial to the practitioner, and highly prejudicial to the individual.[57]

Diarrhoea and dysentery might be treated the British way with water arrowroot flavoured with port wine or cognac, but red gum broken off a local tree and dissolved in water worked as well as any remedy.[58] An effective emetic after 'the free patronage given to the Alcohol' could be made in a kitchen from mustard and water, while fevers were starved, or raw egg and brandy, or toast water given. Typhoid patients sipped diluted milk and in convalescence were given port wine, whisky or brandy.[59] The colony's surveyor-general had his 'sore eyes' relieved by a mixture of alum, salt petre, white Copperas and 'camphire'—a recipe passed down by 'Mrs King's mother', and Mrs Whatley stirred up effective 'eye-water' using zinc sulphate in solution.[60] Later colonists would find that urine relieved Sandy Blight and a dog's lick cured Barcoo Rot.[61] Women played a major part in the colony's alternative medical service through their preparation of kitchen remedies, when they nursed family members and others in the community, and acted as medical advisors. Many

---

[54] *Perth Gazette*, 7 October 1843. Nathanial Ogle writing in 1839 also spoke of reports by the colonial surgeon and military surgeon stressing the 'salubrity of the climate' and the low number of ailments reported in the colony. These included slight eye inflammation and bowel complaints or intemperance. See N. Ogle, *The Colony of Western Australia: A Manual for Emigrants 1839*, 1977. First published 1839, p. 141.

[55] Moore, *Diary*, p. 412.

[56] W. T. Fernie, *Kitchen Physic: At Hand for the Doctor, and Helpful for Homely Cures*, 1901, p. viii.

[57] *Perth Gazette*, 7 October 1843.

[58] Statham, *The Tanner Letters*. P. S. Tanner to mother, 11 April 1831.

[59] Fernie, *Kitchen Physic*, p. viii. See also *Perth Gazette*, 7 October 1843.

[60] Cohen, *A History of Medicine*, pp. 81–2.

[61] C. Polizzotto, 'Jessie Viner's Childhood on the Peel', in P. Hetherington (ed.), *Childhood and Society in Western Australia: Essays in Social History* (forthcoming), 1988.

became adept at midwifery. On one occasion, Eliza Brown at York was delivered by Mr Bland's housekeeper—'a very experienced nurse', and Eliza in turn attended to 'two women of the labouring class who were without Nurse, Doctor or neighbour or any female but myself within several miles at the time of their illness'.[62]

If trained doctors resented the patients who practised folk medicine, they bitterly denounced the 'quacks'. As anyone could claim to be a medical practitioner, and registration was not introduced until 1861, there were inevitable conflicts between the trained professional and the untutored, asserting their right to heal. The bodily illnesses of the Reverend Mr Brown's isolated flock in Busselton seemed as urgent as their spiritual afflictions, and for many years the minister and his wife were requested to treat the sick among them. The families even established a medicine fund through voluntary subscription to keep the Browns supplied with drugs. Content with the only treatment available to them, these patients did not seek the professional services of Dr John Rosselotty when he arrived in the area. In 1870 Rosselotty complained to the Colonial Secretary:

> . . . Of course I am aware that Mr Brown is at liberty to quack if he will, but I think he would only be doing his duty as a neighbour if he attended to the spiritual wants of the people and left me to attend to the bodily ones.[63]

Even though medical men were required to be registered, the colonial secretary responded that: 'the giving of medical relief in certain cases by the clergymen is strictly in accordance with the usage of clergymen in the Mother Country . . . and with that of the Chaplains in similar Districts out here'.[64] Interests between temporal and spiritual ills were close and more than one priest practised medicine, while more than one doctor became a spiritual mentor.[65] Because it was a large centre of population, medical and ecclesiastical interests were always served separately in Fremantle.

Fremantle doctors prescribed pills, wine and other spirits for patients, but it was also a time when 'emetics, warm bathing, leaches [sic] and occasionally blisters' were believed effective.[66] Poverty, however, could cause a condition that no pills or leeches could remedy. It was not uncommon for those out of work to require treatment for debility and one colonial surgeon said of such a patient that 'he had got gradually into his present state . . . from having no work and want of food and is now unable to work . . . he does not require medical aid but will die if he does not get proper nutriment'.[67] In accident cases amputation was common, although where

[62] P. Cowan (ed.), *A Faithful Picture: The Letters of Eliza and Thomas Brown at York in the Swan River Colony 1841–1852*, 1977, p. 76. See also E. O. G. Shann, *Cattle Chosen. The Story of the First Group Settlement in Western Australia 1829–1841*, 1978, p. 125.

[63] CSO, Vol. 660 Fol. 57, 58, 64, 65, 1870.

[64] *Ibid.*

[65] Drs H. Wollaston and M. Griver gave up medicine for ecclesiastical work. R. Salvado was a Bishop who practised medicine and F. W. Waldeck, the Methodist missionary, did all the medical work at Geraldton for 30 years until a qualified doctor arrived. Dr Louis Guistiniani also preached and practised medicine. See appropriate references in Cohen, *A History of Medicine*, and *Dictionary of Western Australians*, relevant volumes.

[66] CSO, Vol. 142, Fol. 171-3. Colonial Surgeon Joseph Harris to Colonial Secretary, 'Medical Report on the State of Health in the Colony during the past year', 1844.

[67] CSO, Vol. 129, Fol. 44. Harris to Colonial Secretary, 15 March 1843.

possible the body was left to its own healing process of exfoliation. At the Colonial Hospital in 1846, one man with compound fractures of his leg and foot was allowed moderate exercise with occasional rest during the day, while over a period of months 20 pieces of bone worked their way to the surface and were removed.[68]

The area by the sea which was marked by little more than a huddle of tents in 1829 changed, but not dramatically, over the next 50 years. By 1832 in Fremantle 'many pretty tolerable houses had been built of stone and brick', and by 1872 there were some 'handsome and substantial houses belonging to either the government or to some of the principal inhabitants'; others were less substantial, all 'glaring in white-wash' and blinkered by green verandah blinds.[69] There were shops—some large, but more small, rather scattered and many selling fish or fruit. A new sea jetty and a river pier were centres of activity as people and cargoes were transported to or from Perth. There were sailors finding land legs, merchants despatching and disposing of cargoes, a handful of Aborigines, now looking very out of place and often finding themselves gaoled after achieving a kind of peace in the white man's liquor.[70] Children ran and played as they always had, especially near the jetties, and they often worked in shops and family businesses. Women, large with crinolines, swept over half-completed streets and unpaved footpaths, sometimes shopping, sometimes visiting and sometimes on their way to the immigration depot to hire female domestic servants. Labourers, artisans and, between 1850 and 1863, convicts in chain gangs, government officials, the poor who were often hungry and who sometimes found comfort in the bottom of a glass—all were a part of the life of Fremantle in the 1870s.

While the town changed, most of the afflictions listed by Dr Harrison in 1829 did not, but with increased medical knowledge and experience gained with time, diagnosis became more specific. Some of the causes of death in Fremantle between June 1873 and June 1875 included 'disease of heart and spinal cord', 'disease of liver with dropsy', 'haematosis', 'disease of kidney', 'inanition aggravated by neglect' and 'whooping cough' for an infant of six months. Convulsions, scurvy, dysentery, bronchitis, tonsillitis and 'softening of brain' were diagnosed. One 65-year-old died from 'natural causes accelerated by drink' and one of three who died after childbirth was 14 years old. Three children under 12 months were reported to have died from 'teething'. During 1874, 60 of the 95 who died in Fremantle were male.[71]

Although the town boasted a lunatic asylum by 1865, patients requiring hospital treatment still had to be sent to the Colonial Hospital in Perth, but could be admitted only if there was a spare bed. Only accident cases and those unable to pay for private medical treatment and classified as 'paupers' were accepted as patients, which meant that most people were nursed at home. In 1888, while walking from North Fremantle to Miss Thorpe's, where he ran errands, nine-year-old Thomas Robinson was asked by a man trying to drive his cart over a bridge to take the whip

---

[68] CSO, Vol. 152, Fol. 131. Harris to Colonial Secretary, 9 February 1846.
[69] Cottesloe, *Diary and Letters*, p. 87; Mrs E. Millett, *An Australian Parsonage, or the Settler and the Savage in Western Australia*, 1980, p. 15; H. Taunton, *Australind, Wanderings in Western Australia and the Malay East*, 1903, cited in Ewers, *The Western Gateway*, pp. 74–5.
[70] *Evening Times*, 20 March 1888.
[71] Register of Deaths, Fremantle District, 1875–1884, Acc. 2799, BL. (Includes 1873.)

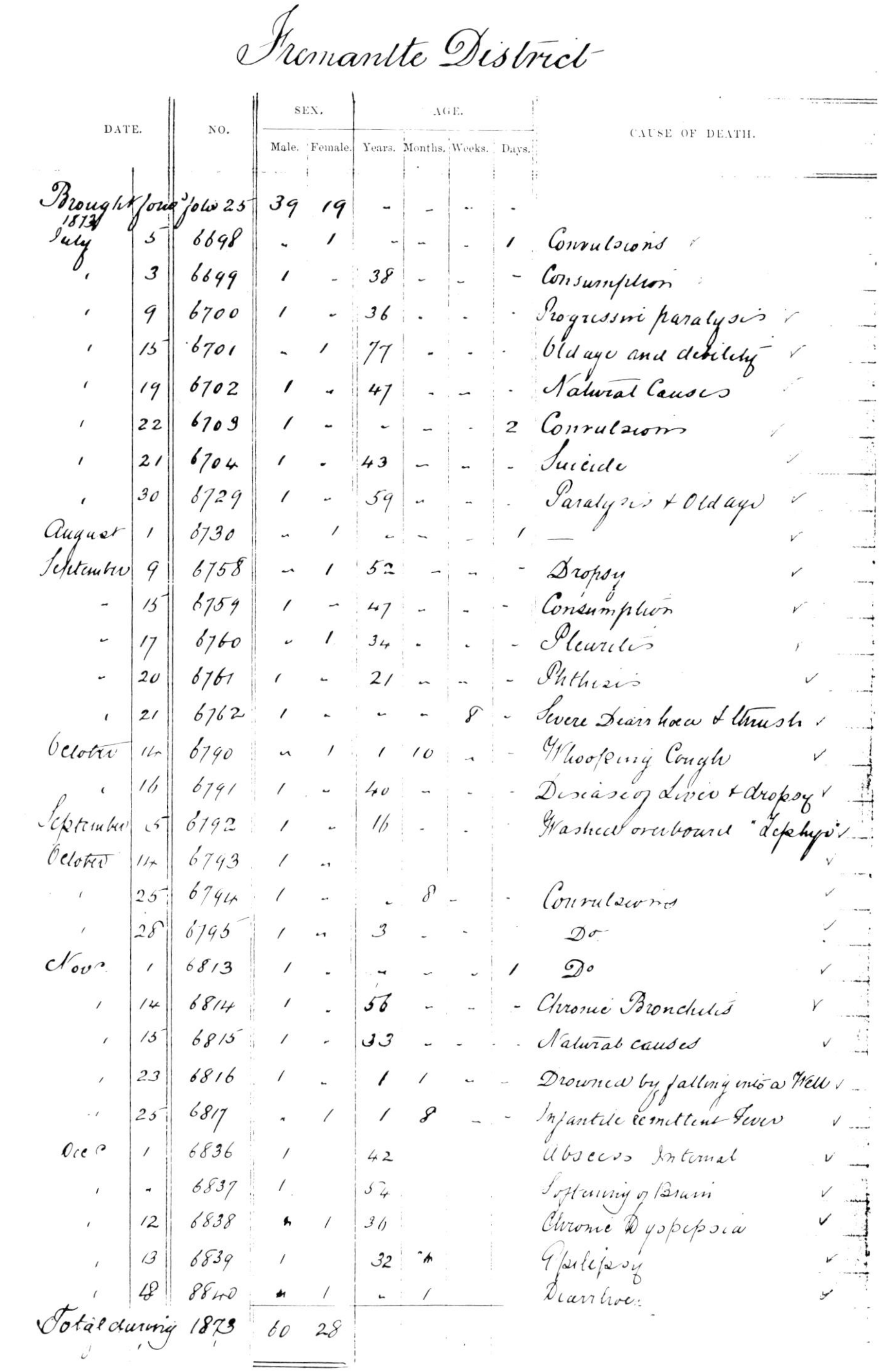

Fremantle District

DATE.	NO.	SEX.		AGE.				CAUSE OF DEATH.
		Male.	Female.	Years.	Months.	Weeks.	Days.	
Brought forward July 25 1873		39	19	–	–	–	–	
July 5	6698	–	1	–	–	–	1	Convulsions
" 3	6699	1	–	38	–	–	–	Consumption
" 9	6700	1	–	36	–	–	–	Progressive paralysis
" 15	6701	–	1	77	–	–	–	Old age and debility
" 19	6702	1	–	47	–	–	–	Natural Causes
" 22	6703	1	–	–	–	–	2	Convulsions
" 24	6704	1	–	43	–	–	–	Suicide
" 30	6729	1	–	59	–	–	–	Paralysis + Old age
August 1	6730	–	1	–	–	–	1	—
September 9	6758	–	1	52	–	–	–	Dropsy
" 15	6759	1	–	47	–	–	–	Consumption
" 17	6760	–	1	34	–	–	–	Pleuritis
" 20	6761	1	–	21	–	–	–	Phthisis
" 21	6762	1	–	–	–	–	8	Severe Diarrhoea + thrush
October 14	6790	–	1	1	10	–	–	Whooping Cough
" 16	6791	1	–	40	–	–	–	Disease of Liver + dropsy
September 5	6792	1	–	16	–	–	–	Washed overboard "asphyxia"
October 14	6793	1	–	–	–	–	–	
" 25	6794	1	–	–	8	–	–	Convulsions
" 28	6795	1	–	3	–	–	–	Do
Nov 1	6813	1	–	–	–	–	1	Do
" 14	6814	1	–	56	–	–	–	Chronic Bronchitis
" 15	6815	1	–	33	–	–	–	Natural causes
" 23	6816	1	–	1	1	–	–	Drowned by falling into a Well
" 25	6817	–	1	1	8	–	–	Infantile remittent Fever
Dec 1	6836	1	–	42	–	–	–	Abscess Internal
" –	6837	1	–	54	–	–	–	Softening of Brain
" 12	6838	–	1	36	–	–	–	Chronic Dyspepsia
" 13	6839	1	–	32	–	–	–	Epilepsy
" 18	8840	–	1	–	–	1	–	Diarrhoea
Total during 1873		60	28					

Fig. 4. Some causes of death in the Fremantle district 1873.

and encourage his obstinate horse. The animal reared and struck Thomas so heavily that little hope was held for the boy's recovery. Another lad, riding on the shafts of a cart laden with wood, had both legs broken when he fell and the cart ran over him. Both boys were taken to their homes where they were treated by one of the Fremantle doctors.[72]

Acceptance at the Colonial Hospital was neither assured nor immediate. Fremantle patients eventually admitted for treatment at the Colonial Hospital were first examined by a local doctor who recommended their admission in a letter to the Fremantle resident magistrate. He in turn advised the colonial secretary, who consulted the colonial surgeon for his advice. If admission was agreed to, the decision filtered back through the same clumsy hierarchy of reference. Often the Superintendent of Poor Relief was involved and the patient was taken to the Poor House at Mount Eliza. The resident magistrate could send a man directly to hospital on a court order. Fred Stephens fell off a horse in the Ashburton, breaking his arm, dislocating his jaw and breaking three ribs. He travelled to Fremantle and applied for treatment at hospital through the Fremantle Police Court, where Resident Magistrate Fairbairn gave him the necessary letter of authority to present at the Colonial Hospital.[73] At times the local doctors felt frustrated by the system and their lack of influence. William Birmingham wrote to Fairbairn in 1891:

> The bearer is a sailor, and is ill, he has no place to go here and I thought if I brought his case before you, you would interest yourself sufficiently in him to give him a recommendation for admission to the Perth Hospital. I would not trouble you but I find that my own recommendation carries no weight with the authorities of the Perth Hospital.[74]

The police at Fremantle were often involved in assessing a patient's financial position and in transporting the sick. Mrs Reilly's daughter, Louisa, suffered old and extensive leg ulcers which prevented her working and her mother wanted the girl to be admitted to hospital for treatment. The police found that Mrs Reilly was a widow living in a cottage off Packenham Street, unable to work because of 'rheumatics' and subsisting on the income from one boarder. Her family helped with food and clothing when they could, but daughters with large families of their own or who were 'in service' had limited means themselves. Fifteen-year-old Louisa was sent to the hospital.[75] Rose Smith was also admitted suffering from 'lung disease' and needing 'nursing and good food'. As a destitute single woman with no friends in the colony, there was no dispute about her need.[76] Neither was there debate about Mrs Hanham 'in a state of much debility suffering from gastric disease and great haemorrhage from the rectum'. Her husband was out of work and assisted his wife as best he could but, police reported, their landlady refused to allow the couple stay in the 'dirty hovel' in which the sick woman lay. So serious was her condition that permission to enter hospital was telegraphed to the resident magistrate.[77]

[72] See *Inquirer*, 17 March 1888; *Evening Times*, 7 January 1888.
[73] *Evening Times*, 13 January 1888.
[74] CSO, Vol. 1668/91, 25 August 1891.
[75] CSO, Vol. 2769/90, 1 October 1890.
[76] CSO, Vol. 1414/91, 22 July 1891.
[77] CSO, Vol. 834/88, 22 March 1888.

Less benevolence was shown to patients suffering the effects of old age or infirmity. Such patients needed 'comfortable quarters and good food' as much as medical treatment, but because they were likely to remain in the hospital for many weeks, they were usually sent to the Poor House. Such was the fate of Andrew Hanson of Fremantle, who was receiving assistance as a pauper, suffering a 'rheumatic affection' and was finally asked to leave the boarding house where the owner was supporting him.[78] It was almost the fate of a strong young man named Thomas Cunningham who came to Fremantle following an accident while working on the Great Southern Railway Line. An ulcer on his leg prevented the man from working, but he was only seen by a doctor after he was gaoled for seven days for disorderly conduct. The colonial surgeon thought the man should go to the Poor House, but the superintendent there thought otherwise, as the depot was not a convalescent home. As a government pauper, Thomas was given food for a time, but a month later police were instructed to take him to the Colonial Hospital.[79] There were many Louisas, Roses and Thomases among the colony's first generations and it was not uncommon for a Fremantle request for an admission to the Colonial Hospital to be returned marked: 'There is no room'.[80]

For those accepted into the Colonial Hospital, treatment was often lengthy, as a Fremantle lad with a fractured arm found in 1845. He was admitted in early April but was still a patient in September, able to do spade work and handle a light wheel barrow, but still waiting for the broken pieces of bone to work to the surface and be removed.[81] As medical patients were generally paupers, and accident cases often sailors, their discharge from hospital often meant a return to conditions which promoted ill-health rather than recovery. Two seamen returned to their ship after hospitalisation were reported to be worse than ever. 'As long as they stay on ship exposed to cold and wind which is unavoidable, they are not likely to be restored to health or become fit for duty'[82] reported Dineley. With nowhere to convalesce, the solution to both the problem of a sick sailor and the expense to the colony of his upkeep, was to return him to his port of embarkation.[83]

Hospital funding was a concern to the government of Western Australia. By the 1880s the provision and upkeep of hospitals in Britain rested in the administrative hands of individual subscribers who nodded obediently at the ideal of Christian charity. In the United States of America, hospitals were financed by public philanthropy in the interests of the poor. In Sydney, Melbourne and Adelaide government initiative in hospital concerns was limited and each looked with appreciative eyes to the overseas models of public beneficence.[84] In Western Australia, where population

78 CSO, Vol. 1979/88, 10 July 1888.
79 CSO, Vol. 3391/89, 27 November 1889.
80 When recommending Andrew Hanson to the Colonial Hospital in July 1888, Barnett fumed '... for a long time past I have had only one reply—"There is no room"'. CSO, Vol. 1979/88.
81 CSO, Vol. 142, Fol. 140, 1845.
82 CSO, Vol. 139, Fol. 250, 18 July 1845.
83 An American seaman from the *Guyon* was treated at the Colonial Hospital for general debility. On his discharge the ship's captain was paid to ship him back to Singapore 'to defray the cost of his becoming a burden', CSO, Vol. 500, Fol. 214, 18 September 1862.
84 Bolton and Joske in *History of Royal Perth Hospital*, pp. 2–3, point out the difference between Western Australian and overseas and interstate hospitals and government involvement in establishing

and riches were less than in other states, the government's involvement in hospital care was essential but reluctant, and it actively discouraged the medical drain on its limited and limiting budget. The official disinclination to provide and extend hospital care, even for the needy, directed the onus of medical care to the individual and the family.

It was not surprising that commercial remedies promising relief for all mortal ills were popular. Weston's Wizard Oil taken internally and massaged externally could relieve all 'nervous diseases and inflammatory aches and pains, curing rheumatism, sciatica, gout, neuralgia, cholera, spasms, headache, coughs and colds, tumours, ulcers, scrofula, a diseased liver, piles, swellings or wounds'. Only a little less ambitious were the makers of India and Eno's Fruit Salts who promised 'It keeps the blood pure' and 'aids the organs of digestion, absorption, circulations, respiration, secretion and excretion.' Holloway's Pills could be taken to purify the system, and to aid indigestion, sick headache and female irregularities, venereal affections, scrofula or King's Evil, fever, gout and ague while Ayer's Cherry Pectoral was for coughs, croup, colds and bronchitis. Dr J. Collis Brown's Chlorodyne promised quiet refreshing sleep, relief from pain and the healthy functioning of the secretions of the body 'without creating any of those unpleasant results attending the use of opium'.[85] Some hopeful colonists were relieved of ill health, but others were not. Yet a time of medical progress was at hand. In the context of decades and centuries it was close, but in terms of generations there was still much to be learned. Many in the colony went to chemists and general stores for proprietary relief. The accompanying hefty dose of hope was perhaps as effective a cure.

---

the Colonial Hospital. See also, B. Abel-Smith, *The Hospital 1800–1948: A Study in Social Administration in England and Wales, 1964; A. M. Mitchell, The Hospital South of the Yarra: A history of Alfred Hospital, Melbourne, from foundation to the nineteen-forties*, 1977, pp. 3–11; D. Rosner, *A Once Charitable Enterprise: Hospitals and Health Care in Brooklyn and New York 1885–1915*, 1982.

[85] Newspaper advertisements for proprietary medicines were common in the 1880s. Those mentioned can be found in *West Australian*, 22 May 1886, 7 March 1888.

*'... let me urge on each and all that they use every means
in their power, individually and combined and do not cease
till we have both the Asylum and an hospital, a credit
instead of a standing disgrace to the colony.'*
Inquirer, 17 March 1893.

The introduction of convicts in 1850 was a boulder dropped in the pond of Western
Australian society; it affected many areas of colonial life, including the state's
medical services. Between 1850 and 1868, convicts contributed 9,700 of the 17,000
growth in population.[1] Most convicts, with the establishment personnel their
presence entailed, were concentrated in Fremantle. For the first time, the idea of a
hospital for the port promised to become reality.

Shipton pointed out the need in December 1851:

> I would also take this opportunity of respectfully pointing out to the Government the
> necessity of a Seaman's Hospital at the Port; as ships are now daily arriving, and it
> entails a great expense upon the ships, the Medical Officer having to pay daily visits
> and also the great difficulty of my finding time, to do so, owing to the great prefs [*sic*]
> of duties, at this time.
>
> I would also beg to point out the great loss of time, in having to communicate with
> the Col. Surgeon, previous to admitting a man into [the Colonial] Hospital.[2]

In 1852 the Fremantle government resident was invited to accompany the Superintendent of Public Works to select a site upon land reserved by the Governor for
the erection of a wooden building to be used as a hospital.[3] Plans were drawn up for
a rectangular wooden building 32 feet long by eleven feet wide, with two wards each
ten feet square, separated by an attendant's room with a fire at one end for heating
and cooking.[4] Perhaps the project lapsed when the first stage of the convict depot
was constructed in 1853. By 1858 when the depot was completed with a surgery,
fever ward, extensive cell accommodation, a 'dead house', and a general ward, it is
likely that the convict hospital provided accommodation as good as that at the new
Colonial Hospital in Perth, which until 1855, had no building and was probably
combined with the military hospital.[5] In times of 'extreme emergency in Fremantle',

---

[1] Figures from R. T. Appleyard, 'Western Australia: Economical and Demographic Growth, 1850–
1914', in C. T. Stannage, *A New History*, p. 212.
[2] CSO, Vol. 221, Fol. 36, 31 December 1851.
[3] CSO, Vol. 34, Fol. 110, 26 May 1852.
[4] PWD Map 653, 27 May 1852.
[5] See Bolton and Joske, *History of Royal Perth Hospital*, p. 12. For plan of the 'Old Hospital' at the
Convict Establishment, see PWD Map 654, 21 January 1888.

however, free men could be taken to the convict hospital for treatment before being taken to the one at Perth and the practice continued after the convict establishment was handed over to the state in 1886, when the sprawling stone prison overlooking the town became the Imperial gaol. It was not a habit which was encouraged, for as John F. Stone explained:

> There are ... many grave difficulties to contend with in [this?] opening the Prison doors to the Public, one of the greatest in my experience being in regard to Visitors (especially females) to the Patients, and the opportunity afforded of communicating with the Prisoners.[6]

Rules were made by which only males were allowed to visit and only with the permission of both the officer in charge of the station and the medical officer. In all but a few cases of emergency, patients requiring hospitalisation continued to be sent directly to Perth.

Many years later in 1869, the question of a hospital for Fremantle was broached again. The Fremantle resident magistrate whose task it was to refer the sick poor to the Colonial Hospital, urged the establishment of a hospital ward for free colonists at the port. When asked for his opinion, William Dickey, as the acting assistant colonial surgeon in place of Shipton, effectively quashed the idea. He thought that while it would be occasionally advantageous to have a ward in Fremantle where a sick person could be received and attended, the expense of equipping such a ward with suitable furniture, bedding and utensils and the cost of a dispenser and nurses, not to mention 'a means of cooking etc.' outweighed any advantage. If the government wished to go to the expense of providing accommodation for just two patients while there were that number of spare beds at Perth, Dickey would be prepared to organise and maintain it. However, he reasoned, more than half of those sent to Perth were seamen from the merchant shipping who had always been sent to the Colonial Hospital. What was really needed was an improved means of transporting urgent cases.[7] The basic frugal sense of the argument appealed to a government preoccupied with costs, and the perceived medical need was deferred.

The number of sick and injured at Fremantle increased with the population growth. Less serious cases were still nursed at home where possible, and the indigent sent to Perth when beds were available. No matter how ill or how much the pain, patients for Perth had to endure a long wait for the daily steamer before they were laid on its deck, or experience the agonising jolting of a cart ride over rough roads which often must have seemed endless. From 1881 there was the option of a faster, rattling ride by train to Perth station and a short trip to the hospital on a stretcher.

Subdued and periodic muttering about the need for a hospital in Fremantle was ignored by the government for over ten more years until W. E. Marmion, M.L.C., on behalf of his constituents in Fremantle, moved in parliament that a sum should be placed on the 1883 Estimates for a casualty hospital. The present state of affairs was a disgrace to both the town and the colony he declared on 29 August 1882, and

---

[6] CSO File 1259/88, 7 September 1882. See also CSO File 9556, Fol. 13. Circular issued by Comptroller General's Office, 19 May 1870.
[7] CSO, Vol. 638, Fol. 154.

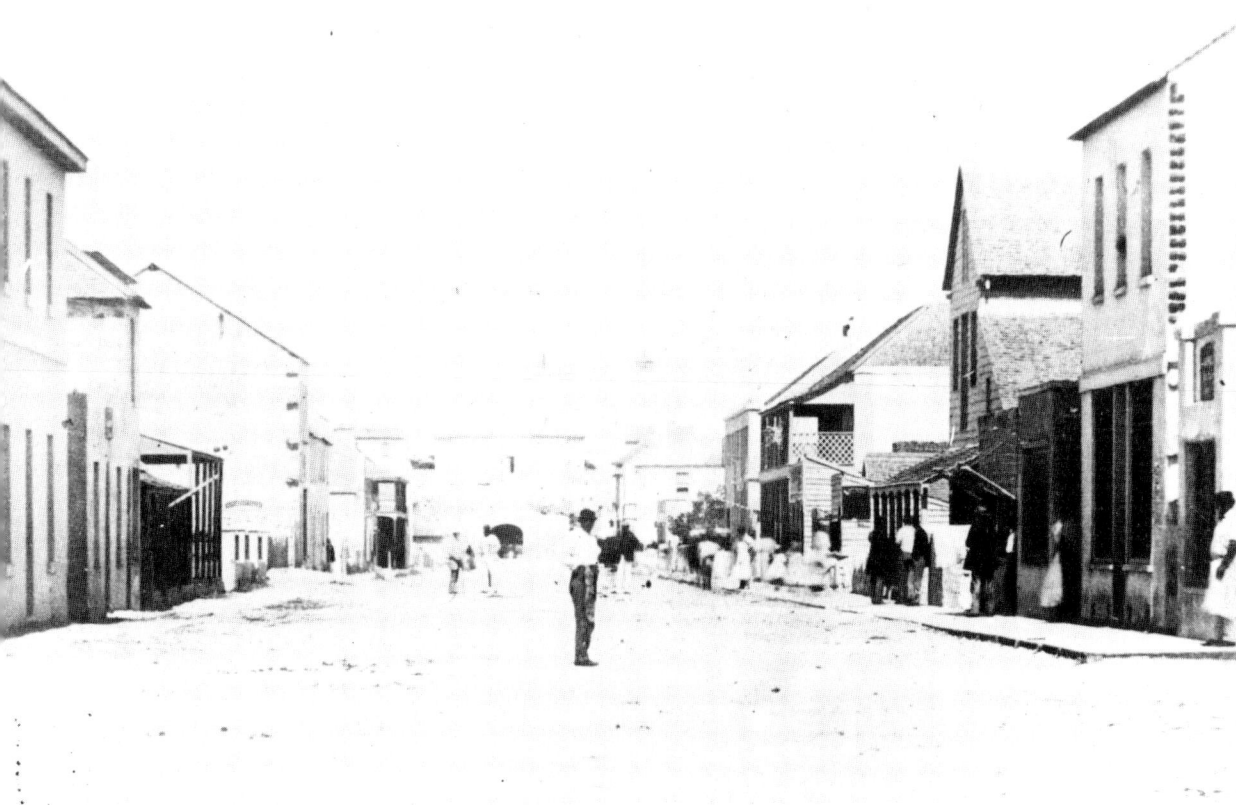

Photograph courtesy Battye Library

Plate 3. High Street, Fremantle, looking towards the Round House, *c.* 1870s–1880s.

> ... such a hospital was absolutely necessary in the cause of our common humanity, there being no place at present in the town—the second in importance and in number of population in the whole Colony, and its principal seaport—where persons meeting with accidents could be conveyed and attended to.[8]

The project was agreed to unanimously, although the Governor later wondered if the gaol hospital might not continue to be used for urgent civilian cases.[9]

With the question of funding settled, the next task was to find a suitable building. Marmion favoured the old guard room opposite the water police quarters just near the South Jetty. While suggestions were exchanged, Richard Birch, a Fremantle druggist at Lot 423 (now No. 71) in High Street, heard of the plan and with enterprise offered both his services and part of his premises as a casualty hospital 'to

[8] *WAPD*, Vol. 7, 29 August 1882, p. 215.
[9] CSO File 1259/88.

attend to and dispence [*sic*] for the sick'.[10] The offer had merit and was approved by both Alfred Waylen as the colonial surgeon, and by the Fremantle medical officer, Henry Calvert Barnett, who inspected the premises. Birch explained that right across the back of his place of business was a large room 20 feet by 12 feet, with a separate entrance fronting High Street and access to both the front and back yards. The premises were centrally located and the room could accommodate three patients. While he would provide food, drugs and attendance for patients, Mrs Birch would look after bed linen and the cooking and cleaning. All these services would be provided for £60 a year and the ward could be ready in a little over a week. 'I can only add that for years I have longed to see such a ward established in the port; and should enter on such service more as a labor of mercy than for the profit of the undertaking', enthused Birch early in October.[11]

The offer was too good to ignore. The walls of the large room which had been used as a kitchen and dining room were whitewashed and the ceiling coloured; a revolving ventilator was placed in the back wall and a window installed. The large fireplace was contracted and a new family kitchen run up between a back sitting room and the ward. Outside on the door, a brass plate inscribed 'Government Casualty Ward'[12] was attached 'so that the spot should be well known where to take patients at once'.[13]

Furnishing the ward proved less costly than was at first feared by Colonial Secretary Gifford. Two narrow iron bedsteads each measuring six feet, six inches by two feet, three inches, with palliasses to fit, plus two mattresses and pillows, sheets, blankets, pillowslips and a mahogany commode threatened to total £13.12.0 until it was thought that furniture from the prison could be used. The pillow slips were of coarse weave, but as patients were not likely to be Fremantle's élite and were expected to be discharged or sent to the Colonial Hospital as soon as possible, the economy seemed worth the short discomfort. Labour to make palliasses and mattresses was readily available with the gaol close-by and, towards the end of 1882, some of Fremantle's prisoners found themselves detailed to the painful and monotonous task of unpicking the fibre from worn ropes to make up the palliasses, and carding horsehair to make the larger mattresses. The finished bedding was carted down the hill to the town and taken into the Casualty Ward, with its new brass plaque on the door. Richard and Eliza Birch were enthusiastic about their new responsibilities, although the loss of the area across the back length of the house made living with seven children and a new baby a little cramped.[14] However, the

[10] CSO File 1259/88, 22 September 1882. Information on the location of Birch's shop was provided by Larraine Stevens from Rate Books at Fremantle City Library. Between 1880 and 1881 the druggist occupied Lot 409 (presently No. 66 High Street) on which was a shop and dwelling. Between 1882 and 1889 his family moved to Lot 423 High Street and then back to Lot 409 between 1890 and 1899. In 1891 until 1898, Alfred Edwin Webster, an English-trained chemist, joined in a business partnership with Birch. Both were foundation members of the Pharmaceutical Society of Western Australia. See references in *Dictionary of Western Australians*, Vol. 4, Parts 1 and 2, for Birch and Webster; *Western Mail*, 2 July 1910.
[11] CSO File 1259/88, 4 October 1882.
[12] *Ibid.* Agreement between Richard Birch and the Colonial Surgeon Alfred Waylen, 30 November 1882.
[13] *Ibid.* Birch to Colonial Secretary, 4 February 1882.
[14] *Dictionary of Western Australians, 1850–1914*, Vol. 3. Reference R. Birch.

first yearly fee was very welcome, as Richard's lack of enthusiasm in his duty as Fremantle's stamp vendor had just led to a transfer of the right to the storekeeper Joseph Doonan.[15]

During the following six years to 1888, the town's serious accident cases were taken to the small High Street Casualty Ward for treatment. Sometimes it was considered necessary to transfer the patient to the Colonial Hospital and the injured person would be carefully carried on a stretcher to the railway station for the trip to Perth. Other patients were nursed at the ward. While many of them, no doubt, remembered the Birch children who sometimes seemed to travel through the ward in a never-ending procession to get to and from their play in the backyard, the children also recalled their special boarders:

> The patients might be in the ward for several days before their removal and were looked after by ... father and mother. The patients were always attended to by Dr. H. C. Barnett, a one-legged doctor and the patients always knew when he was coming by the sound of his crutches.[16]

If patients always knew when the doctor was coming, the druggist and his wife were less sure of knowing when patients would arrive and, with a large family and a business to attend to, may not always have been prepared for their boarders. By agreement, Birch was required only to provide the single room and to keep it clean and in good order, to serve a plain hospital diet, to give prescribed drugs and to nurse the patients admitted. No agreement covered anaesthetics or surgical instruments, which were not provided. The ward was indeed a medical stop-gap and the community, which on occasions witnessed injured men carried in great pain through their main street to the Casualty Ward or who spoke with the doctors who patched the wounded as best they could, knew it.

The second boulder to hit the smooth waters of Westralian society in the nineteenth century began to fall in the mid-1880s. It glittered yellow with the promise of riches with the opening of goldfields in the Kimberleys and it splashed down in the early to mid-1890s with the Yilgarn, Coolgardie and Kalgoorlie finds. Many of the travellers who came to the state were funnelled through the port, and its population floated with the arrival and departure of sailors, with settlers introduced through the Board of Immigration, and gold seekers. The numbers were also swelled by railway and harbour workers and by builders and traders following extensive expansion in these areas in the 1880s.

While population increased and inadequate medical facilities at Fremantle were merely noted by the government, the problem was voiced by the *West Australian* in 1886. It directed attention to the unsuitability of the Casualty Ward as a medical centre for the people of Fremantle and urged that before the need became too great, provision should be made for the care of those 'lower class' residents 'who are poor,

---

[15]   CSO File 1342/88, 1 August 1881.

[16]   Recollection of George Birch, cited in A. McWhinney, *A History of Pharmacy in Western Australia*, 1975, p. 241. So proficient did the thickset doctor become on his crutches that once, during a conversation after a lad tried to 'pinch' one, Barnett '... took a few quick strides with his crutches and kicked himself out at right angles and horizontal to the ground. This feat greatly impressed me ...', recalled L. Manning, notes, FH.

and in sickness', and for those of any class away from home. 'The want of foresight and provision usually leave only regret for what is beyond remedy ... Among the arrangements, therefore, which are now being made in Fremantle for the supply of other needs a hospital should not be overlooked.'[17] As he was assistant to the Fremantle Medical Officer, Dr James Hope, in 1886, Frederick Ingoldby knew well the need. Because the medical facilities at the chief port of the colony were so limited, had he not helped carry injured men in great pain to the railway station to await a train to Perth? Drawing on both his experience of voluntary hospitals in Britain, where regular subscribers formed a board to manage a hospital, and his recent experience in Western Australia, where the government funded and ran the Colonial Hospital, he proposed a synthesis of the two systems:

> I think a public hospital, governed by a local board would meet the difficulty best and the necessary funds to be found partly by voluntary subscription and partly by a Government grant. The patients too should have a small tax put on them as there are few really destitute poor. I know that my brother practitioners here would be just as heartily glad to give their services as I should be to give mine to such an institution and I am sure that with the valuable aid of the press, a scheme could soon be set on foot to provide the want.[18]

Although nothing had been done when he left for Albany two years later, Ingoldby's scheme bore a remarkable similarity to the one eventually adopted.

Stronger moves for a hospital were made early in 1887 by a band of 'concerned ladies' in Fremantle following a serious harbour accident when a sailor named Kayander had both legs badly crushed. Again the 'want of foresight and provision in hospital accommodation' was made very clear when no suitable place could be found at which an amputation could be performed, and the sailor had to be carried to the train for the trip to the Colonial Hospital. The ladies who met in concern believed that something had to be done to 'supply a want which would disgrace any civilized community, implying as it does a quite barbarous indifference to suffering'.[19] Fremantle was coming of age. No longer was suffering an inevitable prelude to either healing or dying in a colonial outpost; now there was communal outrage and compassion for the sick or injured. The ladies prepared to petition the Legislative Council to request a sum sufficient to provide a cottage with an attendant until a proper hospital was approved, but the mayor assured them that the matter was in his hands and that it would be better and wiser to let him carry it through.[20]

With the celebration of Queen Victoria's Jubilee imminent, in early June 1887 William Wells Leach, a well-known bootmaker and currier in High Street, sat down with paper, and hands more comfortable with tools than a pen, and shared with Governor Broome his plan to celebrate the Jubilee:

> I am embolden to write to your Exellency confident if you or Lady Broome could see any way of rendering assistance to the distressd or needy you are always Willing.

[17] *West Australian*, 19 May 1886.
[18] *Ibid.*, 22 May 1886.
[19] *Inquirer*, 7 March 1888. The writer was reminding of events which had taken place eight or nine months earlier.
[20] *Ibid.*

In this mornings paper I see Lady Broom is starting a fund to assist Necessitus Woman on discharge from hospitable. This emboldens me to make the following suges- tions. The nesecity of a Cottage Hospitabal in Fremantle and the Good it would be for the [interests] of the port and those who come to the Port as Sailors.

This is the suggestin if you could see your way to set apart a Cottage or three or four rooms to be called Victoria Cottage Hospitable. It would be a great blessing to the town. only about three weeks ago a poor man ran over by the train laid on stretcher in the street for more than twenty minites crying with pain. Wailing until the Dr. came as there was no place to take him to he was then moved to the Prison Hospitible and shortly died. I am [not an] advocate for either Rich or Poor hanging upon Govement for all they require but I think in this case the Govement could assist the inhabatants. First the Govement by giving the use of Cottage or rooms with any spare Medicine or Surgical instruments secondly those better off in the town subscribe the mony to furnish the Drugs and funeture, and also subscribe say from 10/– to any sum per annum for which they might have tickets in proportion to what they subscribe to give to there neubours who may be in need.

Thirdly by the poor themselves paying a small sum weekly or monthly so that if they feel sick could have the benefit of Medicial advice arrangements being made for a Dr to call at a certain hour to give advice thus saving them from being paupers.

I think the different churches would [be agreeable to] collecting? On one Sunday in the year for the same purpose I also feel convinced Mr Congdon the Mayor or the [?] Rv Watkinss with others would do all they could for such a purpose. Your Exellency and Lady Broom with experience I am sure will sugest some better way than I can explan by writing-but if your Exellency thinks by seeing I could give any sugestion I should be most happy to wait upon you. I have resided in Fremantle nearly thirty years.

Yours Exellency
Faithful Servant
W. Leach

Home Cottage
Fremantle

I have huredly writin the enclosed letter as I thought if it was possable to mature any plan by the day of opining the Town Hall Your Exellincy could announce it and it would be a blessing making the Jubilee Day remembered by rich & poor.[21]

This letter joined a growing number of letters and petitions for a hospital in the government files. The Town Hall was opened by the Governor on 22 June 1887 after a long celebratory procession of lodge members and school children. Sports events followed, with a grand ball at night and a children's fancy dress ball on the follow- ing evening. There was no mention of a hospital for Fremantle, although the shoot- ing of Councillor Snook by the landlord of the Victoria Hotel following the chil- dren's ball was an eloquent testimony to the need which was 'under consideration'.[22]

The matter was introduced in the Legislative Council in August of 1887, when there was serious talk about the hospital at the Convict Establishment being made

---

[21] CSO File 2354/87, Leach to Governor Broome, 9 June 1887.
[22] See Ewers, *The Western Gateway*, p. 83. The landlord William Conroy was subsequently hanged for the murder of Councillor Snook, who had refused to admit Conroy to the celebration because he was drunk.

over to the community to serve as a general hospital. The colonial secretary, Sir Malcolm Fraser, thought that the walling-off of the hospital from the gaol was rather impractical but that he would 'consider the matter'. However, it was commonly known that Mayor Congdon favoured turning the old building, which had housed the comptroller-general of convicts, into a hospital if alternative accommodation could be found for the invalids now residing there, and Malcolm Fraser privately agreed: 'The Knowle could be converted easily and would serve the purpose for years'. If the council had been more aggressive in its agitation for a local hospital the question may have been resolved quite quickly. The mayor was asked by the government to write his views on the subject, whereupon they would be duly considered, but perhaps other issues seemed of greater importance at the time, for a few days later Malcolm Fraser observed laconically that: 'Probably the Municipal Council will move again in the matter ere long!'[23]

A move was not long in coming, but it was not from the council. On a Friday in mid-February 1888, a lumper named Regan was working on South Jetty, slinging goods on board the hulk *Eliza Blanche*. The labour of hand loading ships was hard and dangerous. As the vessel dipped gently with the swell, a case of galvanised iron swayed, slipped, and crashed loudly onto the wharf, sending gulls screeching into the air and pinning Regan beneath the load. Workmates carefully carried the injured man along High Street to the Casualty Ward while others went to call Drs Hope and Birmingham. The casualty room was in anything but a satisfactory condition with no equipment for performing surgery on Regan's injured leg. As best they could, the doctors bandaged the crushed limb and Regan was sent by train to Perth.[24] Indignation increased a week later when George Cooke, a sailor on the *Gemma*—a small lighter used to land cargoes from large steamers anchored out from the port in Gage Roads—also had his leg broken while landing two heavy, unwieldy bundles of wire.[25] Barnett attended to him, although on this occasion the ward was better prepared.

If interest in the Casualty Ward was intermittent in early 1888, it was not surprising. Growling threats of war in Europe were heard as far away as Western Australia and there was rumbling talk of self-government for the state.[26]

In Fremantle there was some concern about poverty, which inevitably affected some far more than others. Those who experienced it would not have wholeheartedly agreed with the sentiments of the telegram sent to Queen Victoria on the people's behalf to celebrate her Jubilee, recognising 'with infinite thankfulness the many blessings which under Providence have accrued to them during the sixty years of your Majesty's most glorious reign'.[27] By 1888 there was a sense of despair as people looked to the future. The proposed harbour works seemed little more than wishful thinking, there was much unemployment and the issue of responsible government

[23] CSO File 2354/87. Letters by J. Arthur Wright, director of Public Works, 25 June 1887, and Malcolm Fraser, Colonial Secretary to the Governor, 27 June 1887, considering the provision of a hospital for the Port. At this period, The Knowle was in use as the Invalids' Depot.

[24] *Inquirer*, 15 February 1888.

[25] *Ibid.*, 22 February 1888.

[26] *Ibid.*, 15 February 1888.

[27] CSO File 1988/97.

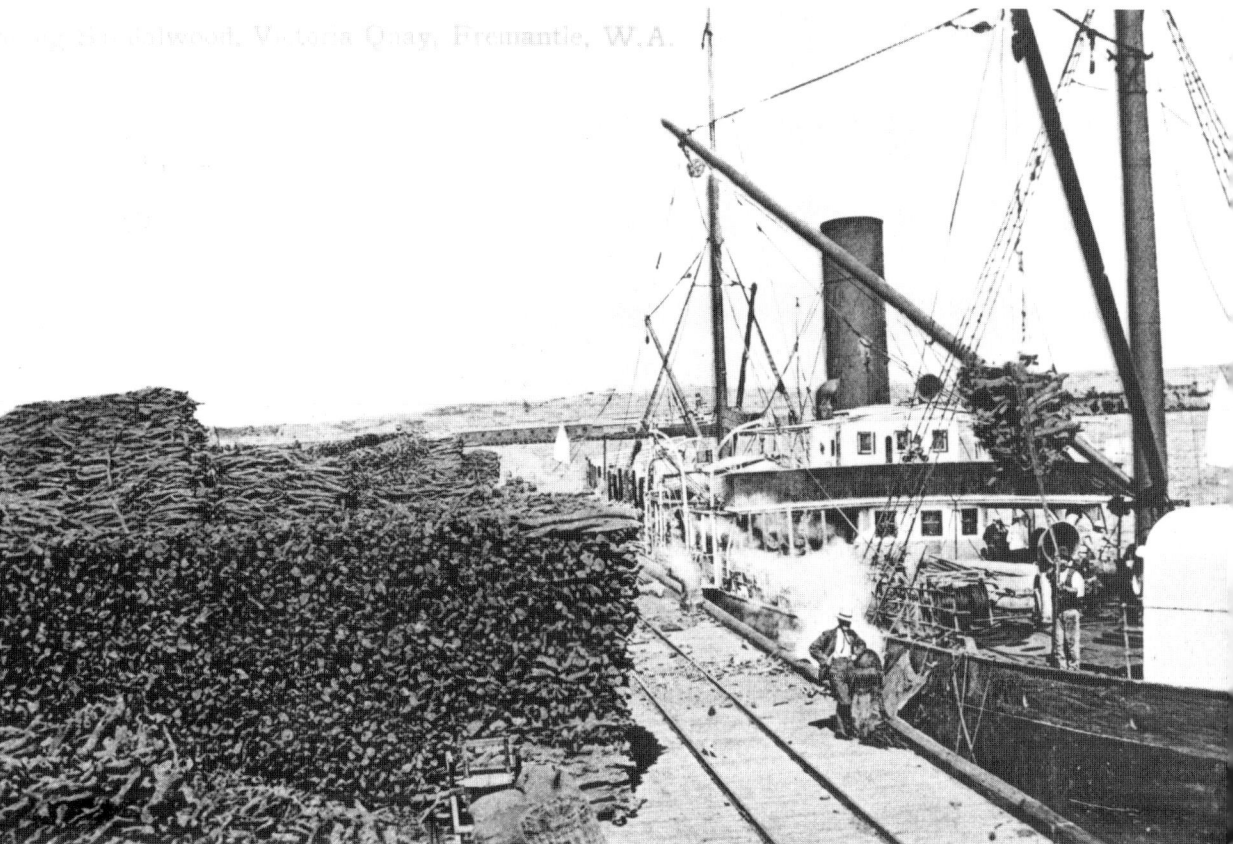

Photograph courtesy West Australian Newspapers

Plate 4. While loading sandalwood at Fremantle, lumpers frequently had accidents on the wharves:

> A lumper ... fell down one of the steamer's holds last evening ... /unloading a truckload of piles on the South Mole when one of the piles rolled off the truck and fell on his right leg.../the tackle broke, striking Laurie who was knocked thirty feet down into the hold .../ by some means a heavy piece of oregon fell on his left foot, crushing it badly ... /a sling of twelve planks slipped ... and [each] was taken to the Fremantle Hospital.

The *West Australian* (various)

for Western Australia remained unresolved. There were also deep private despairs. Afghan camel drivers with a consignment of camels from Karachi for the goldfields found their employer so far in debt that the animals were seized under a bill of sale. There was no pay, no accommodation, no return passage, and for three days, out in the bush near Albert's piggery at Fremantle they deliberated and hungered before applying at the police station for rations of bread and tea. A week later, the Afghans fought out in the paddock at Albert's—and smiled as they were made to understand that they were under arrest with food and shelter provided for seven days, albeit in gaol.[28] In January a quite sober, elderly bootmaker named William Sherry, who had been unable to find work, staggered into the Fremantle police station from the bush where he had been sleeping and begged to be placed in prison rather than suffer his present misery. Dr Barnett was called, but Sherry could not swallow the soup which was cooked for him. He lay down on the rugs and blankets the police provided and quietly died. Barnett grimly recorded the cause of death as 'failure of the heart's action and debility, caused by the exposure in the bush and want of food'.[29] Two days earlier, a hawker with a small shop had taken his own life after his business faltered and failed.[30] Six weeks later the resident magistrate was told that a woman who had not eaten for four or five days had collapsed after begging a housewife in Bannister Street for a glass of water. The householder regretted that 'she had enough to do to keep herself' and would have to turn the woman out, but that 'it was a great shame to leave the woman starving'[31].

Little consolation was extended to the impoverished through the editorial of the *Evening Times* on 27 February 1888, which explained that in the United Kingdom there was now an increase in the diffusion of wealth and, although there was still poverty, its origins no doubt 'would be found in circumstances within the control of the sufferer himself'. A Fremantle storeman named H. Goldsworthy took up the cause of the poor through the port's evening paper.[32] Readers of the *Inquirer*, however, thought the whole poverty issue 'the fabrications of a diseased imagination'.[33] While Fremantle, as in other places, had its poor, they were not considered to be starving—the hungry had only to go to the mayor and the government resident, who would authorise relief; the homeless could get shelter at the depot through the resident magistrate; sick paupers could be sent to the Colonial Hospital and, of course, there were the good ladies of the town who on being acquainted with a case of need would pay a personal visit to the home of the distressed to render assistance. But there were some too proud to submit to the indignity of a personal investigation of their morals and circumstances by police and government officials, and others knew that they would not pass the 'worthiness to receive relief' test.

Just a month after the publicity on poverty, Ada Towser applied to the Fremantle police for assistance. Although obviously ill and only a year in the colony, Ada was 18 years old, unmarried and pregnant. The case was referred through the resident magistrate to the colonial surgeon and then to the colonial secretary in Perth. Not only was reception at the poor house or the hospital denied to the young woman, but also food. Police and the resident magistrate took the only course of assistance open to them and used the gaol as a refuge. Ada was kept in a cell overnight. The following morning she was brought before the resident magistrate and sentenced to 14 days' imprisonment for vagrancy.[34] While the *Inquirer* thought that 'the disease'

[28] *Evening Times*, 16 January 1888, 17 January 1888, 19 January 1888, 25 January 1888, 21 February 1888, 27 February 1888. The Afghans became a familiar sight in Fremantle streets and were eventually given shelter in the immigration depot.

[29] *Ibid.*, 6 January 1888.

[30] *Ibid.*, 4 January 1888.

[31] *Ibid.*, 23 March 1888.

[32] *Ibid.*, 27 February 1888.

[33] *Inquirer*, 29 February 1888.

[34] *Ibid.*, 21 March 1888.

from which Ada suffered should have suggested special treatment, official judgment was otherwise. Humanity after all, did have its limits. Sometime later Ada stowed away on the *Rob Roy* to Bunbury with the daughter of a Fremantle blacksmith.[35] There the resident magistrate found work for them.

Community concern for the afflicted 'worthy', however, was open and unmeasured. While Ada's distressed condition was seen as a result of a logical justice, the suffering of the citizens of Greenough in the 1888 floods was through an act of God and the hearts and purses of good Fremantle people opened in response. The conduct of the town's regular business almost came to a halt on 21 February 1888, when a Fancy Costume Cricket Match in aid of the Greenough Relief Fund was played by some of the leading citizens. Dr Ingoldby cancelled his practice for the day to dress as a French jester and joined the procession, led by a drum and fife band, that formed at Messrs Farmer and Imray's. With children running in excited circles and adults barely less disciplined, the cricketers marched to the station to await the 1.15 p.m. train from Perth. The band played negro melodies until the travellers arrived, then all moved on to the cricket ground:

> On Wednesday in Fremantle Park, a cricket match was played
> By wielders of the willow, in most varied dress arrayed;
> Thirty six, with umpires two, paraded round the town
> And many hearty laughs were raised, at the antics of the clown.[36]

The Chinese tobacconist, F. Imray, led the first team to bat. Rules were bent and invented and one player who could not be bowled out was carried off the field to the delight of the crowd. 'To stimulate to prompt and healthy effort becomes a duty in those who should be leaders of public opinion,' urged the *Inquirer*, and these leaders of public opinion in the town took their duty seriously:

> The object was a good one, t'was to help those in distress
> And the people of Fremantle, all were ready you may guess,
> To help the kind promoters, though the day was hardly cool,
> And many prominent men were not too proud to act the fool.[37]

As he had been Dr Hope's assistant since 1881, Frederick Ingoldby was well known in the town, and popular as a doctor. His enthusiasm as the clown was appreciated both by those who had benefited from his professional advice and others who used the freely-available proprietary medicines for their ailments. However, most ills were forgotten in watching Ingoldby in one of his last appearances with a Fremantle cricket bat before leaving for Albany.

> ... No nervousness or fear is seen, as the clown steps to the ground,
> Who carefully throws his medical eye upon the fielders round
> For every ball that's bowled he runs, now one, now two, now more,
> New bowlers must be tried, fat boy, so quickly mounts the score.[38]

---

[35] *Dictionary of Western Australians 1829–1914*, Vol. 4. Entries for Ada Tozer and Adelaide Stevens.

[36] Verse, 'The Chinkees's Side', by Billy Green, in *Inquirier*, 22 February 1888; see also 19 February 1888. *Evening Times*, 14 February 1888.

[37] *Inquirer*, 22 February 1888.

[38] *Ibid.*

The event was a great success. Ingoldby was presented with the cricket bat, and the victims of the flood at Greenough with £89. As W. E. Marmion had predicted, 'Fremantle people were never behind in showing their sympathy and giving their substantial aid and assistance when required'.[39] Perhaps young Ada Towser forgot the cramps of a hungry belly for a while with the music and merriment; the day was a welcome respite for those caught up in the continual concern about food and shelter and survival. Perhaps, too, on that Wednesday afternoon in 1888, George Cooke was aware of the laughter from the cricket field as he was carried from the jetty to the Casualty Ward to have his broken leg set by Dr Barnett.[40]

When the winter rain started in Fremantle, it fell on the roof at the Round House, soaked the convict gaol on the hill, and splashed over the new courthouse. It rolled down the steeple at St John's Anglican Church in King's Square, off the new Wesley Church in Cantonment Street and along the shingles of the Adelaide Street Roman Catholic church. In the town some shopkeepers set buckets under leaks and at warehouses and merchant houses windows were quickly shut. At the lunatic asylum, with its soaring turrets and barred windows, some cowered at the rain's drumming, and Richard Birch in High Street checked that the doors of the Casualty Ward were shut against the weather. Travellers at the railway station scurried for cover, as did pupils at Fremantle Boys' School and the grammar school. Drinkers at the hotels ambled inside, while workers at the railway workshops and lumpers on the wharves watched their step on ground made slippery. It rained on the convict-built traffic bridge across the river and trickled off the gas and kerosene street lamps. Up near the gaol, water gurgled down The Knowle which was in use as an Invalids' Depot, while in the town, consternation was felt at the new Town Hall when rain penetrated the imposing clock tower. In 1888 Fremantle was a complacent town, a town proud of its substantial architectural expressions of civilization and the civility of its more prominent citizens. There was room for improvement which the council was working towards—and which would come with time, people reasoned, but in an unlisted scale of wants and needs a hospital was not a priority before 1888.

If good came from the misfortunes suffered by Regan and Cooke on the wharf in February it was the rekindled interest for a port hospital. One of the 'concerned ladies' of early 1887, under the pseudonym 'Rusticus Expectat', wrote to the *Inquirer* on behalf of the group to enquire what had been done in the matter during the past eight or nine months. 'Yet again', they protested,

> . . . a victim of the gross callousness of men in health and comfort, had to be jolted up to Perth with limbs crushed—in agony terrible to even witness—to the the hospital which still remains the one hospital for Port and City, and which is moreover, now, full.[41]

The press urged that the fervour generated by the 'band of ladies' should not be allowed to cool without anything practical being done by the town's leaders, who celebrated anniversaries with expensive festivities but deferred decisions about a

---

[39] *Inquirer*, 19 February 1888, 22 February 1888.
[40] See footnote 25.
[41] *Inquirer*, 7 March 1888; see also 15 February 1888.

necessary hospital.[42] Under pressure from the publicity, the mayor accompanied the Governor and several members of parliament to look at available premises which might provide casualty ward accommodation.

When the Legislative Assembly sat in the following week, Sir Malcolm Fraser moved that £300 should be placed on the Estimates to secure and supply a room with appropriate surgical instruments for a cottage hospital at the port; a portion of the immigration depot could be set aside for the purpose, he suggested. The resulting debate about the state of government finances on one hand and a regard for 'common humanity' on the other, was animated and divided. The representative for Fremantle, William E. Marmion pointed out that the present emergency medical accommodation at the principal port of the colony was 'utterly unfit to enable cases to be attended to in a manner consonant with the dictates of humanity'. William Pearse, M.L.C., and Mayor Daniel Congdon (also representing Fremantle) agreed and told of accident victims from the wharves and workshops 'writhing in agony' on their journey to Perth because 'the miserable room' now used in an emergency had no 'comfort or convenience, and there were no surgical appliances—not even a bandage—at hand to enable the simplest operation to be performed'. But the Attorney General, the Honorable C. N. Warton, who had visited Birch's 'little den' and seen the room's inadequacies when he had gone with the Governor and others to look into the hospital situation at the port, thought that: 'It was not a Fremantle question at all; it was a question, as had been already said, of humanity.'[43]

Humanity, however, had a price and experience had suggested to these men juggling the public purse, that the price tended to escalate. Young Dr Edward Scott, M.L.C., representing Perth, joined with his brother-in-law, Robert F. Sholl, M.L.C., and Alexander Forrest, M.L.C., in thinking that the £300 grant was only the thin edge of the medical wedge, but Harry Venn was willing to vote a lump sum provided there were no annual increments. Scott's motives were no doubt shaped by his moves to enlarge the Colonial Hospital's capacity from 37 beds[44] and to introduce private subscription, as in England. His entry into parliament in 1886 and involvement on the select committee into the working of the Colonial Hospital had raised an awareness in parliament of medical needs. When put to the vote, finance for the Fremantle Cottage Hospital was included in the Estimates for the following year. It was a jubilant Mayor Congdon who met with his council that month.

While most residents welcomed the news about the proposed hospital in Fremantle, the area's colonial surgeon was less elated. Henry Calvert Barnett was a realist and not backward about stating his concerns, whether about public health or other matters. As the son of well-to-do parents who provided a tutor for his education in Belfast, a youthful Barnett found an outlet for his energy when he went to Canada. In Quebec he witnessed the devastation and anguish of cholera when hundreds of Irish immigrants died daily and were buried in mass graves.[45] It was not an experience easily shrugged off and although shipwreck delayed his return home, Barnett channelled his enthusiasm into study for a doctor's qualification, which he

[42] *Ibid.*, 14 March 1888; *Evening Times*, 8 March 1888.
[43] *WAPD*, Vol. 13, 21 March 1888.
[44] Bolton and Joske, *History of Royal Perth Hospital*, pp. 39–44.
[45] Cohen, *A History of Medicine*, pp. 83–5.

gained in 1860 at the age of 28. Barnett travelled and adventured for eight years before accepting the position of colonial surgeon in the Swan River colony's York district. This period proved difficult for the young doctor who suffered so badly with a knee injury that in 1869 he required three major operations before his leg was finally amputated. For another year he carried on his medical practice at York, often in as much pain as the patients he was called to see: 'the condition of my stump at present is such that there is no possibility of my being able to use an artificial limb without previously having some portion of the end of the bone removed'.[46] At Fremantle in 1870, that operation was performed. In 1872, when Dr Dickey left the port and his position as assistant colonial surgeon, Barnett accepted the post and was also appointed superintendent of the lunatic asylum, a position which he retained for the next 25 years.[47]

Knowing well the parsimonious tendency of government thinking, Barnett realized that the decision to equip a cottage hospital in Fremantle would only result in more work for him as the assistant colonial surgeon, and he promptly protested to the Governor the extent of his important asylum work—always arduous, always increasing and with no assistance. Then there was his

> ... ordinary Government work [which is] incessantly increasing notably in the Railway Department where, instead of 6 or 8 as formerly, I have now a list of 108 persons, residing all over the place, and claiming from me constant attendances though I have neither forage or assistant ... My official work is now so great and increases so rapidly that *it is* not *possible* for me to undertake charge of the intended *Cottage Hospital* in Fremantle.[48]

The colonial secretary thought otherwise. Between Barnett and Dr James Hope, who served as the gaol surgeon, as medical officer at Rottnest and health officer at Fremantle, the government was paying £700 a year to the two medical men in the area, and work-load aside, the sum was 'quite sufficient for such duties as have to be performed'. Waylen thought that the responsibility for treatment might be shared by the doctors, each of whom would treat the patient he had admitted, but with cooling enthusiasm for the project, Malcolm Fraser pointed out that the 'cottage hospital is only a casualty ward' and while he hoped that there would be no patients to attend to, that the colonial surgeon of Fremantle was the logical man for the job.[49]

Enthusiasm for the hospital dwindled further and Malcolm Fraser's proposal to use part of the immigration barracks as a casualty ward did not eventuate. With the end of transportation in 1886, the massive convict establishment retained its basic function as a prison, but was administered by the colonial government instead of British control, and the surrounding auxiliary prison buildings were adapted for different uses. To help meet the needs of the ailing and the aged, the comptroller

[46] CSO, Vol. 660, Fol. 49, correspondence January-June 1870. Legend has it that Barnett amputated his own leg, but as yet no direct evidence has been found to verify this. See further biographical notes in *West Australian*, 4 November 1897; *Possum*, 25 Feburary 1888; *Inquirer*, 2 April 1890; Kimberly, *History of West Australia*, Biog., p. 88.

[47] See Ellis, *Eloquent Testimony*, pp. 26-41.

[48] CSO File 1069/88, 11 April 1888.

[49] *Ibid.*

general's once-beautiful old house, The Knowle, was used as Fremantle's Invalids' Depot. The No. 2 Pensioner Barracks on South Terrace were altered and added to by J. Banfield at a cost of £685, to provide an immigration home for the girls who arrived by ship[50] and who were welcomed as domestic servants and potential wives in the predominantly male population. Already over 30 years old, and built as convict gaolers quarters, the rooms were not suitable as a hospital. In any event, arrangements were made with Richard Birch to continue the lease of his room, but only on a monthly basis until arrangements for the new ward could be completed.

By January 1889, Fremantle's new Casualty Ward had been opened. Phoebe Stewart, the wife of the harbour crew's coxswain, who lived adjacent to the ward, was appointed caretaker and undertook to supply ward patients with food for the sum of two shillings and sixpence a day each. Like the colonial secretary, Barnett hoped the patients would be 'few and intermittent', and so they were for a time.[51] The ward was well located for the treatment of accident cases, as it was situated near the waterfront and railway yards and close by the tunnel which had been gouged from cliffs under the Round House in whaling days. However, its existence was not well known. In August a notice was placed in the *Government Gazette* reassuring that the ward was 'open for the reception of urgent cases'.[52]

While agitation for a hospital in Fremantle continued, the government did move to secure land for a hospital in 1890.[53] North-east of the town and further from the town centre and the wharves and railway yards than even the lunatic asylum, lot 1362, a plot of about five acres, was bounded by Skinner (now Burt), Tuckfield and Quarry Streets. As it was adjacent to the quarry, where accidents were frequently of a serious nature, workers there welcomed the choice of land. Perhaps it was not by chance that the site was also only a block away from the town's cemetery in Skinner Street which was used from 1852 in place of the old one in Alma Street.[54]

With land as the incentive, a hospital fund was discussed and the Reverend A. T. Boas, a well-known lecturer visiting from Adelaide, offered to give a lecture to commence fund-raising. On 30 July 1891, his lecture on 'Proverbs and Sayings, Ancient and Modern' raised £15, none of which the Fremantle Council deducted for the use of the Town Hall as they usually did.[55] By 1891, gold and politics were of greater interest than hospitals as immigrants poured to the 'fields and John Forrest took his place as the state's first premier. It was over a year before the hospital funds again received a boost with the proceeds from a lecture by J. P. T. Caulfield on 'The Working of Responsible Government in Australia'.[56] Not surprisingly, when the Fremantle council tried to enlist the support of the Colonial Hospital in its bid for a hospital which would inevitably vie for government funds, there was little encouragement. Council was assured that only 20 of the 37 beds at Perth were usually occupied and emergency beds were always available. Nevertheless, Fremantle's

[50] *Western Australian Government Gazette*, 4 March 1886, 25 March 1886, 1 April 1886, 10 June 1886, 24 June 1886, 15 July 1886.
[51] CSO, Vol. 274., Fol. 89. The exact location of the building is unknown.
[52] *Western Australian Government Gazette*, 1 August 1889.
[53] Minutes of FMC, 2 December 1890.
[54] Ewers, *The Western Gateway*, p. 46.
[55] Minutes of FMC, 17 July 1891.
[56] *Ibid.*, 16 September 1892.

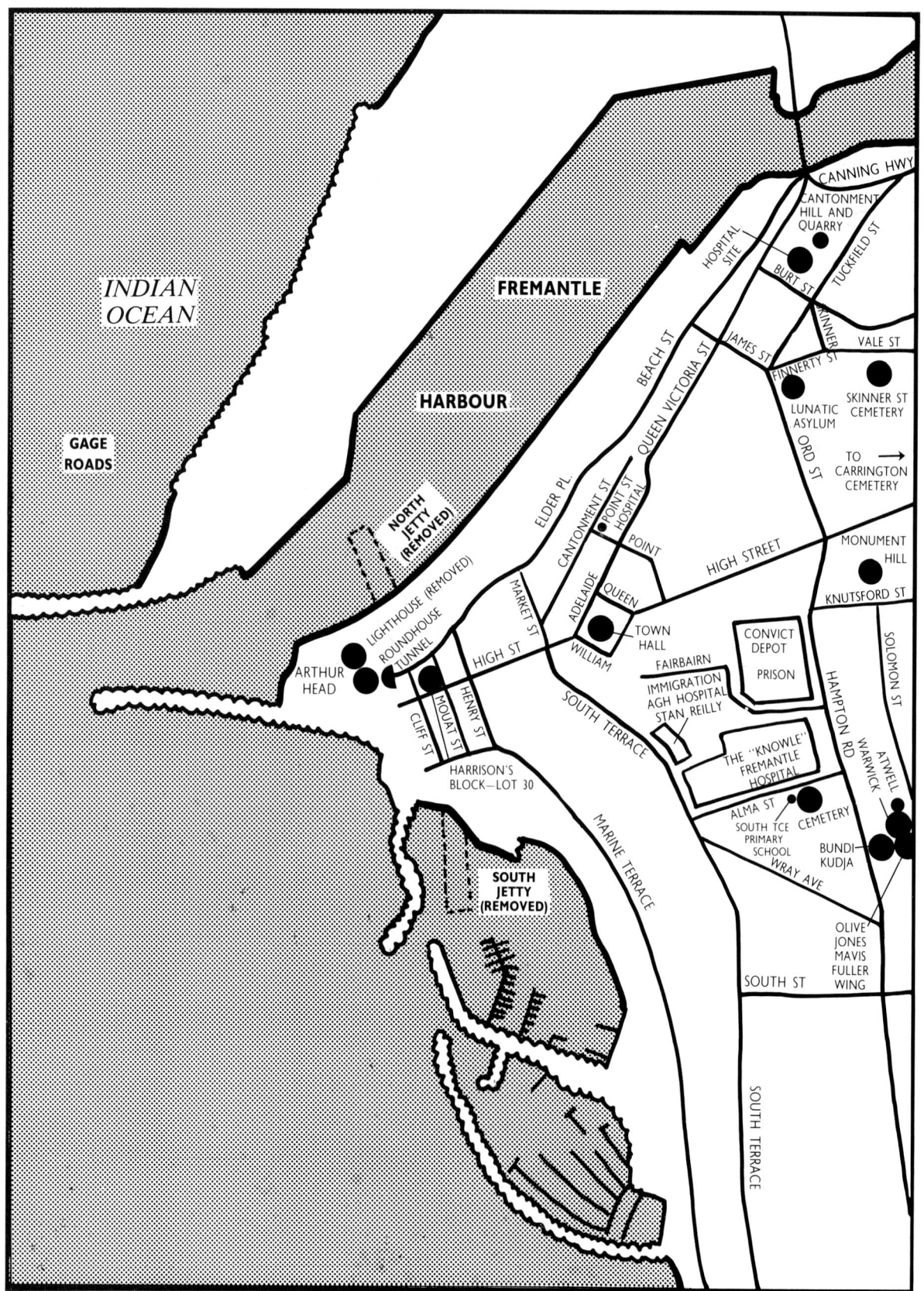

Fig. 5. Map of Fremantle district.

Mayor William F. Samson and Dr James Hope continued to work towards a hospital for the port and as they felt concerned about the position of the Casualty Ward in an area where railway development seemed likely, both urged that The Knowle should be retained for hospital purposes when required.[57]

In September 1891, the acting colonial surgeon was called to the Casualty Ward to treat a man named Martin from the S.S. *Bullara* who was in great pain from a broken right leg. Hope set the leg and, recalling past precedents and the function of the ward as a 'casualty station', sent the man to the Colonial Hospital. The journey was premature, for Martin's leg was further injured through the move. Without giving reason, Waylen, now nearly into his twentieth year as colonial surgeon, testily admonished Hope for sending the patient to Perth and advised him that future cases were to be kept at the Fremantle ward and not sent to the capital. In the following month a man suffering perforated lungs and several broken ribs was admitted to the ward after a dynamite explosion. Hope kept him at the ward but when Colonial Secretary George Shenton heard of the case he wondered why the patient had not been sent to the Colonial Hospital. Again the function of the Casualty Ward was examined and its need debated by Waylen, Hope and the colonial secretary. Aware of his parliamentary influence in setting up the present ward and conscious of his authority, Shenton had the last word. The ward was to continue, but all serious cases were to be sent to Perth as soon as practicable.[58]

Between 1881, when the railway between Perth and Fremantle was opened, and 1891, the Fremantle railway workshops had become, with the wharves, major industries in the town. Both needed land on which to build and extend.[59] On a day in late October while Phoebe Stewart was nursing the patient from the dynamite accident, she heard a great knocking and banging at the wall surrounding her small backyard. Gathering up her skirts she ran outside to remonstrate with the men who were hammering at the blocks of limestone. When they refused to stop she hurried to Dr James Hope who was deputising for Barnett on his first extended holiday in 20 years. The acting assistant colonial surgeon wrote directly to the colonial secretary: 'Some notification of intended alterations should have been sent to me ... I think the townsfolk of Fremantle will think the premises ought not to be interfered with'.[60] Despite Hope's indignation, Phoebe and her husband received notice from the chief harbour master to leave their quarters, which were to be pulled down, and the nurse had no alternative but to write to the colonial surgeon that '... myself who has acted as caretaker to the casualty ward for three years will have to resigned as their [*sic*] is no quarters here to go to'.[61]

Over seven months later the problem of accommodation for the caretaker was still not resolved. The ward remained empty and almost intact, shouldered on one side by the harbour crew quarters and free standing on the other, where the Stewart's old

[57] Minutes of FLBH, 24 August 1891.

[58] CSO File 2060/91, 7 November 1891.

[59] The people lost their large expanse of public riverside recreational land named The Green to the railway by the mid-1880s. R. Reece and R. Pascoe, *A Place of Consequence: A Pictorial History of Fremantle*, 1983, p. 43.

[60] CSO File 2060/91, 29 October 1891.

[61] CSO File 2171A/91, letter written 14 November 1891. See also Minutes of FLBH, 5 November 1891, 27 November 1891, 8 January 1892.

quarters had been demolished and the railway had taken over the land. With the town full of 'eastern staters' trying to escape the Depression of the 1890s and out-fitting themselves for Coolgardie; with entrepreneurs and workers gathering in an effort to meet the new demand for supplies, transport and equipment; with labourers hoping for work engendered by C. Y. O'Connor's new plan to open the river's closed mouth to form a safe river harbour for shipping, accommodation near the Casualty Ward was not to be found.

In mid-September 1892, the colonial secretary declared flatly to Hope that: 'Some arrangement must be made to open this ward. Being on the spot and knowing what is wanted you are best able to do so'.[62] No government building was available for use as a ward, including The Knowle, which Hope had suggested as a town hospital and which was about to be used as a branch of the lunatic asylum for 'imbeciles and other harmless male patients'.[63] Then Hope thought of a solution. As the Casualty Ward comprised one small and one larger room, '. . . let the small one be used for accommodating a man as caretaker. He could live in it and cook and perform work . . . necessary.'[64] A ticket-of-leave man named Frederick Bevan who had been trans-ported for stealing a purse and 12 shillings was suggested. Not only had he worked for two years as an orderly in the Fremantle Prison Hospital, where he earned Hope's approval for his care and kindness to patients, but he was a sober man. For 30 shillings a week, Bevan commenced work as caretaker and Hope announced with satisfaction that 'the ward is now open'.[65] But as locomotives continually passed and repassed just outside the ward, patients found no rest and quiet, and as space was limited, at least one man carried to the ward with a broken leg had to be passed in through the window.[66]

Bevan had been at the ward for only six months when one of the worst building accidents in the colony's history occurred at Fremantle. The new brewery under con-struction in Beach Street on the eastern river bank, with a central tower four storeys high and two wings each of two storeys, had taken shape after four months' work. Limestone blasted from the site as building progressed was the major building material. There had been some talk of cracking in the walls and questions raised about the quality of the cement mortar, but as the building rose around the connect-ing arches it seemed a fine asset to the five partners in the brewery venture and to the town as well.

At five past twelve on Saturday, 4 March 1893, as all the walls reached nearly to their completed height, the 13 builders were preparing to 'knock off' when with a great rumbling, the whole body of the middle structure crumbled, and walls, beams, scaffolding and men crashed together to the ground.[67] Miraculous escapes were quickly compared by the men suffering mainly severe bruising until it was realized that two of their number had been working in the basement. One was J. Costigan, the other a newly-arrived Englishman named Arthur Westwood, whose wife and

[62]   CSO File 1058/92.
[63]   Minutes of FLBH, 22 June 1892, 5 July 1892; W.A. Blue Book, 1893 (deaths).
[64]   CSO File 2060/91, 11 September 1892.
[65]   Ibid. See also CSO File 1490/92.
[66]   Inquirer, 17 March 1893.
[67]   Ibid., 10 March 1893.

family were due from London any day. Frantic efforts to cut through timber and remove the stone and rubble covering the groaning men were hastened by many of the hundreds of townsfolk who left their businesses and occupations and gathered at the site, but it was an hour before Westwood was found pinned under a beam and large blocks of stone, and a little longer before Costigan was uncovered lying face downwards with a joist on the back of his head. Dr Barnett, now back in the colony, directed the medical treatment and Hope and White assisted. Barnett looked at Westwood's broken legs and crushed torso and instructed some men to carry him to the Casualty Ward. But the two-bed ward was already occupied. Although one patient was 'nearly well', the other bed held a man 'in a frightful condition'.[68]

When the first of the brewery casualties was carefully carried in, Barnett instructed: 'We have no bed; lay him on the table.' On Westwood's arrival there seemed no option but to order: '... take him to the train, we have nowhere to receive him'.[69] The terse words were likely a result of ill-concealed anger at inadequate conditions long endured as Fremantle's colonial surgeon, but they were no consolation to Westwood and the men who accompanied him on the train, trying to quench his thirst with the little water they carried. Costigan also was taken by train to the Colonial Hospital, but no brandy given to the two injured men could dull their pain. Only Costigan survived. Of the two other men carried to the Casualty Ward, young Rollinson, a stone mason and the chief support of his mother and family, was treated for broken ribs; the other labourer suffered bruising, a gash on his forehead, and part of a lip torn off. Another worker, Silas King, was able to walk to the Casualty Ward for treatment before going home. To the small community, the occurrence was nothing short of a disaster and great indignation erupted about the inadequate medical facilities at the port.

The indignation took a positive form when 300 ratepayers gathered in the Town Hall the following Friday in response to a public announcement convening the meeting. Most Fremantle notables were there—Mayor William Frederick Samson, the Honorable William Marmion, William Pearse, Elias Solomon, the Honorable Daniel Congdon and the town councillors. Archdeacon Watson conveyed his support and an apology for his absence. Feelings ran high among citizens who knew and saw or had assisted the injured. Past efforts to obtain a hospital were reviewed, the inadequacies of the Casualty Ward discussed and opinions about the doctors exchanged. Some suggested The Knowle as a hospital, and Dr Hope, speaking from the body of the Hall, told how Messrs. Masters and Reynolds had offered to supply plans and specifications for a hospital, free of charge. One suggested that working men could contribute 10 shillings each to raise most of the £3,000 required for building, but more agreed with Congdon that 'the town needed a place where the poorer class could obtain medicine and medical advice gratis, and for which they had a perfect right to look to the Government'.[70] Walter Padbury renewed a previous offer to donate £50 when building commenced. The enthusiastic meeting concluded with the formation of a deputation of the town's most respected citizens which planned to

[68] *Ibid.*, 10 March 1893; for report of the inquiry, see *Inquirer*, 17 March 1893.
[69] *Ibid.*, 17 March 1893.
[70] *Ibid.*

meet with the Premier, Sir John Forrest. One resident, mindful of the sporadic nature of agitation for a hospital, wrote to the press urging everyone to band together and not rest until just rights were granted:

> It is at such times as this when the late sad fatality is fresh in the minds of all that people are apt to agitate and say what should be done, but when the nine days' wonder ceases they fall back into their normal lethargic state and let things jog along in their old groove.[71]

The deputation of 13 men met the premier at the Treasury but could not agree on their objectives. They were divided in opinion about the suitability as a hospital, of the immigration depot, which they had visited. Some wanted a public dispensary for the many who were too poor to pay for medicines. There was dispute about whether a cottage hospital or a casualty ward was preferable. With the convenient solution of the depot in mind, Forrest calmed the waters of dispute with sympathy and the promise of a building already in existence until a hospital could be built on the land set aside for it near the bridge. The Knowle could not be used as it had been earmarked for recreational purposes for the town, but the temporary use of the immigration depot, Forrest assured, would not prevent the building of a new hospital.[72] It was a return to the familiar old groove.

Henry Barnett was determined that his town should have better emergency medical accommodation, but when he limped through the old No. 1 Barracks on a tour of inspection in mid-July and saw the rooms that had been erected for convict guards and recognised their disadvantages, he knew the immigration building was not suitable. He submitted an adverse report to the colonial secretary and the Fremantle Council and invited them to 'inspect both the present and the proposed Ward and discuss the subject'.[73] The matter was left in abeyance for six months. Accidents kept pace with the growing population, and at the Casualty Ward near the tunnel, the caretaker was rarely unoccupied for long. After a year, Bevan was replaced by Henry Gibbs at the same salary of £78 a year.[74]

On the goldfields, fine fortunes were sometimes made in the dust and heat, but often misfortune was a miner's lot as the result of typhoid. In the decade from 1893 until 1903 nearly 2,000 died from the disease and another 8,000 suffered its symptoms.[75] Many sufferers and carriers returned to and through Fremantle which eventually stirred the council to action. Most councillors were content with the old plan to use the immigration barracks as a place for the sick, but Barnett still persisted in his opposition, with the colonial surgeon now in support.[76] When Mayor Congdon met the fiery doctor at the No. 1 Barracks on 15 January 1894 and saw conditions through the doctor's eyes, he also tempered his view. At the following

---

[71] *Ibid.*, Letter to the Editor by 'One Who Has Derived a Benefit From a Well-Appointed Hospital', 17 March 1893.
[72] *Ibid.*, 31 March 1893.
[73] Minutes of FMC, 14 July 1893.
[74] CSO File 1584/93.
[75] D. Snow, *The Progress of Public Health in Western Australia 1829–1977*, 1977, pp. 70–82.
[76] Minutes of FMC, 5 January 1894.

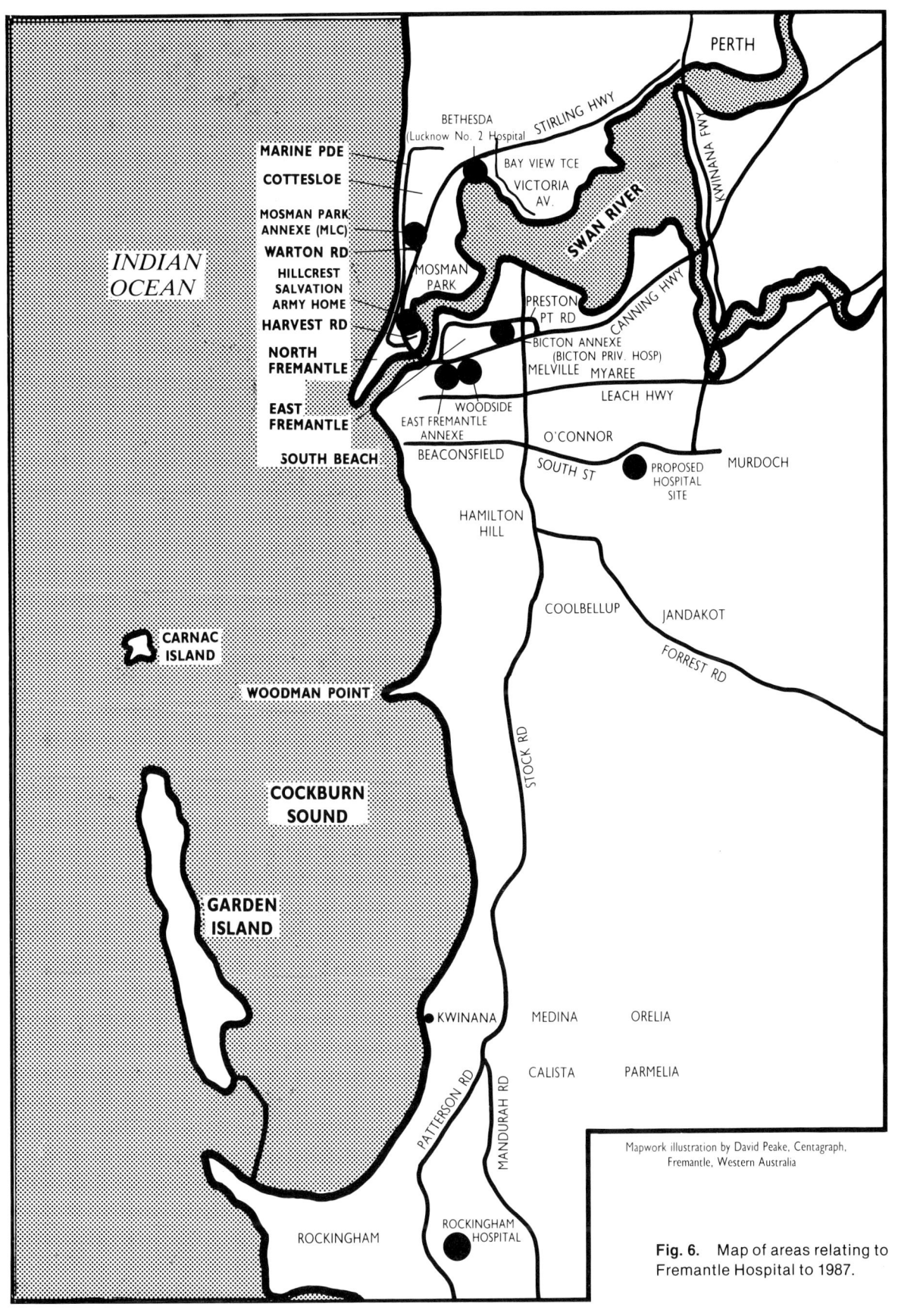

Fig. 6. Map of areas relating to Fremantle Hospital to 1987.

INDIAN OCEAN

PERTH

BETHESDA
(Lucknow No. 2 Hospital)

STIRLING HWY

MARINE PDE

COTTESLOE

BAY VIEW TCE

VICTORIA AV.

SWAN RIVER

KWINANA FWY

MOSMAN PARK ANNEXE (MLC)

WARTON RD

HILLCREST SALVATION ARMY HOME

HARVEST RD

MOSMAN PARK

PRESTON PT RD

CANNING HWY

NORTH FREMANTLE

BICTON ANNEXE (BICTON PRIV. HOSP)

MELVILLE   MYAREE

LEACH HWY

EAST FREMANTLE

WOODSIDE
EAST FREMANTLE ANNEXE

O'CONNOR

SOUTH BEACH

BEACONSFIELD

SOUTH ST

PROPOSED HOSPITAL SITE

MURDOCH

HAMILTON HILL

COOLBELLUP

JANDAKOT

FORREST RD

CARNAC ISLAND

WOODMAN POINT

STOCK RD

COCKBURN SOUND

GARDEN ISLAND

KWINANA   MEDINA   ORELIA

PATTERSON RD

MANDURAH RD

CALISTA   PARMELIA

Mapwork illustration by David Peake, Centagraph, Fremantle, Western Australia

ROCKINGHAM

ROCKINGHAM HOSPITAL

council meeting, all joined with Barnett in requesting the government to allocate between £1,000 and £1,500 from the next Estimates for the construction of a cottage hospital .[77] To reinforce the decision, councillors visited the hospital reserve and selected a site set well back on the block facing Skinner Street.[78] Use of the old Casualty Ward continued, but as patients in a position to do so were required to pay three shillings a day for attendance and maintenance on top of the colonial surgeon's operating fee, it is likely that workers preferred to complete their recovery at home as soon as it was possible to do so.[79]

When parliament sat in August 1894, the colonial secretary assured that £2,000 had been budgeted for a hospital at Fremantle. The hospital was to be a 'capacious one' having 16 beds for men and eight for women, with all the requirements of a hospital. Congdon's satisfaction was marred only by the fact that Fremantle's new member, T. H. Marshall, M.L.C., had anticipated the issue prematurely and suggested that the municipality should receive the funds to build.[80] While the council wanted a hospital, its upkeep and administration was not a responsibility they wished to undertake.

The discovery of gold made its inevitable and irrevocable mark on inland areas, but the port was no less affected. The hopeful and the desperate from the Depression-hit eastern states arrived by steamer in their hundreds, and then their thousands. In 1881 Fremantle's population had been 3,641, in 1891 it was 5,607. By 1896 the number had increased to 13,000 in Fremantle town with another 2,000 at North Fremantle and Plympton.[81] So busy was pedestrian traffic in High Street that a notice had to be erected: 'Keep to the Right'. Roadways were equally congested. Traffic at the station and in the main streets—especially on Saturdays—increased to such alarming proportions with assorted horse-drawn carts and cabs, hawkers selling their wares, carriages, hand carts, dogs and other stray animals, that a traffic ranger had to be appointed. Signs were erected at major intersections advising traffic to 'Walk Round This Corner' but 'furious driving' continued to be a problem. By the end of 1896, all street names had been signposted to guide newcomers around the town. The horse-pulled hackney buses were provided with a stand and a new rule decreed that they were to leave if full after three minutes and in ten minutes whether full or not, and also that they were to keep to a certain route instead of leaving the general public in order to pursue something more remunerative. Another rule forbade the passage of cattle through the town outside the hours of midnight and five in the morning, but stray beasts still roamed about, making walking a definite hazard and causing great destruction to property.[82] Slow-moving trains of tall camels driven by Afghan keepers were often seen passing through the main streets. The two boys employed by the council with pan and broom to keep High Street free from dung were kept constantly busy; two bins for manure had to be placed in busy Market

[77] *Ibid.*, 23 January 1894, 6 February 1894.
[78] *Ibid.*, 19 July 1894.
[79] *WAPD*, Vol. 6, 1894, pp. 188, 227.
[80] *Ibid.*, pp. 133–4.
[81] Ewers, *The Western Gateway*, p. 101.
[82] Minutes of FMC, 2 August 1892.

Street and the council's own town scavengers were sometimes still working at 9.30 a.m. when business for the day had begun.[83]

The ladies who swept over the mosaic-like footpaths made of jarrah paving blocks, tar, asphalt, gravel, tan bark or paving stones freighted from England, averted their eyes when passing prison parties working on roads with their council paid and appointed warder. Sand continued to be a bane for householders, and British marram grass from Warrnambool, seaweed, broken brush and the planting of rye were tried to stop the drift which at times undermined houses and fences and covered the railway line. It seemed that sand threatened to 'engulf the whole town in time, and to cause more serious destruction of property'.[84] *The Sand Drift Act* of 1889 had encouraged measures to arrest the problem, but children kept stealing the brush for firewood and there were people like Mrs O'Halloran who reasoned about sand blowing from her allotment that 'Providence has placed it there, and some day He may see fit to remove it'.[85]

But sand-drift and traffic were minor problems compared to those of public health. While sweet-scented handkerchiefs were held over noses passing Chester's and Ferris' piggeries and the warehouses and woolsheds and tanneries, they were also needed in streets to alleviate the 'sickening smells arising from the drains'.[86] All the activity and excitement, the expansion of the town, the shopping, checking into hotels, and opening of new businesses was conducted beside and between surface drains and open cesspits in which bodily wastes, food scraps and bathwater mingled and matured. Periodically the pits were emptied at a cost to the council of between 10 shillings and 20 shillings a load. One cesspit in the town's main street was

> ... a hole 10 feet by 4 feet, several feet deep, overflowing with an accumulation of garbage of every sort and kind, the refuse of about half a dozen cottages, the inhabitants of which continually throw from their kitchen slush and slops of the baser sort into the mixture just to keep it fermenting ...[87]

As it was illegal to run household drains into the streets, kitchen slops and bathwater were supposed to be emptied into backyards. In low-lying areas the ground became so saturated that it could not absorb the waste and in cottages below street level and those with basements, the problem of flooding was almost unbearable, although children often enjoyed paddling in the foul water. Houses in Henderson, Adelaide, Cantonment and Packenham Streets were particularly affected. There was talk of 'building yards up and cutting channels to sandy soils'[88] but no real moves were made to extend the limited number of underground double nine-inch

---

[83]   Information for this glimpse of Fremantle was gleaned from Minutes of FMC. See particularly 29 December 1895 (High Street traffic), 1 May 1894 ('furious driving'), 6 September 1898 and 5 October 1897 (hackney buses), 2 August 1892, 18 June 1895 (cattle and camels), 6 September 1898 (horse manure). See also Ewers, *The Western Gateway*; Reece and Pascoe, *A Place of Consequence*; J. K. Hitchcock, *The History of Fremantle: The Front Gate of Australia 1829–1929*, 1929.

[84]   *WAPD*, Vol. 14, 1888, p. 412. See also Minutes of FMC, many references including 10 February 1891, 1 September 1891, 5 April 1892, 3 March 1892, 5 July 1892, 7 February 1899, 28 March 1899.

[85]   Minutes of FMC, 31 January 1899.

[86]   *Ibid.*, 31 March 1897.

[87]   *Messenger*, 15 November 1895, cited in Reece and Pascoe, *A Place of Consequence*, p. 62.

[88]   Minutes of FLBH, 5 July 1895.

pipe drains that led into the river. With the population increase, coffee houses and hotels were severely affected by the lack of drainage. Miss Costello, an eating house proprietress from Market Street, was told that she could not run a pipe to a drain in Leake Street, but that she must store drain water in a tank and have it carted away. The new tank filled within an hour—an impossible situation. Miss Costello then offered to pay to have the street drain flushed daily but again permission was denied by council. 'Well, then instruct your officers to prevent people all over the town from running water into the street channels,' the woman flared. When the problem was brought up in council, the meeting was adjourned. There were no easy answers.[89]

Although Fremantle had an abundant supply of waste water, clean drinking water was less easy to find. Residents in the West Ward had water pumped from prison mains from the mid-1880s but even here, some householders drank well water 'not at all good . . . yet preferred to that supplied by the prison',[90] or could not afford the cost of connection. Some wells were built within feet of cesspits; many remained as uncovered as the dust bins alongside them and some residents cared little into which opening their rubbish was tossed. One well had water contaminated by 'animal cula, feathers and other foreign matter'.[91] Others were similarly fouled.

Nightsoil disposal was also a problem. Alongside many wells, gardens flourished with the help of untreated human wastes dug into trenches by householders. Both Hope and Barnett advocated the practice at the asylum in 1894, for without the manure, inmates could not be supplied with the vegetables they grew, and would have been deprived of the 'healthful occupation' the labour of gardening provided.[92] Throughout the first half of 1890s councilmen disagreed about sewage disposal. In the West Ward, dry earth closets were tried, and in other areas the bucket system, while two councilmen pressed for the retention of cesspits, regularly cleaned and the contents taken to the sewage farm. Hope advocated the bucket system, whereby ashes, sand or sawdust were sprinkled over the contents of a used bucket. 'If the system seemed offensive,' explained the doctor, 'it was through people's own carelessness.' Not until 1896, under Mayor Solomon's influence, was the more satisfactory covered-pan system introduced.[93]

Pollution was a problem throughout the town and on the sea. Prosecutions were launched for dumping onions or fish on the road, running bathwater into streets, depositing rotten eggs on allotments, and dropping dead oysters from oyster beds onto the street. Alongside ships, carcasses of dead horses and cattle bobbed, thrown

---

[89] *West Australian*, 17 February 1897.

[90] Minutes of FLBH, 9 August 1889; see also 38 June 1889. Ewers, *The Western Gateway*, pp. 85-6.

[91] Minutes of FLBH, 5 February 1891. For an excellent article on water supply and sanitation, see S. Hunt and G. Bolton, 'Cleansing the Dunghill: Water Supply and Sanitation in Perth 1878-1912', *Studies in Western Australian History*, Vol. 2, March 1978, pp. 1-17.

[92] Minutes of FLBH, 30 January 1894, 7 February 1894.

[93] Ewers, *The Western Gateway*, pp. 86-90. See many references to sanitation in Minutes of FLBH, including 15 February 1887, 8 January 1891, 5 February 1891, 29 December 1893, 16 May 1895, 27 October 1898. See also Public Health Dept File 750/08, on sale of nightsoil by Council to Chinese market gardeners near Hamilton Hill in 1909. Dan O'Connell complained, 'The effluvium was most offensive and must be disgusting in the extreme to people travelling on the road and dangerous to the health of both travellers and residents'. (The nightsoil was first treated by heating to 212 °F for 15 minutes.)

overboard from steamers at anchor to be washed up on beaches to putrefy, while condemned cargoes of beef and rotten fruit shared the same watery fate.[94] The public health problem was not new. Barnett had been campaigning for better conditions for over 20 years. In a perceptive paper published in 1876 containing 'Suggestions Respecting Sanitary Improvement in Western Australia', he argued that the experiences of other countries concerning sanitary matters should be adopted where successful, and enforced in the colony to avoid 'the punishment of some terrible epidemic visitation'.[95] As a commissioner called with Waylen and others to enquire into the sanitary condition of the City of Perth and the Town of Fremantle in 1885, Barnett found identical conditions to those he had observed in the 1870s.[96] Only the extent, not the nature of the problem had changed. Frustrated beyond endurance in 1895, he sent the council a letter written to him by the colonial secretary absolving him from any blame should an epidemic occur.[97] Nowhere was the editorial of the *West Australian* more apt than at Fremantle:

> Every day the ground beneath us becomes more polluted, and fuller of disease germs, gathering its poisons into a concentrated form, which may at any moment burst out into a pestilence which will awaken us so thoroughly and rudely to a sense of the terrible dangers, worse than any volcano, slumbering beneath our feet ... The wonder is that epidemics are not always with us. In all probability they will be in a short time.[98]

The whole Fremantle public health problem was aggravated by the large number of people arriving in the town. With space in hotels and boarding houses at a premium, and some too poor to afford the fees, tent cities mushroomed on hills around the town and grew on any available spare ground. There were 100 tents at Willis' Point, occupied by men, women and children and no sanitary or rubbish facilities. Afghans camped on the beach near the courthouse. Hessian and canvas huts appeared on Monument Hill, on Lighthouse Hill, at Fremantle Park, on the rifle range and by the end of the century, out on the commonage. Councillor J. J. Higham visited the new occupants on Monument Hill and found them 'far from being cleanly', and in their 'habits', much wanting.[99] The tent-dwellers at the rifle range petitioned the local board of health for assistance in carrying out sanitary arrangements, which the board blindly declined to do, reasoning that if the tent-holders were uncleanly 'THEY' should be removed.[100] There was talk of a typhoid

[94] See, for example, Minutes of FLBH, 5 July 1895, 17 October 1895, 28 September 1896, 17 May 1889; Minutes of FMC, 3 March 1896 (oysters). See also Reece and Pascoe, *A Place of Consequence*, pp. 39–41.

[95] H. C. Barnett, 'Suggestions Respecting Sanitary Improvement in Western Australia', 1876, p. 4.

[96] *WAPD*, 1885, No. 20. Report of the Commission to inquire into the sanitary condition of the City of Perth and the Town of Fremantle. See especially p. 9 on wells, cesspits, lack of ventilation, drainage and rubbish.

[97] Minutes of FMC, 18 June 1895.

[98] *West Australian*, 22 March 1895.

[99] Minutes of FLBH, 21 March 1895. See also *ibid.*, 18 July 1895 (Afghans), 29 August 1895, 19 September 1895; *West Australian*, 23 March 1895. Harbour employees occupied the tents at Willis' Point, 20 February 1896, 19 March 1896, 2 March 1898, 4 January 1899, 17 January 1899, 7 March 1899.

[100] *West Australian*, 19 March 1896.

epidemic if the government did not either order the tents moved or provide sanitary facilities.

By 1895 the rumbling fear about an epidemic promised awful fulfilment. In 1888 the town had been pronounced 'in good health although with the usual influenza'.[101] In 1889 there was some diarrhoea and a little fever but no typhoid. The influenza epidemic of 1890 left some with chest complications and there was some dysentery through people 'drinking bad water and not taking care of themselves'.[102] In 1891 influenza was again severe and serious, and there were two cases of typhoid, one suspected of having been introduced through a ship's passenger and the other thought to have been caused by bad smells or bad water. Hope was optimistic in thinking that the district was not likely to suffer from typhoid fever but, in 1892, friends of typhoid patients were requested to burn, boil or bury infected excreta, and to use strong disinfectants to prevent the spread of the disease. By 1895 in Fremantle, Drs Hope, White, Birmingham, Lotz and Wheeler were reporting typhoid fever cases—eleven in May, and 18 in April alone.[103] Clean water, proper sanitary arrangements and town drainage were called for to prevent the spread of the disease, but some residents preferred the protection from typhoid and fever promised by the makers of Chateau Tanunda Brandy.[104] In December there were six cases of typhoid—one local and five from the goldfields; in January 1896, nine of the 12 typhoid patients were from the 'fields; in February there were 12 cases—with nine from the Fremantle community and in March ten of the 18 reported typhoid patients were from Fremantle.[105] Despite its floating population, the settled core population of Fremantle was still a close one and no further identification was needed when Hope reported to the council, the 'Death of Fred from Typhoid'.[106] Due to inconsistent reporting by doctors and the fact that patients did not always seek professional treatment, the number of typhoid cases in the town was in reality much greater than statistics suggested. The perennial problem of the sick poor, boosted in number by typhoid sufferers, could no longer be ignored.

Although rejected by Barnett and the council, the immigration depot boasted four walls and a roof, and it was available. In an unprecedented step, the government offered, as a private hospital from the end of December 1894, eight rooms and a bathroom at the depot to a Miss Borough, rent free. It was a measure born of necessity rather than magnanimity: 'Patients come from the goldfields and must be located somewhere,' sighed Hope to the under secretary.[107] Most patients paid for their treatment and hospitalisation, but occasionally a critically ill pauper would be ordered into the private hospital on the recommendation of a doctor, an action dis-

[101] See Minutes of FLBH, 24 October 1888.
[102] *Ibid.*, 26 June 1890.
[103] See minutes of FLBH, 8 May 1891, 6 June 1891, 5 October 1891, 31 May 1892, 18 April 1895, 16 May 1895. Between 1893 and 1894, influenza, measles and mumps appear to have been the main concerns.
[104] *West Australian*, 23 March 1895.
[105] Minutes of FLBH, 16 May 1895.
[106] *Ibid.*, 29 August 1895.
[107] CSO File 268/95, Acc. No. 527. See also *Daily News*, 5 February 1895. The barracks building was variously referred to as the Pensioner Barracks, the Immigration Depot or Barracks, the Immigrants' Home and, with its new function in 1895, as the Barracks Hospital. It would become the No. 8 Base Hospital in World War I.

couraged by the government who bore the expense. In the first six weeks, 39 patients were admitted to the hospital. Most came from the goldfields, and nine deaths were recorded. Bond and Jeffrey from Southern Cross; Fordham, Martin and Power from Coolgardie; Miss Lyons of Perth and Harman from Fremantle, all died as a result of typhoid; the only cases to die from other causes were Mr Loan from alcoholism, and Miss Cox with pneumonia.

Miss Elizabeth Cox was one of only three paupers admitted at the barracks. Her circumstances were shared by many who lived in Fremantle in a hand-to-mouth existence where illness meant destitution. Elizabeth worked as a domestic servant and had been employed at the Commercial Hotel for three weeks when she was taken sick. When her condition worsened, Dr White was called to see her and he had little doubt that she was 'too ill to survive the long trip to the Colonial Hospital'. The police summoned to investigate her circumstances found that the 22-year-old had neither friends in Fremantle nor means. Her mother in Newcastle, a sister in Albany and a brother on the goldfields, were in no position to help either, so the doctor ordered Elizabeth's admission to the Barracks Hospital. There she was accepted only after some dispute with the caretaker, who was assured that her treatment would be paid for by the government. This proved of no concern to the young woman, who died and was buried as a pauper in mid-January of the new year 1895.[108]

Luckier than Elizabeth was another domestic servant named Annie Gould, who worked at the Freemason's Hotel for eight weeks before experiencing the headache and pea-soup diarrhoea of typhoid fever. While she worked for her 17 shillings and sixpence a week, Annie left her illegitimate child with Mrs Ritchie in Essex Street and although her long working hours prevented her from seeing her child often, it was the best she could do under the circumstances. The five shillings contributed by the child's father helped Annie to pay the required ten shillings a week for the child's care, but there was little left to live on and nothing to save. For a week Annie became increasingly ill, until Dr Lotz was called. As her only family was a sister in service receiving fifteen shillings a week, and a brother in poor circumstances who could offer no help, the critically ill young woman was classified as a government pauper and carried on a stretcher by police down to Miss Borough's hospital. Dr Lotz attended his patient free of charge and Mrs Whesstedt from the hotel kindly sent a pound with which to buy some nourishment. After a long illness, Annie's account, totalling £19.8.0, was paid reluctantly by a grumbling government.[109]

Much to the colonial secretary's chagrin, another pauper was admitted to the private hospital within the week. Mrs Varrell and her five children were among the tent-dwellers at North Fremantle trying to keep cool in Western Australia's fierce January heat. The family's breadwinner was looking for work at Southern Cross, but had not been successful. Early in the New Year which they hoped would bring a change of fortune, the Varrell's seven year-old son displayed the unmistakable symptoms of typhoid. With few resources with which to buy medicine and invalid food, and the cost of a doctor high, Mrs Varrell nursed her son for a week through

108   CSO File 119/95, 14 January 1895.
109   CSO File 66/95, 10 January 1895.

the heat of fever and summer before calling a doctor. William Birmingham examined the lad and assured police that '. . . the tent in which Mrs Varrell is living is not a fit place for the child to remain in—and the other children coming in contact with it [as well]'. Although the boy needed proper care, he was too sick to survive the journey to the Colonial Hospital. On receiving Sergeant Taylor's report: 'Mrs Varrell is in poor circumstances and cannot afford to pay the expenses attached to the child going to hospital', Resident Magistrate Fairbairn ordered the boy's admission to the Barracks Hospital, and in due course again received the censure of the government and the Superintendent of Poor Relief for his part in extending the 'large expenditure now incurred'.[110]

The involvement of police in health and other matters increased throughout the 1890s. Citizens of means continually argued for greater police protection of person and property and in a crisis a caller could be told that there was no man in the station to send.[111] As the decade passed, police were also increasingly involved in shaping the ruling-class idea of community morality, mingling with the crowd at the oval or the bicycle track to detect those smoking or betting and using foul language. They investigated the shocking practice of mixed bathing and were stationed at the ladies' bathing site to discourage objectionable young larrikins.[112] In matters of health they provided stretcher transport for the ill and injured, and a police cell was often used as a medical centre until persons felt well enough to care for themselves, or a decision was made by the health hierarchy as to hospitalisation. Theirs was the important responsibility of investigating a pauper's family and financial circumstances to prevent an unnecessary claim on the government for medical care. The police were also asked to help detect persons breaking health laws.[113] Michael Garry was charged at 3.30 one morning by Constable McTavish after emptying foul water from the Fremantle Club into the street drain in Henry Street, 'creating a fearful stench',[114] and Mr Brown was fined for dumping fish on a grant in Packenham Street. Not even a sharp-eyed policeman, however, saw the person who left a bucket of nightsoil on the Dixon's verandah one night.[115] In 1895 the police strength of the town was increased to 20, which the minister hoped would be sufficient for all requirements.[116]

The presence of extra police could bring a certain peace of mind to more affluent citizens, but not surprisingly, considering the fear disease engendered, the opening of the new hospital at the barracks with all its typhoid cases caused some uneasiness. There was talk as early as January about untreated excreta from typhoid patients being removed by the nightman, but concern was muted until George Summers of nearby Norfolk Street expressed his concern publicly through the *Daily News*.[117] As the resident medical officer for Fremantle, James Hope investigated the allegations

[110]　CSO File 119/95, 16 January 1895.
[111]　Minutes of FMC, 16 March 1897.
[112]　*Ibid.*, 26 July 1898, 23 August 1898, 27 January 1899, 27 January 1899 (mixed bathing), 4 July 1899 (smoking and betting).
[113]　*Ibid.*, 31 January 1899.
[114]　*Ibid.*, 31 January 1899.
[115]　Minutes of FLBH, 29 December 1893.
[116]　Minutes of FMC, 2 January 1895.
[117]　*Daily News*, 5 February 1895; Minutes of FLBH, 25 January 1895.

but found patients well cared for and the rooms clean. No dirty bedding was hung on clothes lines as had been claimed, and soiled linen was disinfected by nurses as soon as it was removed from patients, and boiled as soon as possible. A 'great pool of dirty stagnant water' proved to be clean washing water overflowing a washing trough.[118] While Hope refuted Summers inflated claims (some increased attention to cleaning buckets was recommended), he did share the resident's concern at the government's rumoured resumption of the depot. 'Where will the Government house the immigrant girls in future?', Summers had asked.[119] Hope's concern was for the nurses. Unable to rent accommodation because townsfolk boycotted them, Hope queried, 'What is to become of them?'[120]

The government wondered the same question in early February. Already a boat was due to leave London with passengers for the immigrants' home. A number of such girls had once been accommodated at the old Perth Club buildings but the practice had not been satisfactory as 'men could not be kept out of the place'. Where men outnumbered women two to one,[121] such considerations were important. Perhaps, said another, some tents could be loaned to Miss Borough and erected on some vacant government land near Fremantle. No reasonable solution was found and the matron received notice to empty the establishment by the end of March so that the depot could be properly disinfected. Great was the necessity to 'get rid of Miss Borough'.[122] The last patient at the Barracks Hospital was a young Englishman named Brendon Hames who had no friends to care for him. By 27 March 1895, he was nearing convalescence after typhoid, but Dr Birmingham asked the colonial secretary if his patient could remain for another week or ten days after the hospital's closure as moving him could cause a relapse and probable death. Hames was a paying patient and was granted permission to stay.[123]

Patients who tossed in delirium at the Barracks Hospital in February 1895 cared little for anything outside their immediate hell, but in the town it was a momentous month for the council and townspeople. Feelings ran high, as the plan to move the railway workshops from Fremantle to Midland Junction, in order to permit wharf development on the river's southern foreshore, appeared conclusive. The move had been explored since 1892 and although a Vigilance Committee suggested new sites for the 'loco' workshops at Plympton, Rocky Bay, Richmond or even Claremont, midway between Perth and Fremantle, it was of no avail.[124] Premier John Forrest refused to meet the huge deputation of workers and protesters that planned to travel from Fremantle by special train to Perth, but he did receive a smaller group of 20 'influential citizens', to inform them that the decision to relocate had already been made.[125]

Perhaps it was merely coincidence that the long-awaited plans for a hospital began

[118] CSO File 268/95, 6 February 1895.
[119] *Daily News*, 5 February 1895.
[120] CSO File 268/95, 6 February 1895.
[121] Appleyard, 'Western Australia: Economic and Demographic Growth, 1850-1914', in Stannage, *A New History*, p. 220.
[122] CSO File 334/95.
[123] CSO File 159/95, 29 March 1895.
[124] Ewers, *The Western Gateway*, pp. 111–12; Minutes of FMC, 24 July 1894, 3 August 1894.
[125] Minutes of FMC, 7 March 1895, 11 March 1895, 18 March 1895.

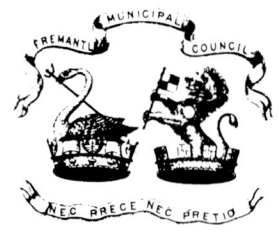

Town Hall.
22nd March. 1895

Sir.

<u>"The Knowle" as a Hospital for
Fremantle.</u>

I have the honour by direction to acknowledge the receipt of your letter No 88/620 of the 9th inst. informing the Council "that the Government has now decided to hand over the site "known as "The Knowle" as a Hospital for Fremantle, and so soon "as possible steps will be taken to effect the necessary ad- ":ditions and repairs to the building to render it suitable for "the purpose". This welcome intelligence is most gratifying to His Worship the Mayor. and the other members of the Council, and I am sure, meets with the wishes of the general public of Fremantle who are exceedingly grateful to the Hon: the Minister in this behalf. It is also gratifying to the Council to note, that in the meantime, and as a temporary measure the Governmt have secured the whole of "The Wesley Home" in Point Street for twelve months together with the furniture as a tempora hospital for Fremantle.

I have the honour to be.
Sir.
Your obedient servant.

Geo Bland Humble
Town Clerk.

The Under Secretary
&c &c
Perth

Fig. 7. Letter from George Bland Humble to colonial secretary, 22 March 1885.

to take shape in that same February. Each of the 'Medical Gentlemen' of the town was asked to submit his recommendations for the hospital's bed capacity and requirements.[126] Young Louis Wheeler, who had qualified as a doctor in 1891, responded immediately. William Birmingham, with seven years' residence in the town, and his scholarly associate of three years, Henry Lotz, soon followed. On 5 March 1895, when the Fremantle Local Board of Health met to consider the replies, Hope's ideas differed from those of his colleagues. With his 20 years of dealing with the government on medical matters and knowing well the needs of the community for a centrally located building without delay, Hope once more suggested The Knowle.[127] Fremantle Council agreed. The following day, Mayor G. A. Davies met the premier on the railway workshops issue and took the opportunity to advise Forrest of the council's wishes about a hospital. The decision was almost immediate:

> ... the Government has now decided to hand over the site known as 'The Knowle' as a Hospital for Fremantle, and so soon as possible steps will be taken to effect the necessary additions and repairs to the building to render it suitable for the purpose.[128]

The hospital sop did not console railway workers who were faced with moving to the other side of Perth, but George Humble, retired headmaster of Fremantle Boys' School and town clerk, felt sure that the decision met with the wishes of the general public of Fremantle.[129] They did not meet with the wishes of Henry Barnett. As superintendent of the overcrowded lunatic asylum, he strongly opposed the loss of the facilities the building provided:

> The patients and staff at Knowle—already—number 38 and are constantly being added to—They could not be crushed into Asylum, when increase, and not reduction of space and accommodation is needed—As population flows in, insanity of course increases fast ...[130]

Nine months later, in December 1895, patients from the lunatic asylum were still at The Knowle. In May the following year, the council strongly censured the government for its delay in converting the building to a hospital.[131] Not until December 1896 did the council finally receive word that the renovations and additions were nearing completion.

It had been a long haul. The moves to secure a hospital in Fremantle had involved many people in an 'emergency response' cycle of concern and agitation for many years. In the end the real impetus proved to be a goldfield far to the east, that beckoned a new population and rewarded it indiscriminately in gold and fever. Perhaps a decision to build a new hospital may have gained the town its hospital more quickly than the renovation and extension of The Knowle. As it was, at the end of 1896, the land at the Skinner Street hospital site stood empty—except for a cow belonging to A. W. Armstrong the licensee of the town's Commercial Hotel.[132]

[126] *Ibid.*, 19 February 1895.
[127] Minutes of FMC, 5 March 1895.
[128] CSO File 643/93; Minutes of FMC, 19 March 1895.
[129] CSO File 643/93, 22 March 1895.
[130] CSO File 543/95. Barnett to Colonial Surgeon, 7 March 1895.
[131] Minutes of FMC, 21 May 1896.
[132] *Ibid.*, 24 September 1895.

Chapter III

'On the 31st December, 1895, there were eighteen
hospitals and one casualty ward in the Colony,
the Fremantle casualty ward having been changed
into a Hospital.'
W.A. Year Book 1894-95.

In November 1894, when the government was considering granting K. Borough the use of the barracks as a private hospital, Fremantle Municipal Council received notice from the Wesleyan minister that he had taken over the boarding house known as Keirle's cottages.[1] Built on Lot 318 at the north eastern corner of the junction of Point and Cantonment Streets in 1891 for the mason Isaac Keirle, the accommodation comprised a large main building and three cottages.[2] The Reverend William Andrew Potts, who had recently arrived from Guildford, requested the council to lay kerbing and repair a footpath near the property. Then he enthusiastically built a bathroom out over the pavement at the 'Wesley Home', as the place soon came to be known. However, at the next council meeting, members agreed that despite Potts' ignorance of the building regulation which had been broken, the new room would have to be pulled down.[3] It was an eager if inauspicious beginning to the church's tenure.

The activity had not gone unnoticed and with accommodation in the town so scarce, news of a large premise for rent interested a number of townspeople, but none more so than Henry Calvert Barnett. He stumped over to the building and with the Reverend as guide, inspected the three cottages which were to let on the site and his fertile mind leapt. With the casualty ward still under threat through railway land expansion, he enthused 'that with two or three alterations, the place would suit better as a Casualty Ward for a year or two, than any other place in Fremantle'.[4] One of the cottages could be adapted for a surgery, the other as quarters for a caretaker, he reasoned, and the two large detached rooms could serve as casualty wards. The colonial surgeon, Alfred Waylen, went to inspect the buildings with James Hope and was less impressed. Although well situated and adequate in size, the rooms were 'unventilated and I should say damp in winter—being a lean-to'.[5] Considering that the cottages had been let and occupied but condemned by the council the previous year as 'unfit for human habitation', the opinion was no doubt

---

[1] Minutes of FMC, Letter Rev. W. A. Potts to Council, 2 November 1894.
[2] Fremantle City Library, Ref. B/O'Reilly.
[3] Minutes of FMC, 14 December 1894.
[4] CSO File 2111/94. Barnett (the Colonial Surgeon, Fremantle) to Waylen (Colonial Surgeon), 8 December 1894.
[5] CSO File 334/95.

warranted.[6] The main boarding house, however, was large and clean with 12 furnished rooms capable of holding between 24 and 30 patients, and it also had sleeping accommodation for nurses. Waylen murmured about expenditure in the light of the decision already taken to build a new hospital, but the urgency to clear the Barracks Hospital before the arrival of the immigrant girls now on their way, overrode quibbles about costs. It was decided to ask the Wesleyans for the use of the entire accommodation: the cottages, boarding house, and the 'lean-to' which had already been decided on as a casualty ward. The 12 months' rental of £450 seemed reasonable to both parties. Once more the Wesleyans set to work, improving the ventilation in the casualty ward and providing 'suitable privy accommodation', and on 21 March 1895, it was announced in the Fremantle Local Board of Health meeting that: 'The Wesley Home has been secured by the Government as a temporary hospital'. The first patients were carefully transferred on stretchers from both the Barracks Hospital and the old casualty ward by policemen.[7]

Miss K. Borough came straight from the Barracks Hospital to serve as matron. Well placed to hear of the vacancy in the proposed new hospital and having proved her dependability in charge at the Barracks, she wrote succinctly to the colonial secretary:

> Dear Sir,
>   I hear you are about to put up a public hospital in Fremantle. I should feel obliged if you would put my name down for Matron.[8]

The application was accepted at least a month before one received from Mary Nicholas with her years of nursing and administrative experience in England and at Alexandria, who would serve as matron at the Perth Public Hospital for three months in 1896.[9] Miss Borough hesitated at the proffered salary of £90 a year, when at Perth the matron received £150, but accepted the position after a government assurance of an increase to £100 after three months' employment.

Work at the hospital proved arduous and the pay inadequate for nurses and domestic staff alike. One of the hospital's first cooks was Elizabeth Shuffleton, employed at £36 a year.[10] On her resignation two months later, she was replaced by Emily Johnson.[11] Although the laundry was sent out, both women single-handedly cooked for the patients and staff and were responsible for all housework as well. When visitors and tradesmen, who constantly interrupted the cook's routine by knocking at the door, received a cool reception, it was not surprising.

If cook was hard-working, the nurses were equally burdened. Only two were employed to care for the 25 or so patients. One worked a 12-hour day shift, the other for the 12 hours of night. Their pay was only £40 a year. Nell McCarthy and Minnie

6   Minutes of FMC, 2 May 1893.
7   Minutes of FLBH, 21 March 1895. See CSO File 2111/94; CSO File 334/95 and *West Australian*, 28 March 1895.
8   CSO File 283/95, 7 February 1895.
9   CSO File 761/95, 26 March 1895.
10 CSO File 1586/95, 18 June 1895.
11 CSO File 2479/95, 8 August 1895.

Compton objected and then resigned in October 1895 in the only real recourse they had at 'salaries not being large enough for them'.[12] Private nursing, although less secure, could be as well paid and was certainly less strenuous. In their place and on the strength of their good testimonials, Hope was fortunate to engage Winifred Harris and Cassie Hamilton on the following day at the same salary. Even with the best of nursing intentions, it was inevitable that patients suffered through the lack of staff employed to treat them.

The appointment of nurses and domestic staff was by recommendation of the matron, but James Hope, the Fremantle medical officer, made the final decision. In turn the colonial surgeon and the principal medical officer were advised and the appointment was referred through the under secretary to cabinet for its confirmation. It was a clumsy system and it meant that Hope, and not the matron administered the institution.

After eight months at the hospital, in November 1895, Hope was moved to appeal against the unsatisfactory conditions at Point Street. Twenty-two beds were occupied by patients, half of whom were surgical cases requiring heavy nursing. Two of these were amputations of the forearm, another had fingers so badly crushed that they had to be amputated and one patient suffered a compound fracture of his leg.[13] It was impossible for one woman working for 12 hours a day to nurse this number of patients. Just a few days earlier there had been 24 cases. After his 20 years of government service, Hope was careful to couch his requests in terms of financial stringency and when he asked for permission to employ a probationer nurse and a laundry kitchen-maid, he suggested that the maid's employment would save the weekly cost of between 12 and 18 shillings to a washerwoman, and she could help the cook as well. For £3 a month, persuaded Hope, 'we could get more work and assistance at a trifling additional cost'.[14] It was a valid point. Mary Jane Harman was appointed as the hospital's first laundry maid, and Delia King its first probationer nurse. The former received £36 a year, the latter just £15, but as those in the profession knew, she would receive a certificate of competence at the end of two years and probably eternal reward through her ministering to the suffering poor. Delia learned the skills of nursing and worked the long, hard hours required until August 1896 when she became 'much indisposed'. There was no sick leave. At last, unable to work at all, she took her 14 days' annual leave to recuperate.[15]

Towards the end of December 1895, when carols were ringing from the churches and tradesmen in the town were counting increases from sales, Cassie Hamilton painfully but providentially burned her foot.[16] For nearly 12 months the kitchen and nursing staff had carried out their tasks of cooking, cleaning and patient care, sharing one small stove and boiler, and all hot water had to be carried from the kitchen.[17] Under threat of complete disruption to the hospital through the loss of one in a skeleton nursing staff, Hope was able to arrange the appointment of Mary

[12] CSO File 3015/95, 6 November 1895.
[13] *Ibid.*
[14] *Ibid.*
[15] CSO File 3110/95; CSO File 2800/96.
[16] CSO File 18/96, 1 January 1896. The accident had occurred 10 days earlier.
[17] CSO File 797/96.

Hillman and Miss Johnson as nurses, and George Kinnaford as a much-needed orderly to help with the heavier lifting.

It had been a hard year for Miss K. Borough. Not only had she come straight from the Barracks Hospital but she had been responsible for setting up a new hospital, instituting routines, seeing that the doctor's orders were carried out and that patients were fed, cleaned and made as comfortable as possible under trying conditions. She had arbitrated in staff disputes and dissatisfactions and probably assisted at operations, and had done so at the minimal rate of £90 a year. On 11 January 1896, she wrote to Hope from the hospital:

> I have been nearly a year as Matron in the hospital and feel very much in need of a rest. I do not know what time is allowed, but should like my leave as soon as convenient.[18]

The district medical officer supported her request in strong terms, urging that: 'Leave is absolutely necessary for these people—in the case of the present applicant she has an anxious and arduous battle and now requires rest and change'. On 1 February 1896, Miss Borough left for a welcome break and was temporarily replaced at the same rate of pay by Vashti A. Stewart, a qualified nurse. Benefited by the change, Matron Borough tackled Hope on her return about conditions which had not improved during her absence. 'Nothing could be more opposed to my wishes than to make any complaints with regard to the Hospital but I feel I would be wanting in duty if I were not to represent to you the dissatisfaction existing here at the present amongst the servants and nursing staff.'[19] She spoke of inadequate staff numbers to efficiently carry out necessary hospital work, of the want of ordinary conveniences such as hot water which made duties so heavy, of the cook having to do all the housework and cooking without assistance and answer the doorbell as well. Nurses demanded a guinea-a-week pay—understandable when temporary nurses appointed by the government in times of emergency received that amount—and K. Borough reminded him about the increase in her pay, promised but never received.

Again Hope supported the matron, urging the payment of her salary increase as 'she well deserves this amount'. He stressed the unsatisfactory working conditions and the lack of staff at Point Street:

> We also require a night orderly, another nurse or probationer and a scullery maid who will each want about £3.0.0 per month. At this time and for sometime past we have had 30 patients ... Amongst the surgical cases are Fractured pelvis, Compd Comm[td] fr leg. Amputate[d] leg ... Fracture of fibula and crushed foot. [injured] knee joint, Injury to head &c. This last case has necessitated the nightly attendance of a couple of convalescent patients ... otherwise someone would have had to be engaged and this is properly the work of a night orderly. The cook has to cook for 38 persons and the various extras for patients makes the work so heavy that we cannot get a woman to stay unless she has a scullery maid to help to wash up &c. Wages are too small all around, the Matron says she cannot get women with experience to come ... at the rate of pay offered which is only as much as an ordinary servant gets.[20]

[18]   CSO File 423/96.
[19]   CSO File 797/96, February 1896.
[20]   *Ibid.*, 2 March 1896

Conditions would have proved difficult in a Nightingale ward for the matron, the three nurses, the probationer nurse and the orderly employed to attend patients 24 hours a day. In a boarding house of separate, small rooms and detached cottages the task was almost impossible. Hope also upheld the nurses' claim for a wage increase. Not only were new areas of employment opening up for these women with their specialised skills he pointed out, but the labour of nursing 'is trying, the hours long and they have given up a great deal of their life and . . . money also to get the knowledge'.

Costs for the hospital escalated as Dr Edward Scott and others had predicted. By the end of April, a night orderly, another nurse named Margaret Grover and a kitchen-maid had been appointed to the hospital,[21] the senior nurses were receiving £1 a week and the matron £100 a year. Encouraged by this success, Hope requisitioned a new five-feet-long kitchen range at a cost of £9.0.0 as 'the one in use belongs to the Wesleyans—it is absolutely worn out and useless—cooking cannot be done with it. A new one is urgently required'.[22] Although there was some discussion as to whether the landlord or the government should pay for it, and whether if the government paid, the new stove could be transferred to the new hospital building, three weeks later at the beginning of May, the cook regarded a newly installed Metters in the hospital kitchen with great satisfaction.

Matron Borough did not share the satisfaction, for in early April she left the hospital to which she had devoted so much energy and for which she had received so little support. Her replacement was an outsider—a Miss Bessie Steele who had trained at Addenbrooke's Fever Hospital in Cambridge, England, before nursing privately in Melbourne.[23] Her coming was not accepted with unanimous favour. Not only was she new to the people of Fremantle but to Western Australia itself, having worked as matron at a private hospital in Perth for just a year, and even Dr Hope could only say of her after her appointment in April: 'I feel sure she is most considerate of the inmates of the Hospital'.[24]

One of the inmates was not so sure. A little over a week after Bessie Steele's arrival he complained anonymously to John Forrest about the new matron 'who is strange to Hospital work and the Colony'. Accustomed by doctor's orders to sitting on the verandah on sunny days with a pillow and rug, the patient was quite put out on the new matron's first day to be forbidden to take 'these necessaries' outside. Food was not only inadequate, he continued, but because there was no fish as usual for the Roman Catholics one Friday, the faithful 'had to be without food all day'. Milk was also scarce, with one tin of condensed milk reportedly watered down to serve all the patients. Perhaps because it was the way things were done, or perhaps because of the government's unwillingness to become embroiled in an area which would entail greater expenditure, only the medical officer for Fremantle was called upon to make enquiries. Not surprisingly, when their tenure depended on Hope's support and approval, both patients and staff denied knowledge of the complaining

[21] CSO File 2032/97.
[22] CSO File 1214/96, April 1896.
[23] CSO File. 2032/1897. For brief history of Addenbrooke's Hospital, see G. S. Haynes, 'Addenbrooke's Hospital Cambridge', in *The Medical Press and Circular*, 4 February 1942, pp. 72–6.
[24] CSO File 1168/96, 15 April 1896.

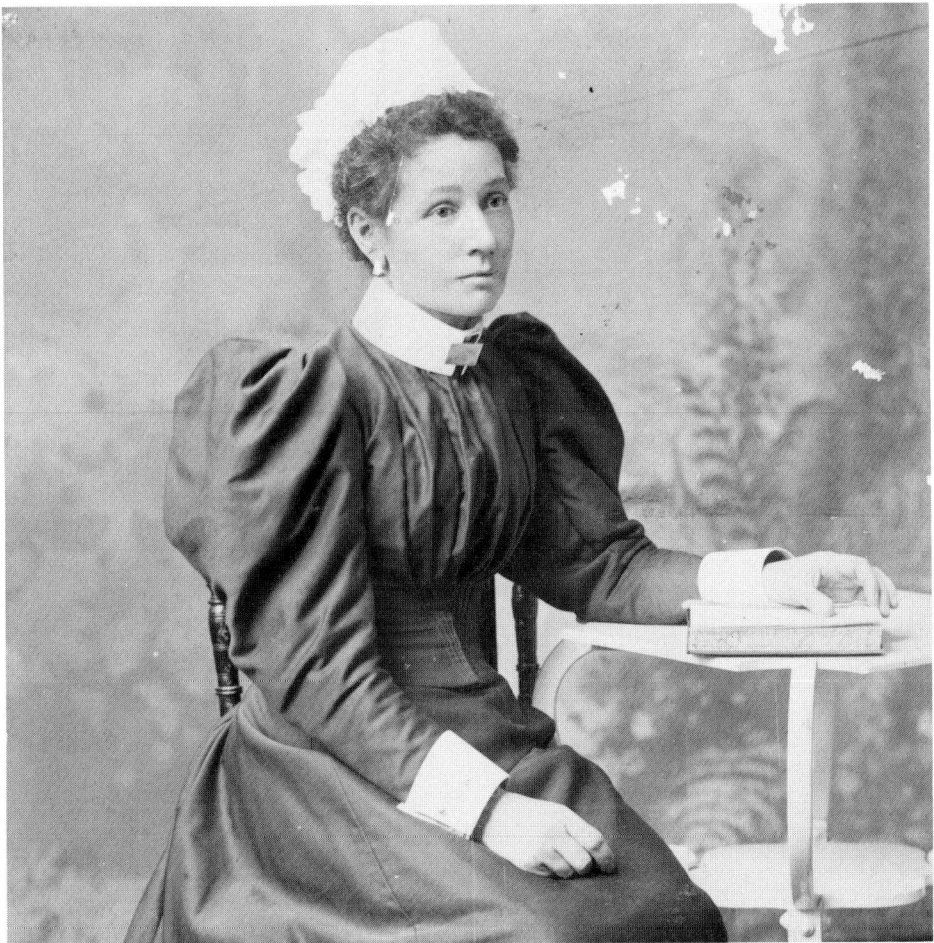

Photograph courtesy Fremantle Hospital

Plate 5.   Bessie Steele, first Matron of Fremantle Hospital, wrote to Dr Hope, the Fremantle Resident Medical Officer, on 21 August 1897:

I beg to report that three nurses in this Institution viz. Fisher, Grover and Crudden have broken the rules by absenting themselves without leave until a late hour at night. It is not the first time that it has occurred but I was not made aware of the fact until this morning. I cannot tolerate such conduct amongst the nursing staff for one moment.

C.S.O. File 2769/97

letter. Much piqued, Hope reported to the under secretary that the anonymous communication was without foundation: 'Patients know that if they have any grievance they should first appeal to me.' Residual grains of truth remained, however. In that month of April, the matron and her ways were new, and it was admitted that the local itinerant fish vendors on whom the hospital depended for supplies sometimes delivered irregularly, particularly at Easter. And even though Hope claimed that there was an abundance of fresh milk for the fever and severe cases on a light diet, convalescents were allowed only condensed milk for their tea. No one could be found to mention the 'other and serious grievances' of the anonymous letter and Hope's report was filed and the matter forgotten.[25]

Many of the patients at Fremantle's first government hospital were elderly men, but of the 32 beds available, six were reserved for women, and one of the cottages housed patients with grossly infected wounds. Pneumonia and typhoid fever were common afflictions. One probationer nurse remembered in her old age, the problem of 'bugs' at the hospital, often due to the sailor patients who had long lain unattended in their ships at sea. 'O'Reilly's Home From Home' as the hospital came to be known, was not the most comfortable of accommodation.[26]

Nor was it for the nurses who shared a single room with a tub for bathing in a screened-off corner. Towards the end of 1896, the number of nurses was increased to five in preparation for the move to The Knowle.[27] A two-year course of training which had been started at the Perth Public Hospital early in the year included lectures by a doctor, but at Fremantle Hospital, probationers were taught only by the matron and learned 'bandaging, dressing of wounds with the use of foot and hand baths, poultice making, and sponging, and bed making'.[28] In their compulsory two hours off-duty on alternate days, the probationers were not allowed to rest but were required to walk in the fresh air for their health. Because the hospital was in a red-light area, the nurses wore their distinctive silver gray uniforms to clearly distinguish them from other women who walked and worked in the area at very different occupations.

In November one of the nurses burned her face and was unable to work. Hope engaged a trained nurse named Emily Duncan who had earlier in the year proved her worth when Delia King took her 14 days' holiday. In this month also, Hope was able to notify the Fremantle Municipal Council that work on The Knowle was nearly completed.[29] Plans to convert the once-beautiful two-storey stone and plaster building—which had been erected by convicts as a residence for Captain Edmund Henderson, the comptroller general of the convict establishment—had been made and discarded and made again in 1896. The final alterations and additions were shaped by an architect named J. Herbert Eales, who married the daughter of James Lilly, first chairman of the Fremantle Hospital Board, appointed in 1897.[30]

From mid-1896, R. Bushby, as the supervisor appointed by the Public Works Department, had faced a difficult task in restoring the building. Doors and windows

[25] *Ibid.*
[26] E. de Moulin (née Woodhead), interviewed by Victoria Hobbs, 1970, cited in V. Hobbs, *But Westward Look: Nursing in Western Australia 1829–1979*, 1980, p. 20.
[27] CSO File 2032/97. See also R. Bottle, interviewed by V. Hobbs, 1975, BL.
[28] de Moulin interview, cited in Hobbs, *But Westward Look*, p. 20. For background of nurse training at Perth Hospital, see Bolton and Joske, *History of Royal Perth Hospital*, p. 61.
[29] *West Australian*, 6 December 1896.
[30] W. Kerr, 'Architecture in Fremantle 1875–1915', Dissertation towards degree, Bachelor of Architecture, UWA, 1973, p. 26. A magnificent plan was also drawn up by Charles Rosenthorpe of the PWD, who would be remembered by posterity as an Army General in World War I rather than as an architect. The ambitious plan, however, guided the first extensions to the hospital. For biographical details, see W. Perry, 'Major General Sir Charles Rosenthal: Soldier, Architect and Musician, *The Victorian Historical Magazine*, Vol. 40, No. 3, August 1969.

had long disappeared from The Knowle and the shingled roof alternately leaked or splashed sunlight through large holes. The house on the hill was thought by many to be 'almost a total ruin'. Bushby renovated, repaired and supervised the construction of a new southern wing, extending the total area of the building by a third. Long French windows led directly to the ten-feet-wide verandah that wrapped around the front and sides of the house, from whence convalescent patients could catch the 'invigorating sea breezes' and watch the activities of the port with its shipping and river traffic. By December there were 15 rooms downstairs, including one for a dispenser, another for visitors, an office, a bedroom and a sitting room for matron, four wards and an 'operating apartment'. A new kitchen with pantry and a larder were also added. Three nurses' bedrooms, four male wards, and women's wards were included upstairs, running the full length of the building. The south and north entrances were linked by a wide lofty hallway and throughout, the jarrah floors were polished until they shone. Two isolation wards were built outside, beside the laundry and wash house. Water was run from the prison pump into elevated tanks to give good pressure and the plumbing was unique for the times—based on principles of underground sewerage, with all drains leading to outside surface sinks and thence into a big dry well in the far corner of the grounds. The transformation by Bushby far exceeded the expectations of the most sanguine and at the close of the council meeting for December, it was suggested that 'as this would be the first hospital worthy of the name that Fremantle had had' the ministry might be invited down to the opening day. As events transpired, only Dr Hope, Mayor Elias Solomon, Councillor J. R. Doonan and the Town Clerk, Mr George Bland Humble, were present to represent officialdom.[31]

On Friday, 22 January 1897, the patients were very carefully carried on stretchers from Point Street to The Knowle. A party of men from the prison, who had been busy putting fittings and beds in position for some days, were still making the carriageway from Alma Street. The other entrance to the hospital was from a private road leading in from John and Fairbairn Streets, across the front of the gaol where the tramway ran. Patients appreciated the large airy rooms, and nurses were delighted with two or three gas stoves to heat water, and the unaccustomed luxury of plumbing to pipe hot and cold water to fixed baths and sinks.[32]

Hospital accommodation was increased from 32 beds at Point Street to 52 at The Knowle, but the old problem of patients distributed in small rooms continued to make nursing heavy. Upstairs there were 25 beds in four rooms, while downstairs, which was always full, 27 patients were nursed in five separate rooms. Although the demand for beds outstripped the availability, preference was given to tent-dwellers, who were always admitted if a bed was available.[33] The first death at the hospital in February was that of a 12-year-old typhoid sufferer named Rose Mason. The second was due to dropsy and the third to die, in mid-February, was William Hayes as a result of pleuro-pneumonia. Hayes, a well-known circus performer and proprietor, was said to have made and lost several fortunes but died a pauper. He was given a

[31] See Minutes of FMC, 15 December 1896; *Morning Herald*, 23 January 1897; *West Australian*, 23 January 1897; Minutes of FLBH, 21 January 1897.
[32] *West Australian*, 23 January 1897.
[33] CSO File 2032/1897.

send-off of which he would have approved when local show people combined to give him a suitable burial. The cortège was led by the united bands of Fitzgerald Brothers circus and the proprietors of the Old English Fayre, followed by tumblers and artists on performing horses.[34] The hospital was still the preserve of the less affluent but if a patient was in a position to pay, a charge of a guinea a week was made.[35]

Hope's administration of medical services at Fremantle continued unchanged with the move to The Knowle. Not only was he the government medical officer with responsibility for patients in the public hospital, but he held the positions of health officer, medical officer to the port, medical officer to the Local Board of Health and was a member of the new medical board set up in 1895 to register the state's doctors. Hope was also medical officer to the police, carrying out post-mortems and attending inquests, medical officer to the gaol, medical officer to Rottnest and he held the private contracts to attend all shipping cases in the port, as well as running a large private practice.[36] It was too much for one man. Following the departure of Hope's assistant, Frederick Ingoldby, in 1888, Arthur Thomas White entered into partnership with the Fremantle medical officer and was often seen at the Point Street Hospital, presenting for surgery 'immaculate in full morning dress'.[37] Council's concern about medical practitioners aiding the spread of disease through carrying 'about with them, the germs of disease unknowingly' on their person may have had good ground.

Hope's position of medical supremacy in the Point Street Hospital before the move to The Knowle had not gone unchallenged; many patients wanted treatment by their own doctor while in hospital, and doctors also expressed the wish to attend their own patients. As the hospital was purely a government institution, funded, administered and controlled by the Medical Department through Hope, the notion was unprecedented. 'It would not work unless the hospital was handed over to a board as was the Colonial Hospital in Perth,' objected Lovegrove, the principal medical officer, and 'I would not recommend this being done at present'.[38] When the move to The Knowle was imminent, Lovegrove and Hope discussed the matter further and were prepared when Fremantle doctors, William Birmingham, Henry Lotz, Louis Wheeler—who had joined in partnership with Barnett in 1893, Owen Paget and Arthur White, suggested the formation of a committee to manage the hospital, and the introduction of a system of honorary medical attendance with each of the doctors permitted a certain number of beds. Thomas Lovegrove had considered it best to restrict the appointments to Drs White and Birmingham as honorary physician and honorary surgeon, and to ask Dr Barnett to act as a consulting surgeon to the institution, so that control of the hospital would be kept by the government, but he agreed to talk with the doctors. Their concerns were a mixed bag—for their patients, their pockets and their prestige. Paget found it 'very unpleasant to the doctor who was attending a patient to get the patient to declare before a magistrate that he is a pauper and unable to pay for advice' and all found it 'very mortifying' to

34   *West Australian*, 1 February 1897, 8 February 1897, 15 February 1897.
35   CSO File 2032/1897.
36   *Ibid*.
37   de Moulin interview, cited in Hobbs, *But Westward Look*, p. 20.
38   CSO File 2763/97, 20 April 1896. See also Minutes of FMC, 28 April 1896.

find there were no vacant beds in the hospital when a patient needed hospital care or an operation. On the other hand, if beds were available, they lost the case and the income to Hope. The doctors wanted five beds each, either medical or surgical as the need arose, and were agreeable to a weekly consultation day to discuss their cases as a source of interest and instruction. As long as they had access to the hospital, board control was not an issue. Hope could remain supervisor, they agreed, and would retain the greater number of beds, but each doctor would have undisputed control of his own patients. Lovegrove's suggestion of specialisation in medical and surgical areas, however, met with great opposition from the doctors. 'No. No. No! That would only cause petty jealousy and would be extremely detrimental to the hospital and would lower us in the eyes of the public'.[39] It was yet a time of the general practitioner in every sense of the word. Lovegrove left the qualification for honorary service to the doctors' discretion and seemed persuaded in favour of their suggested system, but would only promise his consideration, not his consent. He left them with the encouraging admonition that the government did not supply champagne or three-star brandy, and that if these comforts were ordered they would have to be provided by the patients or their friends.

While Lovegrove approved of the doctors' plan to introduce an honorary system of treatment at the hospital, he did not recommend that the hospital should be made a public institution, run by a board as at Perth under *The Hospitals Act* of 1894. Tobias Burt thought that the hospital should be one thing or the other—either a government hospital, pure and simple, or else a hospital under the Act. In the end Colonial Secretary Wittenoom's unfortunate decision settled the dispute: 'Let it remain as at present for a further period.'[40]

Although used to dealing with the Medical Department in practical matters, Hope's first efforts at financial administration caused some tension. His order to England for surgical instruments and 'a dozen catheters, prostatic and a'boule', earned him a reprimand and an order to direct future requisitions through the department. Perhaps it was as well, as only one of each of the catheters was sent, the remaining eleven having to be made and sent at the earliest opportunity. The 'Colgates Perfume and Rinse Bouche' were not available, and the 'Lanolin with Cucumber Cream' had not even been heard of.[41] Another censure followed Hope's order for a case of champagne from Faddy and Knight. Medical comforts had long been given to patients to aid recovery but Lovegrove persisted in his belief that it should not be given at the country's expense. 'It is only rarely I order this wine,' replied Hope, 'I think that sometimes it is necessary—and aids a patient's recovery. I shall be sorry not to have the power to prescribe it.'[42] His greatest unauthorised expenditure was the hospital fowl house, installed in an effort to get a few fresh eggs for supper time. Richard Honey, timber merchants of Packenham Street, and Sandover and Company, delivered the material and Hope had a prisoner from the gaol build both an enclosure for the hens and a coal bunker. There was talk at the government

[39] CSO File 2763/97, 10 March 1897.
[40] *Ibid.*
[41] CSO File 1066/97. The instruments were ordered from Ferris and Company wholesale and export druggists and surgical instrument makers in Bristol, England.
[42] CSO File 2545/97.

level of the fowl house being disposed of at public auction but it was eventually paid for and Hope was again reprimanded.[43]

After the old Point Street premises, the stately building set high on a rise over-looking terraced lawns, with views of the ocean, seemed like 'heaven'[44] to the new occupants, a condition which did not last long. With summer came typhoid sufferers in unprecedented numbers. On 1 February 1897 there were 28 hospital patients, a week later 39, and by 15 February the number totalled 48. In March there was an average of 43, more than half of whom had typhoid, and the increase continued in the intense heat which followed light rain during April, with 45 or 46 patients remaining at the end of each week after the convalescent had been discharged. By May, 27 out of the 40 patients were still typhoid victims.[45] If anything, the typhoid position was worse at Perth, where victims had to be treated in tents in the hospital grounds or at the old Isolation Hospital at West Subiaco.[46] Some of the Perth patients were sent down to The Knowle. The resulting 'congested state of the hos-pital' meant that the Fremantle sufferers could not be moved from the public board-ing houses where they lay and the local board of health deeply resented the 'outside patients'.[47] The board optimistically requested the erection of a temporary conva-lescent hospital planned by Hope and the town's surveyor. The need was emphasised later in the month. A middle-aged man from Victoria named William Crofton came down with typhoid on his way to the West and spent seven weeks in the Fremantle Hospital. He came through the crisis of the disease, but during convalescence, because of the great need for hospital accommodation, he was discharged. The few shillings he had, sustained the man briefly but he was too weak to work. In a desper-ate move to obtain food and shelter, Crofton took a stone and broke a street lamp glass outside the Court House. The resident magistrate ordered 21 days of imprison-ment and the nurses who had come to know their patient so well, were distressed to recognize him a few days later as a member of the prison gang clearing and cleaning in the hospital grounds.[48] A little over a week passed before another typhoid patient, John Walin, collapsed and died while working on the wharves after being discharged from the hospital in a weak state. At the inquiry into his death, the jury found that Walin had returned to work too soon after his illness. Hope took the opportunity to emphasise the town's need for a convalescent home for the indigent, to which Love-grove and the jury to a man added their voices.[49]

On 1 May 1897, the Ministering Children's League Convalescent Home at Cottes-loe, which quickly became known as the M.C.L. Convalescent Home, was officially opened. Through the efforts and foresight of Mrs Marian Holmes, who organised a strong branch of the league in Western Australia, the beautiful sandstone building with a 12-bed ward, dining hall, sitting room and staff quarters, all shaded by veran-dahs and overlooking the sea, was built. Some Fremantle Hospital patients went to

[43] CSO File 3972/97.
[44] de Moulin interview, cited in Hobbs, *But Westward Look*, p. 20.
[45] Weekly hospital reports, published in *West Australian*, 1, 8, 15, 25 February 1897; 1, 8, 15, 22, 29 March 1897; 5, 12, 19, 27 April 1897; 3 May 1897.
[46] Bolton and Joske, *History of Royal Perth Hospital*, p. 57.
[47] Minutes of FLBH, 18 March 1897; CSO File 250/97.
[48] *West Australian*, 23 March 1897; de Moulin interview, cited in Hobbs, *But Westward Look*, p. 20.
[49] *West Australian*, 2 April 1897.

the home designed 'for those for whom a fortnight's rest and quietness with the bracing air and the comforts of a home are essential before they resume their ordinary occupations' but most did not, as admission was only by the recommendation of a subscriber. The available beds were few and the cost varied between ten shillings and £1 a week, so that many convalescents discharged from Fremantle's hospital were no better off.[50]

Not all patients at The Knowle were typhoid sufferers in 1897. The increase in building, shipping, and trade was reflected in the intensive labour required at the harbour and the railway. It was not unusual for 28,000 tons of cargo to be taken over the jetty in a month and the Fremantle merchants professed themselves 'very much satisfied at the state of things now existing'.[51] Railway employees worked overtime one Saturday and all day Sunday to clear goods, and in a day and a half loaded 406 wagons with 2,800 tons of supplies and equipment. There were stones for road works, timber and firewood for the city, general goods for Perth and the goldfields, and piles for the North Fremantle jetty, part of O'Connor's magnificent inner harbour, which was nearing completion.[52] It was almost inevitable that accidents increased. Men fell down hatchways and holds of ships, were pinned by shifting loads, caught feet in moving chains, were knocked down by a train or fell under one. A 15-year-old labourer at the quarries behind Skinner Street was struck by falling rock, another quarryman suffered severe sunstroke and died. A patron named Patrick Shannon fractured his skull when he fell from an upstairs window of the Club Hotel and a labourer broke his arm when he lost his footing on some scaffolding at a building site in Mouatt Street. A railway guard lost his leg when he accidentally slipped under the wheels of the No. 62 down train as the locomotive shunted some trucks off a line. Like most injured workers, he was taken to the hospital, where Hope took up his much-used, nineteenth century amputation instruments to remove the man's other mangled leg.[53] Through the social changes that accompanied the huge increase in population, through the mobility of people who landed and moved on without making family and community networks of support, and with the availability of a conveniently sited and adequately equipped medical centre, the use of the hospital was becoming more socially acceptable.

Most of the more respected in the Fremantle community were still nursed at home. The owner of the Pioneer Oyster Saloon in High Street, bleeding heavily from multiple stab wounds inflicted by an angry dismissed cook, was taken to his home, not the hospital, to receive treatment from Dr Hope. So too, was the proprietor of the Beaconsfield Newsagency after being knocked down and seriously injured one night by a runaway trap without lights. The 84-year-old chaplain of the Fremantle Prison, Reverend G. C. Nicolay, was also taken to his residence when he fell unconscious in the street with a 'fit of paralysis'.[54]

Some who could pay, were able to go to local private hospitals which were established in the early 1890s. In Fremantle, one such hospital was in Norfolk Street:

[50] *Ibid.*, 14 April 1897, 28 April 1897, 3 May 1897.
[51] *Ibid.*, 22 December 1896.
[52] *Ibid.*, 4 January 1897, 3 February 1897, 30 March 1897.
[53] *Ibid.*, 14, 18, 19, 28 December 1896; 2, 5, 19 February 1897; 1, 30 March 1897; 1 April 1897.
[54] See *West Australian*, 15 February 1897, 5 April 1897, 10 May 1897.

'Private hospitals are springing up like mushrooms around us, and unfortunately they have come to stay, and therefore their use should be recognised', advocated a correspondent to the *West Australian* in 1895.[55] By 1901, another private hospital, run by Eva Gormley, was on Monument Hill, while Mrs Kennedy owned a hospital on Mandurah Road.[56] The Madeleine Hospital for expectant mothers was run by Mrs Jensen, but the best-known in 1897 was Dr White's hospital on Mandurah Road.[57] Mrs H. E. Richardson had permission to operate a private hospital in South Street, Beaconsfield, and Ellen Harrison and Rose Carlton ran the Surgical Sanatorium and Convalescent Home at Monument House on Monument Hill.[58] Objections to private hospitals were common. From his beautiful house near Monument Hill, James Lilly organised a petition against a hospital being erected close to his home. The site was unsuitable and would spread fever germs through the drainage, he thought, but others were in favour of private hospitals and believed that all infectious diseases should be confined to certain areas, lessening the spread of the contagion.[59] But as one woman recalled, most people had to manage as best they could. 'They just sent for the doctor and do what the doctor tells them. Mostly they'd stay at home . . . they just had to cope.'[60]

With the number of injured and the increasing number of typhoid patients requiring long, heavy tending, nursing staff at The Knowle were hard-pressed. First Lillian Webb in January, then F. McIlvaine and Rebecca Crudden in February, were accepted on trial as probationer nurses for the usual three-month term without pay before signing a two-year agreement with the Medical Department. In March, a newly-trained Perth Hospital nurse named Margaret Coombe Birt joined Emma Jane Duncan, formerly of the North London Fever Hospital, on the Fremantle staff. Rosa Snodgrass from Melbourne's Alfred Hospital joined as a senior nurse in May. By July the nursing staff comprised Matron Steele, two orderlies, five trained nurses and five probationers to staff 52 beds for 24 hours of each day.[61] The ratio of trained nurses was not always so high and by September, when Rosa had gone as matron to Kalgoorlie Hospital, the ratio was two trained nurses to eight probationers. The trained nurses received £52 a year. After their first three months without pay, probationers received 30 shillings a month for the rest of their first year, and 50 shillings monthly in the second year of their training.

Nurses worked two shifts, either day or night. Hours were long and the work hard. Probationers rose at 6 a.m. and breakfasted at 6.30 each morning. Although they did not finish work until 8 o'clock at night, a two-hour break was permitted each day and, twice a week if work was done, a three-hour break was taken. Each nurse had one welcome day off a month, but that day would have to be made up by others working in turns through their daily two-hour respite. When a patient was particularly ill, day nurses took it in turns to help during the night; as a doctor

55 *Ibid.*, 1 April 1895.
56 Minutes of FLBH, 30 November 1894, 28 November 1895, 12 December 1895, 20 February 1896.
57 *Ibid.*, 5, 12 March 1896; 16 April 1896.
58 *Ibid.*, 25 January 1901.
59 *Ibid.*, 17 October 1895, 12 March 1896.
60 '. Charlton, interviewed by M. Howroyd, 5 and 19 December 1983, FCL.
61 Western Australian Blue Book 1890–1900; CSO File 1550/97; CSO File 2032/1897; *Morning Herald*, 2 September 1897. For further detail on Margaret Coombe Birt, see Hobbs, *But Westward Look*, p. 8.

pointed out 'this cannot be done frequently without the following day's duties being neglected'.[62] The duties of the nurse varied. The clinical condition of patients had to be observed and the sick had to be prevented from falling or getting out of bed, a task especially difficult with delirium cases. Sometimes these patients, or one in the grip of 'the alcohol' attacked a nurse. 'I often found it necessary to restrain patients as is done here both for their safety and the safety of the nurses,' the matron related in 1897.[63] Fomentations and poultices had to be prepared and applied, beds changed and made, weak patients fed and others bathed with white soap and water. Usually there were wounds to dress and bandage. Bed pans and sputum mugs had to be distributed, collected and emptied. Nor was Florence Nightingale's dictum neglected: 'Keep the air he breathes as pure as external air, without chilling him'.[64] Sometimes a head had to be cleaned of vermin and at times the dead prepared for burial. As no ward-maids were employed, all cleaning and washing-up was done by nurses. Although similar hours and conditions were worked at other hospitals at time of crisis, the nurses at Fremantle felt that it was doubly difficult for them, with their patients spread throughout so many rooms.[65] Because of the pressure of work, no lectures were given to probationers during most of 1897 and their learning was gained from observation and direction by senior nurses. It was noted that 'they were permitted to use their own judgment in dealing with almost any matter with which they were called upon to deal'.[66]

The dreaded month of night duty was done on a rotating basis. Only two nurses staffed the whole hospital; one had charge of the 27 patients on the lower floor, and responsibility for the 25 upstairs was given to a probationer. 'Among ourselves we consider this too many because the beds are distributed among so many wards,' related one nurse.[67] During the hours of night, wet patients had to be washed and changed, dressings attended to if required, medicines and fluids given, but the greatest concern was the typhoid patients whose condition invariably seemed to worsen at night. As in other hospitals, in England, the Eastern States and at Perth, patients in delirium had to be tied down with a wide bandage, usually around an ankle and the upper arms, and narcotics such as opium were sometimes given to restrain violent typhoid patients and prevent them getting out of bed. If a patient succeeded in getting up, the case usually ended fatally.[68] Often, in an emergency, a nurse on one floor had to leave her patients to help the doctor or the nurse on the other floor, leaving her patients unattended for up to an hour at a time. If necessary, the matron or an orderly could be woken to assist, but as one nurse pointed out, 'I have to leave my floor to call for it'.[69] The matron worked as hard as her nurses and

[62] Evidence of Dr Richard Rendle at inquiry into the general working of the Fremantle Hospital, 5 July 1897, CSO File 2032/1897.
[63] CSO File 2032/1897.
[64] F. Nightingale, *Notes on Nursing: What it is and What it is not*, 1974. First published 1859, p. 8. General information also obtained from lecture notes of J. Brown, student nurse at the Fulwood Hospital, Preston, Victoria, 1897, held at Fremantle Hospital.
[65] Information from *Morning Herald*, 2 September 1897; CSO File 2032/1897.
[66] See *Morning Herald*, 2 September 1897.
[67] Emma Jane Duncan, trained nurse. CSO File 2032/1897.
[68] *Morning Herald*, 25 June 1897.
[69] Margaret Grover, probationer nurse, CSO File 2032/1897.

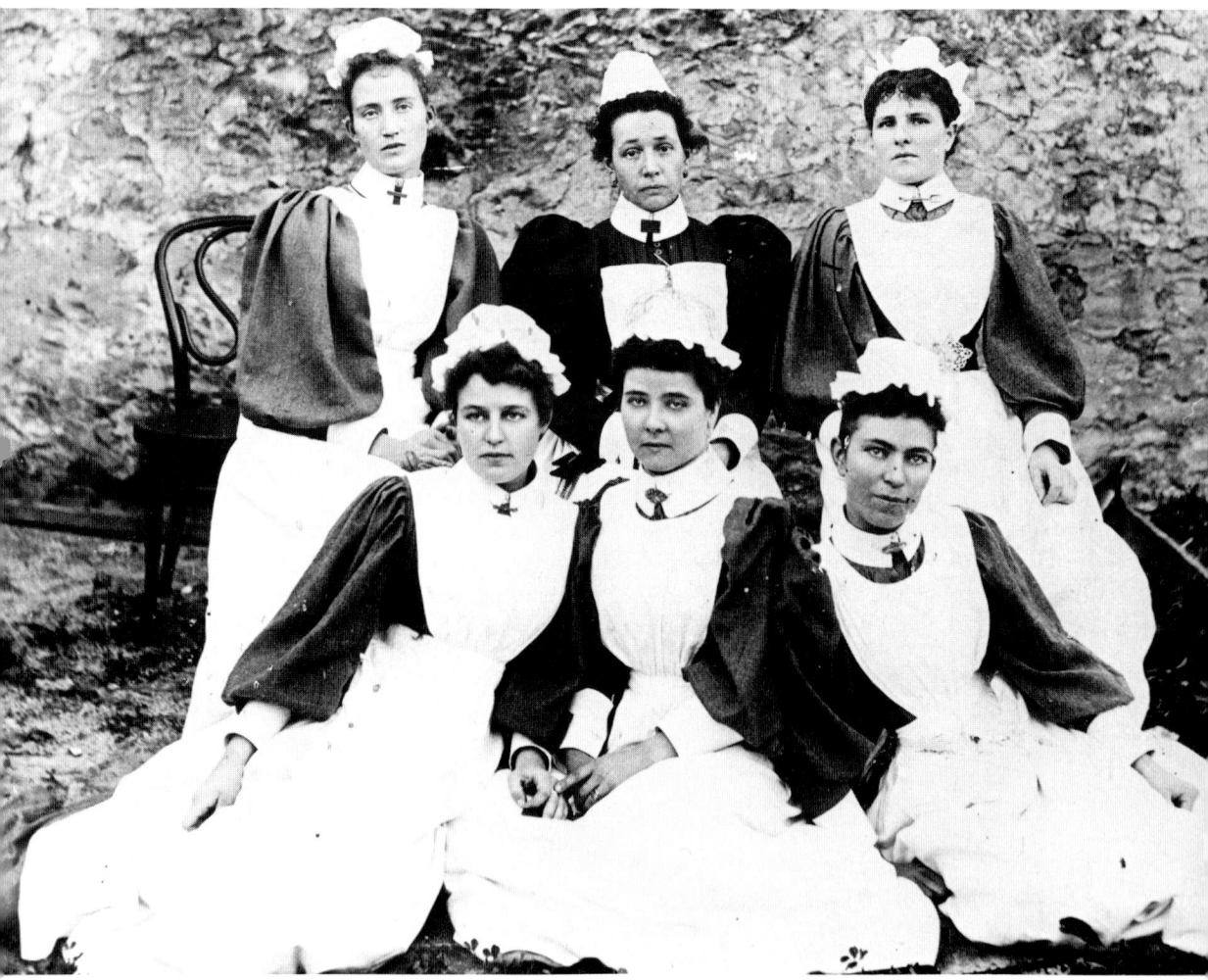

Photograph courtesy Fremantle Hospital

Plate 6. Early Fremantle Hospital nurses.

Back row (left to right): Nurse Mortimer, Matron Bessie Murray Steele, Nurse King.
Front row: Nurse Woodhead, Nurse Price, Nurse Grover. (Nurse Mortimer married the first Fremantle Hospital dispenser.)

apart from her duties as matron, did all the secretarial work for the hospital, dressed wounds, dispensed drugs and often even prescribed for patients. It was not really surprising that one nurse complained that 'I have felt much run down, very often' and matron had to allow nurses time off when they were was particularly 'knocked up'.[70] Townspeople when they met nurses in the street, remarked that 'the nurses

[70] CSO File 2032/1897.

have more the appearance of requiring a nurse themselves than of looking after others'.[71]

In early April, when the hospital was filled to capacity, Hope approached Dr Richard Rendle about him accepting a position as house surgeon at The Knowle, on the understanding that the new doctor would take over Hope's work at the hospital and would be able to conduct a private practice as well. Rendle agreed.[72] It was with great frustration, therefore, that Rendle later found that he was not allowed to see any private patients or even give medical advice to friends to supplement his salary of £250 a year. Neither did Hope surrender his hospital responsibilities. Rendle was a qualified doctor who had been a surgeon at the Seaman's Hospital in Greenwich and at the Royal Infirmary for Women and Children in London and had also taught practical surgery at Guy's Hospital, before working in Brisbane, Queensland, as a private practitioner and hospital surgeon. He therefore keenly felt the loss of status working under Hope's direction in a position much more akin to a clerk and dispenser than a responsible medical officer. Neither did he feel it reasonable or right that Hope should have entire control of hospital cases when he already held ten public appointments and had a private practice as well. Rendle's discontent deepened when Hope expected the house surgeon to visit his own private patients, attend the gaol, and to visit Rottnest on request, without any of the extra remuneration which was usually given for assistance. Perhaps there was also some professional conflict, for Rendle firmly objected to the practice of sedating typhoid patients and tying them to their beds. Hope's 'rude and arrogant manner' also aggravated the house surgeon.[73]

Rendle was an outspoken man, firm in his convictions. In deploring the sanitary condition of the town, which he believed encouraged typhoid, the doctor urged that citizens:

> ... must not like the ostrich shut their eyes to dangers or try to explain them away, but must like an old man kangaroo at bay, stand up, and face them bravely and intelligently, and do their utmost to remedy the evils'.[74]

In May, Rendle wrote to Lovegrove of his dissatisfaction in his appointment and he alluded to 'other matters of public importance connected with the hospital which appear to me to call for an investigation and reform'.[75]

With so many typhoid patients in the hospital, Rendle felt strongly the need for greater public awareness about the disease and on Sunday, May 9, gave a free lecture in the Town Hall on 'What people ought to know about typhoid fever'.[76] In the following month, he agreed to an interview for the *Morning Herald* and submitted some typhoid statistics to the paper which were discredited at the local Board of Health meeting, which considered the paper as alarmist. Rendle wrote to the paper and reiterated the hospital admission statistics which indisputably proved the

[71] *Morning Herald*, 29 June 1897.
[72] *Government Gazette*, 9 April 1897.
[73] CSO File 2032/1897, 25 May 1897.
[74] *Morning Herald*, 22 June 1897.
[75] CSO File 2032/1897, 25 May 1897.
[76] Minutes of FMC, 27 April 1897.

increase of typhoid fever patients at the hospital: one in 13 in 1895, one in eight in 1896 and one in two in 1897—of which two-thirds were of local origin. 'All we wish to impress on the public mind and the Governing bodies . . .', reassured the doctor, 'is that typhoid is rapidly on the increase, so that the causes may be sought out, and preventive measures adopted without further delay.'[77]

If Rendle had confined his comments to those of public health, the matter may have ended there. The town's appalling sanitary conditions were at last being faced by the council in their decision to adopt a covered-pan system, but the doctor addressed other matters alluded to in the Board of Health meeting, substantiating that there was indeed a lack of night staff at the hospital and replying to Councillor John's remark that a towel had been stuffed into a patient's mouth:

> . . . on one occasion only to my knowledge has a towel been held over a patient's mouth, and then it was done by myself in order to lessened the disturbance caused by a noisy patient, and I am quite satisfied that the patient did not suffer more from the proceeding than I did.[78]

On a subject close to his heart, Rendle also advocated the appointment of the city's medical men to the hospital staff. Not only had Hope many demanding responsibilities which made it impossible for him to give adequate attention to the hospital, argued Rendle, but it was 'not just' to other doctors that 'one man should monopolize the whole field of hospital practice'.[79]

Rendle's remarks in the *Morning Herald* prompted a barbed battle with a respondent named 'One Who Knows'. In his first letter the anonymous writer condemned the house surgeon for his reluctance to tie delirious patients to their beds as was usually done to prevent them from getting up. This caused much mental strain for the nurses, the writer claimed. A challenge was then extended to Rendle to give lectures to the probationers.[80] Somewhat 'like an old man kangaroo at bay', Rendle faced his protagonist across the pages of the press and denied having changed the practice of securing and sedating delirious patients, 'for the simple reason, that Dr Hope retains full charge of all cases, and that Dr Rendle has no authority beyond instructions received'. He refuted the claim that there was more than one nurse on each floor during the night and stated his preparedness to instruct nurses if he had the authority and means to do so, 'but at present the hospital is managed by no less than five different persons, whose ideas as to what should be done are so divergent that it is impossible for one to act without friction'.[81] Rendle called for control by a board of management and the establishment of an honorary medical staff and challenged 'One Who Knows' to sign his name instead of 'shooting from behind a hedge'.

In the next skirmish the protagonist retained his cover—'Even from behind a hedge one can shoot straight'. He questioned Rendle's statistics and stated there had

[77] *Morning Herald*, 22 June 1897.
[78] *Ibid.*
[79] *Ibid.*
[80] *Ibid.*, 25 June 1897.
[81] *Ibid.*, 26 June 1897.

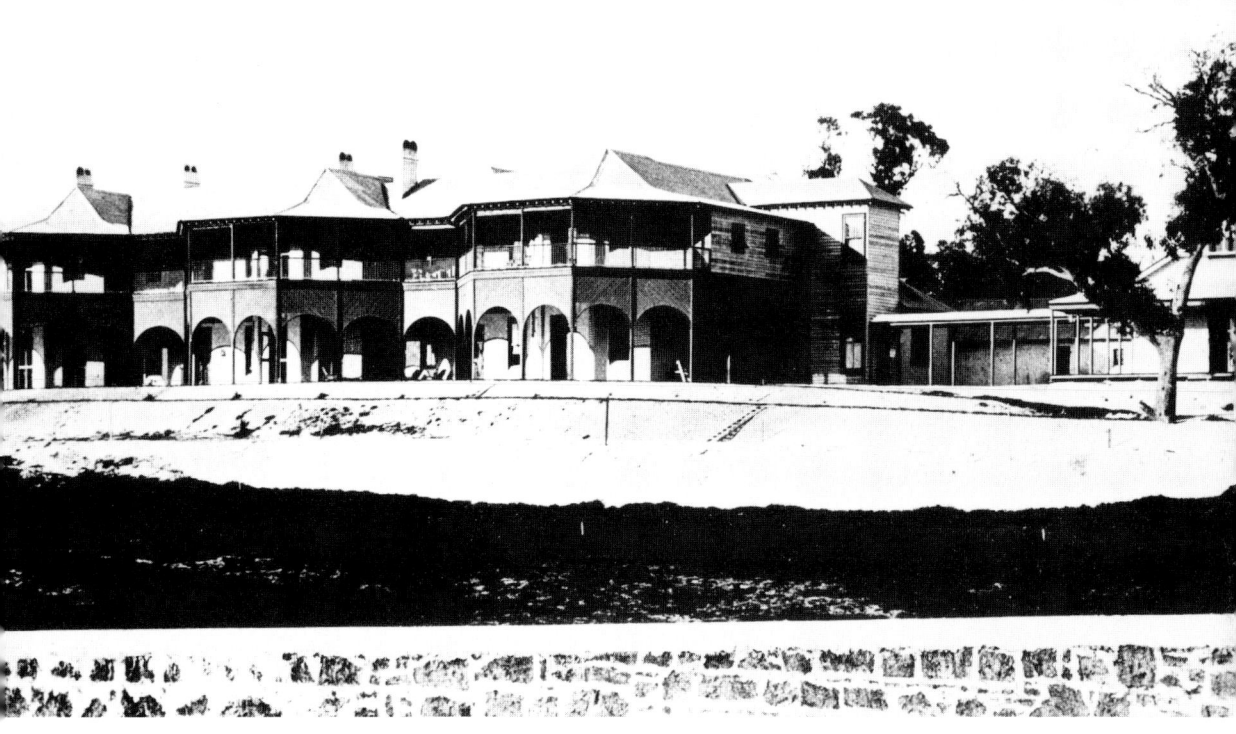

Photograph courtesy Fremantle Hospital

Plate 7.   The Knowle at the turn of the century.

been one, not three deaths from typhoid for the week ending 19 June, and again challenged the doctor to instruct the nurses 'to qualify them for their duties'. The writer then construed Rendle's reference to the 'five different persons' to be Hope and Rendle, the matron and the two staff nurses, and suggested that when doctors differed, nurses should decide the outcome.[82]

In his dissatisfaction with the running of the hospital and his position in it, in defence of his reputation and avowedly 'to help those who suffer', Rendle took up his pen and poured out a volley of words in reply to the writer who had obviously more than a surface knowledge of the hospital's conditions. Rendle defended his statistics which were based on the hospital's weekly records. He defended the matron and nurses whose 'devoted care and untiring zeal' had kept matters at the hospital from worsening. The matron had filled a most difficult post in a manner commanding the highest respect and the 'greatly overworked and poorly paid' nurses who had not sufficient rest, recreation and time to attend lectures or extra instruction—even were the means provided for giving them—were above reproach. It was not only absurd to ask a probationer to nurse 24 patients in four separate

[82]   *Ibid.*, 29 June 1897.

rooms for eleven hours—and to give occasional assistance on another floor—it was downright 'cruel and selfish to demand it'. The doctor defended his reputation and his treatment of typhoid cases. Between March and June 1896, the death rate in the hospital had been 1 in 4.4 of typhoid admissions, while during his period of employment in the corresponding months of 1897 the death rate had dropped to only 1 in every 8.6. '... those who understand the subject will bear me out in saying that it is largely due to my discouragement of large doses of calomel and castor oil, which no modern physician ever dreams of giving in cases of typhoid but which was the routine treatment in almost every case when I came to the hospital'.[83]

The resident doctor had been careful not to offend his peers. 'Hitherto I have avoided hitting [at] individuals or making personal remarks,' wrote Rendle, 'and have pointed out instead "defects in the *system*".' Now he squarely and publicly addressed the issue of the hospital's administration. At the head of the five people said to be in conflicting control of the hospital, Rendle placed Hope, the officer 'who holds all the public medical appointments in the town and who is said to owe his position to political influence'. The others on his list were named as the principal medical officer, himself as the resident medical officer, the matron and the supervisor—with some officers of the Public Works Department and certain members of parliament having influence as well. He spoke of the difficulty of the town's doctors to have a case admitted to the hospital unless it was passed over to Hope or his partner Arthur White. In a final challenge, Rendle called for complete control of the hospital by either the principal medical officer or a board of management, as at Perth Hospital. 'Such a state of affairs as exists at present would not be tolerated in any other colony.'[84]

The state's medical hierarchy shuddered at the ten-day affray but took their time to act. On the publication of his first letter to the *Morning Herald* after the Fremantle Municipal Council meeting, Rendle wrote to the principal medical officer, Lovegrove, submitting his resignation unless his position as resident medical officer was improved. 'The conditions under which the appointment is now held are of a degrading and humiliating character,' he stated. He spoke of a small fixed income unable to be increased, of Hope's attitude and his control of the hospital. 'I submit Sir, that no man of professional ability and standing will continue to hold office under such conditions.'[85]

Lovegrove received a copy of Rendle's first press missive from an indignant James Hope who objected: 'I do not consider the remarks are just, judicious, fair or in good taste coming from an officer attached to the Hospital. I do not remember that he has suggested any improvement in the management of the nursing department verbally to me and certainly not in writing.'[86] At the first response by 'One Who Knows' on 25 June, Lovegrove wrote to the under secretary concurring with Rendle's observations about the difficulty experienced by nurses at The Knowle: 'The real cause of the trouble is the utter unsuitability of the building owing to the smallness of the wards and the way they are arranged which necessitates much run-

[83] *Ibid.*, 1 July 1897.
[84] *Ibid.*
[85] CSO File 2032/1897. Letter, Richard Rendle to Thomas Lovegrove, 25 May 1897.
[86] *Ibid.*, Letter, Hope to Lovegrove, 23 June 1897.

ning about and fatigue on the part of the nursing staff.'[87] However, he felt that Rendle's letters to the press, should not be allowed to continue. Three days later the matter moved to a higher level when Octavius Burt, the under secretary, wrote to the acting premier about Rendle's 'highly irregular' course of action, only excusable by reason of Dr Rendle's inexperience as a government officer: 'I propose causing him to be so informed'.[88] The order to censure Rendle was passed back to the principal medical officer, but his reproof, although curt, was comparatively mild: 'Your action in writing such a letter is inexcusable and can only be condoned on account of your inexperience as a Government officer. Your proper channel of complaint is through the resident medical officer, not the public press. The number of nursing staff is fully up to the required standard.' In a contrite reply Rendle apologised for his correspondence, undertaken in ignorance of departmental procedure, but he remained adamant that 'the present staff is overworked and that it is impossible for the work that is now required to be properly carried out under present arrangements'. He also warned of a forthcoming letter, already on the printing block: 'I am afraid Sir, that my letter in the *Herald* of July 1st will also incur your displeasure. If so I shall be glad to [be] relieved of any duties at the end of the present month or as soon after as you can engage a successor'.[89]

Not surprisingly, when Hope read his paper on the morning of 1 July, he was incensed. His ability as a doctor, his honesty as an administrator and his fairness in admitting patients to the hospital had been questioned and he called for an urgent inquiry. With the delicacy of a sledge hammer, in a postscript to his letter he reminded the principal medical officer that in two of his letters to the press, Rendle had said that he had offered his resignation. Within days Lovegrove arrived at the hospital to interview some of the nurses in the presence of Hope and Rendle, who were allowed to cross-examine the witnesses. With Hope standing by, the matron and nurses were extremely guarded in their replies, although all admitted that night duty was onerous and understaffed.[90] Under cross-examination by Rendle, senior nurse Margaret Coombe Birt related that probationers had no time to attend lectures because of the work that was required to be done each day. Without their outright support, however, Rendle was condemned by the words of the nurses, who justified the conditions at Fremantle as little worse than at other hospitals they had been in. While Rendle's efforts were based in part on personal motives to clear his name, his attempt to improve conditions at Fremantle Hospital was a gallant one. When Hope confronted Rendle at the end of the inquiry, the house surgeon would not retract his press statement that Hope's position was due to political influence: 'It is common talk in the town ... I decline to give any names.' Once more Rendle repeated his observation about Hope's monopoly of the hospital for his own patients. His own defence, the house surgeon said with finality, was in his replies to 'One Who Knows' and 'When I defend myself I don't care at whose expense it is at'.

On 5 July, Lovegrove recommended to Under Secretary Octavius Burt that Dr Rendle's correspondence was 'calculated to awaken a feeling of unrest in the minds

[87] *Ibid.*, Letter, 26 June 1897.
[88] *Ibid.*, Letter, 29 June 1897.
[89] *Ibid.*, Letter, 2 July 1897.
[90] *Ibid.*, Inquiry into the general working of Fremantle Hospital, 5 July 1897.

Dr Lovegrove

Principal Medical Officer

         Perth

                                    Government Hospital

                                        Fremantle

                                        12 – 7 – 97

Dear Sir

        In reply to your favour dated 10ᵗʰ July 1897 received to day I beg to inform you that in conformity with your request therein conveyed I shall move out of residence this evening. The refusal of your department to pay me one months salary in lieu of notice will I think be regarded by the public as it is by me as a very dishonourable action, and one which no court of law would permit any private firm to do with impunity. It is moreover further proof of the vindictive spirit that has been manifested towards me in consequence of my efforts to improve the management of & expose certain abuses in connection with this Hospital.

As however I have neither the means nor the will to fight the Government I must bow to your decision & leave the judgement to the higher courts of Public Opinion and the great Judge of all before to whom even heads of departments & under Secretaries will have to render an account

                      I am Dear Sir

                      Yours faithfully

                      Richard Rendle

Fig. 8. Letter from Dr Richard Rendle to Dr Thomas Lovegrove.

of some people about the general administration of the Hospital' due to Hope's denial to him of a general practice and possibly other personal motives. 'I think Dr Rendle should be called upon to resign. If he is allowed to remain he will only cause more trouble,' he concluded. Burt concurred in a recommendation to the acting premier, if for no other reason than for Rendle's statement that Hope 'owes his position to political influence'. Lovegrove asked Rendle to resign on 8 July, but on the following day, the house surgeon reasoned that as his resignation had been tendered in previous correspondence and had not been accepted, he was entitled to a month's notice or a month's salary. Such impudence could not for one moment be entertained and Rendle was requested to leave Fremantle Hospital on Monday, 12 July.

Before he left, the doctor fired a last spirited round:

> In reply to your favour dated 10th July 1897 received today I beg to inform you that in conformity with your request therein conveyed I shall move out of residence this evening. The refusal of your department to pay me one month's salary in lieu of notice will I think be regarded by the public as it is by me as a very dishonorable action, one which no court of law would permit any private firm to do with impunity. It is moreover further proof of the vindictive spirit that has been manifested towards me in consequence of my efforts to improve the management of and expose certain abuses in connection with this Hospital.
>
> As however I have neither the means nor the will to fight the Government I must bow to your decision and leave the judgment to the higher courts of Public opinion and the great Judge of all to whom even heads of departments and under Secretaries have to render an account.[91]

The man who had stood and faced his opponents bravely and intelligently and who had done his utmost to remedy the evils he perceived, left the hospital to take up a private practice from Higham's chambers in Fremantle. The prevalence of typhoid continued to concern him and in mid-September Rendle announced his intention to run classes in the best methods of treatment. Many lives, he claimed, were lost as a result of the lack of intelligent and trained help in early stages of the illness, and in his classes members would not only be told, but shown, the best methods of treatment and would practise every detail of care on a living model. His method of instruction had been learned as a teacher in Guy's Hospital, London.[92]

In August, Rendle was still writing to the *Morning Herald* in his quest to improve sanitary conditions at Fremantle. No one was too large for his gunsights and even Sir John Forrest and the supposedly responsible medical officers of the government, who were aware of the link between disease and inefficient drainage, came in for attack. The dramatic rise in cases of typhoid reported monthly at Fremantle angered and frustrated Rendle, and he consistently pointed out the urgent need to enquire into causes of the disease, rather than concentrate on the treatment of effects.[93] But the nicknamed 'wait awhile' colony shrugged off the sound logic and dawdled into 1898, dragging its feet through the same foul drains and turning up its nose at the

[91]   CSO File 2032/1897, 12 July 1897.
[92]   *Morning Herald*, 15 September 1897.
[93]   *Ibid.*, 28 August 1897.

unsatisfactory effluent disposal systems. It was easier for the Fremantle flock of the Wesleyan Reverend C. A. Jenkins to respond spiritually to his sermon 'If Thou wilt Thou canst make me clean', than for the council to purge the town of its filth.[94] Rendle would not have been surprised at the increase in the number of typhoid cases in Fremantle in 1898. Eighty-two people died in April and May alone.[95]

Fremantle Hospital's next resident doctor was transferred from Kalgoorlie in mid-July 1897, but his stay was brief, for Patrick Maxwell resigned the appointment in mid-September. He professed that the climate of Fremantle did not suit him, but the Medical Department suspected his proposed return to Kalgoorlie was to enter a partnership there. Through Dr Springthorpe, of Collins Street in Melbourne, Love-grove was able to appoint an outstanding young graduate from the Melbourne University as Fremantle Hospital's third house surgeon. Thomas L. Anderson arrived on the S.S. *Innamincka* and took up his work at the 56-bed hospital as surgeon and dispenser on 20 October 1897, at a salary of £250 a year.[96]

Richard Rendle had not been successful in bringing about improvements at Fremantle Hospital during his tenure but he was a catalyst for change. He could see where improvements were necessary but the Medical Department in their decision to support their trusted long-time employee, Hope, accepted the deplorable conditions rather than using them as a springboard for improvement. Changes most needed, perhaps, were to conditions for the nursing staff. Not only were their days strictly regimented to the degree that they could not converse with each other unless it was about their work, but their evenings were curtailed as well. Matron Steele was a strict disciplinarian. After duty finished at 8 p.m. day nurses were expected to retire to one of the two bedrooms set aside for their use, in each of which four nurses slept. Although there was a need to increase the nursing staff, the move was always delayed because no more beds could be squeezed into the rooms.[97] By a set of rules drawn up by Bessie Steele, nurses were expected to remain 'locked up four together in a small bedroom' until 6.30 the following morning and to extinguish their candles by 10.30 p.m.[98] The rules forbade talking in the rooms and visiting between them, no doubt with the best of intentions, as the nurses certainly needed rest and patients were nursed in the adjoining ward. Permission to go out at night was reluctantly and infrequently given; one nurse who wanted to visit her parents was told by the matron: 'You may go this evening, but you must not make a practice of asking such things.'

As Rendle observed, '. . . a woman does not become a mere machine because she undertakes a vocation of nursing' and it was inevitable that probationers took matters into their own hands. Long before the move from Point Street to The Knowle, nurses made clandestine visits to the town at night. One nurse rationalised:

> . . . when we intended to go to certain entertainment we declined to ask the Matron's permission, because we knew that we should not get it, and as we were determined to go

[94] *Ibid.*, 30 July 1897.
[95] Ewers, *The Western Gateway*, p. 89.
[96] CSO File 2863/96; *Western Australian Government Gazette*, 27 August 1897.
[97] CSO File 2032/97.
[98] *Morning Herald*, 2 September 1897.

we should have had to commit a double fault—disregard of the rules and defiance of the matron's orders. We considered, therefore, that it was better to choose the lesser of the two evils, and consequently, when we wished to go out after duty was finished, we took French leave.[99]

One August evening in 1897, Bessie Steele realised that all was not as it should have been in the nurses' quarters and the following day summoned Nurses Fisher, Groves and Crudden to ask if they had attended a certain private party the night before. Not only did they admit that they had, but another two nurses volunteered that they too had made similar excursions. The outraged matron wrote to Hope in the rhetoric of the armed forces but with the expected humility of a woman and subordinate:

> I beg to report that three nurses in this Institution viz Fisher, Groves and Crudden have broken the rules by absenting themselves without leave until a late hour at night. It is not the first time that it has occurred but I was not made aware of the fact until this morning. I cannot tolerate such conduct amongst the nursing staff for one moment and therefore beg you to give this communication your earliest consideration. None of the three nurses have signed their two years agreement. I beg to remain,
>
> Yours obediently,
> B. M. Steele (Matron).[100]

The nurses were eager to retain their positions after the time already spent on minimal pay, so when Lovegrove conducted a searching inquiry into the 'irregularity' all admitted the impropriety of their conduct and apologised to the matron in Lovegrove's presence. The principal medical officer admonished that in future the nurses were to obey their matron in all respects, but in a private recommendation he suggested that the wooden partition between the nurses' room and the corridor be doubled, to muffle the sound of talk or laughter from the nurses' rooms. With relief, Acting Premier Wittenoom sighed to the under secretary: 'it seems to have been satisfactorily settled which leaves nothing further to be done.'[101]

There was no satisfaction for the nurses, however. The lack of instruction which prevented each from obtaining a nursing certificate angered them. Their accommodation and living quarters were insufferable, the deprivation of their liberty unjust, and they rankled under a system where 'the nurses were made to feel that they lived day and night under the immediate supervision and by the express permission of the Matron'.[102] The *Morning Herald* scented a story and in a page-and-a-half column exposed the nurses' situation. Rendle substantiated the claims and aired his past frustrations with the hospital but warned 'it is hardly fair, however, to blame the Matron entirely', as she was 'overworked and often hardly able to keep about, and consequently at times she seemed harsh and unreasonable to those whose duty it was to help her'.[103] The people of Fremantle united in support of their nurses and at a public meeting planned a deputation to the acting premier on their behalf.[104]

[99] *Ibid.*
[100] CSO File 2769/97, 21 August 1897.
[101] *Ibid.*, 13 September 1897.
[102] *Morning Herald*, 2 September 1897.
[103] *Ibid.*, 6 September 1897.
[104] *Ibid.*, 9 September 1897.

Rendle had gone to the press in an attempt to change the status quo. Following his lead, a deputation of nurses went to the champion of the people, young Frederick Charles Vosper, M.L.A., who represented North East Kalgoorlie and was the editor of the new *Sunday Times*.[105] While Vosper thought that his involvement in the affairs of a district already well represented in parliament was inappropriate, he did write to the acting premier about a number of the nurses concerns. Although the nurses had not been dismissed, the rigid control of the matron in 'an absolutely despotic position' demanded change, he urged. So did the system whereby salaries were paid directly into Dr Hope's private account for distribution to the staff, which gave rise to possible serious irregularities; already when Nurse McIlvaine had been ill and unable to work, her salary had been paid under her name to a substitute. Neither was the close confinement of nurses 'calculated to promote their good health or temper, or to improve their demeanour towards their superiors or their patients . . . The position appears to me to be a serious one,' Vosper concluded.[106]

Wittenoom hedged. His ill-health delayed the town's quickly organised deputation. It was an opportune time to press for changes at the hospital. Many of the town's citizens, including members of the legislature, town councillors, ministers of religion, doctors, and representatives of the Friendly Societies and Harbour and Railway Medical Aid Societies, were organised by the chemist Richard Birch into preparing a petition requesting the appointment of an honorary visiting staff to the hospital. Two hundred and thirty-eight petitioners signed. With his long interest in hospital concerns at Fremantle, Birch promised the government that 'should you decide . . . and desire my presence with the signed memorial, I will at once present it to you. Telephone number 570.'[107] The petitioners pointed out that with an increased number of patients following the expansion in population, it was impractical for one medical man to adequately serve the hospital. The Medical Department commented to itself that there was, after all, a resident medical officer there as well as Hope. The townspeople wanted to be able to go to a doctor for consultation and to have that same doctor treat them in the hospital if they had to be admitted, and they wanted the benefit of consultation in serious cases. Petitioners wanted instruction for the nursing staff so that probationers could obtain a trained nurse's certificate. Instruction by whom, mused the Medical Department. The signatories pointed out the benefits of an honorary visiting staff to doctors 'at present deprived of a large field for clinical investigation', and the department was moved to suggest that the doctors were perhaps the cause of the agitation for change. Petitioners also thought that the hospital would benefit financially through increased public interest and support if it was staffed by honoraries, but this notion was rejected by the authorities. Experience at Perth had proved otherwise: 'the Government find the money and the Board spend it—the intention of the Act is not fulfilled'.[108] The last request was for the appointment of a board of management at the hospital. On 7 October, Birch learned that the community's request had been granted and he

[105] For Vosper, see L. Hunt, *Westralian Portraits*, 1979, pp. 104–10; Stannage, *The People of Perth*, pp. 327–9.
[106] CSO File 2763/97. Text of Vosper's letter also in *Morning Herald*, 9 September 1897.
[107] CSO File 2763/97, 18 September 1897. See also *Morning Herald*, 8 October 1897.
[108] CSO File 2763/97.

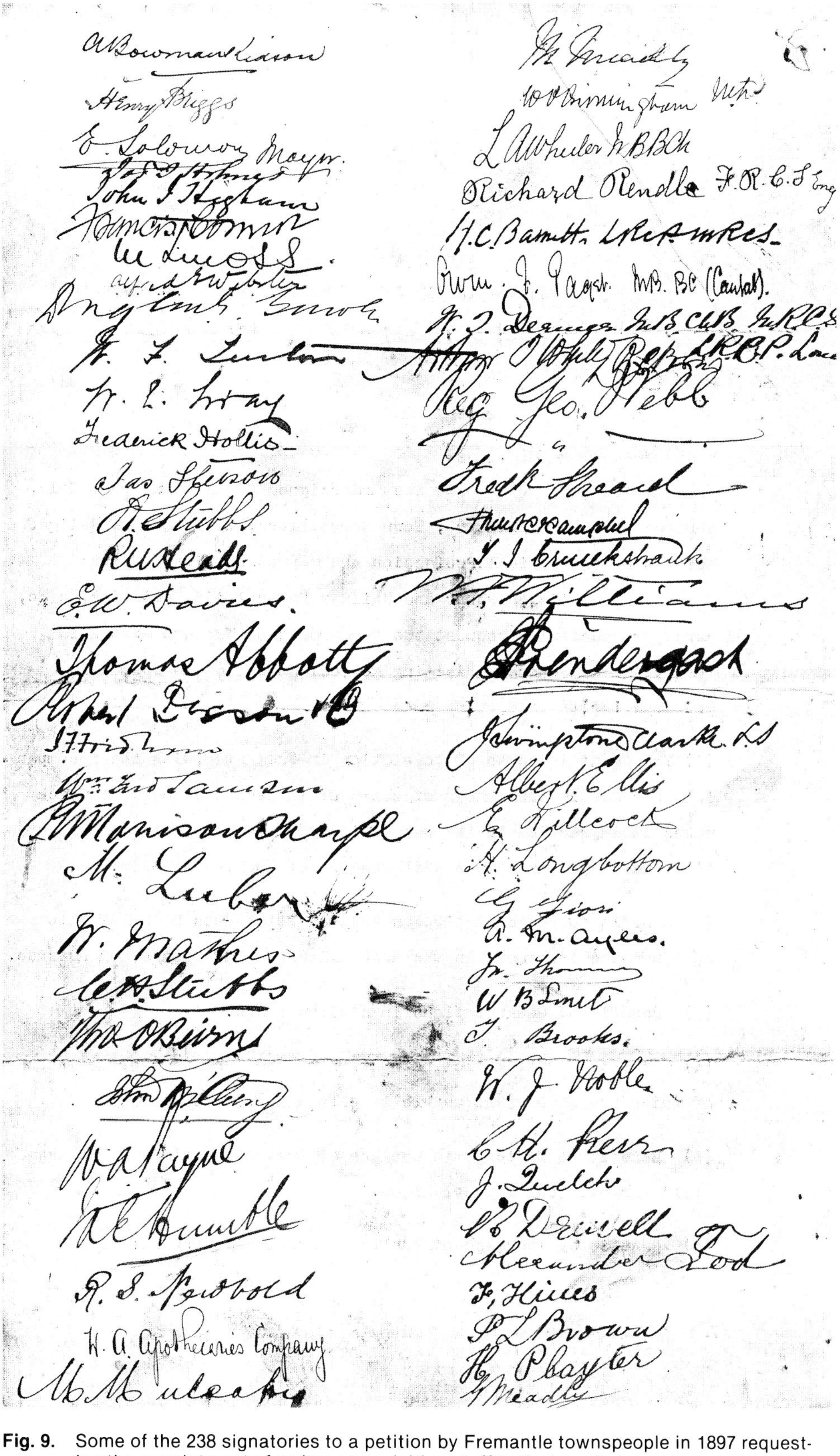

Fig. 9. Some of the 238 signatories to a petition by Fremantle townspeople in 1897 requesting the appointment of an honorary visiting staff to the hospital.

enthusiastically replied: 'your offer will be most gladly accepted, and be in accordance with the wishes of the requirements of the people of Fremantle'. In due course, on 27 October 1897, the hospital was proclaimed a public hospital under *The Hospitals Act* of 1894, the second hospital in the State to be granted such status.[109]

Hospital administration in Western Australia had been different from that in the British homeland and in America where voluntary hospitals had been set up in the eighteenth century by compassionate citizens to help the sick poor whose plight was largely overlooked by the government.[110] It was different from that in Melbourne and Adelaide where the states refused to accept responsibility for the hospitals, which were consequently organised through voluntary public subscription and managed by a committee of the city's worthy citizens.[111] Some subscribers to these hospitals were motivated by pure charity; others derived a certain satisfaction in the promise of eternal rewards and an enhanced temporal status, with their power to recommend a patient for admission to hospital. Under hospital systems in both Britain and the eastern states of Australia, doctors worked in an honorary capacity. From its beginnings, the Western Australian government, like that in colonial Sydney prior to 1840, took on the responsibility of treating the colony's paupers. In both states the initial 'isolation and grinding poverty' made this state involvement necessary.[112] But by 1894, in Western Australia social changes had occurred and administrative changes at Perth Hospital were needed. Under Forrest's prompting and guided by hospital legislation in South Australia and Queensland, *The Hospitals Act* of 1894 was passed in the September sitting of the Western Australian legislative assembly.[113]

Under this Act any hospital could be granted public status by the government. Under the Act a board of management of whom only one-third could be medical practitioners, was empowered to administer all funds and supervise and control staff appointments and discharges, and make hospital rules and regulations. Theirs was the responsibility for patients' moral and religious instruction and their 'discipline, decency and cleanliness'. But there was an optimistic base on which the Act rested. It was envisaged that support of the hospital would be through the voluntary contribution of 'benevolent persons' which would entitle contributors to elect one-third of the board when their combined contributions totalled one-sixth of the hospital's annual costs. Western Australian contributors were never so many or generous that this part of the Act was fulfilled, but many did earn the right to recommend a patient for admission, based on the individual value of their contribution. Most importantly, the regulation spelled out the nature of public hospitals as institutions

[109] *Western Australian Government Gazette*, 5 November 1897, pp. 2, 3, 4, 7.
[110] See B. Abel-Smith, *The Hospitals 1800–1948: A Study in Social Administration in England and Wales*, 1964; D. Rosner, *A Once Charitable Enterprise: Hospitals and Health Care in Brooklyn and New York, 1885–1915*, 1982.
[111] K. S. Inglis, *Hospital and Community: A History of The Royal Melbourne Hospital*, 1958, pp. 2–16; J. Uhl, *Mount Royal Hospital: A Social History*, 1981; A. Mitchell, *The Hospital South of the Yarra*; M. Barbalet, *The Adelaide Children's Hospital 1876–1976*, 1975.
[112] Bolton and Joske, in *History of Royal Perth Hospital*, pp. 2–3, point out the difference between Western Australian and overseas and interstate hospitals and government involvement in establishing the Colonial Hospital.
[113] Victoria Regina No. 20, An Act to provide for the Management of Public Hospitals. The Statutes of Western Australia, 1894. 8 November 1894, pp. 3–8.

Public Hospital at Fremantle.

'٭'٭' PROCLAMATION

Western Australia, } By His Excellency Lieut.-Colonel
to wit.   } Sir GERARD SMITH, Knight Com-
mander of the Most Distinguished
Order of Saint Michael and Saint
George, Governor and Commander-
in-Chief in and over the Colony
of Western Australia and its
Dependencies, &c., &c., &c.

WHEREAS under the provisions of "The
Hospitals Act, 1894" (58 Vict., No. 20), the
Governor, with the advice of the Executive Council,
may, from time to time, by Proclamation in the
Government Gazette, declare any place or places
deemed suitable, and provided for the purposes of an
hospital or institution for the cure of disease or for
the relief of diseased persons, to be a Public
Hospital: AND WHEREAS it is deemed expedient
that the Fremantle Government Hospital should be
proclaimed a Public Hospital: Now THEREFORE I,
the Governor of the said Colony, with the advice
aforesaid, do hereby, by this my Proclamation, declare the institution aforesaid to be a "Public
Hospital" within the meaning of "The Hospitals
Act, 1894;" with effect from

Given under my hand and the Public Seal of
the said Colony, at Perth this 27th day of
October, 1897.

By His Excellency's Command,

GOD SAVE THE QUEEN!!!

Fig. 10.   Proclamation for a public hospital at Fremantle, 27 October 1897.

for the needy. If a patient with means was admitted under a false statement of
poverty, he could be charged for his treatment and the debt recovered by law.

Against the background swell of agitation for responsible self-government for
Western Australia from 1890, Waylen's title as colonial surgeon was abolished and
the position changed to that of principal medical officer. Following Waylen, in 1896
the position was filled by Doctor Thomas Lovegrove, who served until 1908 and was
the government intermediary in the hospital's early years.

The first task following the decision to declare Fremantle Hospital a public one,
was to organize a Board of Management. Influential townspeople on the crest of the
hospital agitation wave suggested a list of suitable members including seven of the
town's doctors and eight of the town's respected men. These recommendations were
heeded, although under the terms of the Act, only one-third of the membership
could be medical. Drs Paget and Lotz were not included on the final list. Lotz, with
probably the largest medical practice in Fremantle and with considerable experience
in at least six different British hospitals, was very put out and surprised: '... there

must be some special reason or an oversight'.[114] It was an oversight—but the mistake was discovered too late to rectify. Other leading Fremantle citizens were no doubt disappointed at not receiving an invitation to board membership.

Apart from Drs Birmingham, Wheeler, White and Hope, the new board consisted of four politicians. First was Daniel Congdon, M.L.C., a successful business man who had married Resident Magistrate Fairbairn's sister. He had been Mayor of Fremantle and retired in 1894 to devote all his time to municipal and parliamentary matters. There was the tall Irishman, Frank Connor, M.L.A., a powerful pioneer in the Kimberley pastoral industry and who, in 1897, was chartering steamers to move cattle by the hundreds to the ready market at Kalgoorlie. The other politicians were solicitor Alfred B. Kitson, M.L.C., and John J. Higham, M.L.A., a genial and kindly cleric who had been a past councillor and Board of Health member at Fremantle. Of the others, Henry Briggs, who had a girth as wide as his popularity, was the able headmaster of the Fremantle Grammar School and was financially secure due to successful land speculation. There was W. T. John and stately James Lilly, J.P., wealthy from shipping and property ownership and renowned as a champion juggler of cusswords. These non-medical men of wealth, status and influence in both Fremantle and the wider business community were numbered among the social élite.[115]

The medical men appointed to the board were of the same social class. After the compulsory registration of medical practitioners from 1869, doctors came from families who were able to support and educate their sons for the period of their training. By the late 1880s, the status of doctors, with their specialised knowledge gained only through long training, was assured. As the *Evening Times* observed in 1888, 'the medical profession is perhaps, before all others, the most important and grave. Anything, therefore, which should take away from its dignity ought to be ostracized'.[116] Western Australia's first historian, W. B. Kimberley, wrote of Waylen that

> officially and unofficially he has well maintained the dignity of medical practitioners, and, moreover, has constantly sought to give a higher status to the profession.

He further declared:

> the profession [medical] must be safeguarded; it must have its special rules of etiquette, its limitations and status; no quacks must enter, and there must be articles of charter under which the practitioners are protected. To negotiate all this work, the pioneer doctors had to exercise caution and judgment. Their practice was an important part of their daily life, but beyond that, they acted as a parent protecting a family in their advocacy of the rights of the profession.[117]

---

[114] CSO File 2763/97, 3 November 1897.
[115] See appropriate references in W. B. Kimberley, *History of West Australia: A Narrative of her Past together with Biographies of her Leading Men*, 1897; *Dictionary of Western Australians 1829-1914*; Truthful Thomas, *Through the Spy-glass: Short Sketches of Well-Known Westralians As Other See Them*, 1905.
[116] *Evening Times*, 28 March 1888.
[117] Kimberly, *History of West Australia*, p. 62.

These Fremantle Hospital board members were leaders of public opinion, men of whom philanthropy for the deserving poor was expected; they represented general not political or factional interests. By the end of November they had voted James Lilly as their chairman and taken up the administration of the hospital with earnest enthusiasm.

During October, pressure on the nursing staff had eased due to staff changes. One of the probationers was replaced by another trained nurse 'to ensure proper supervision'. As a result, the board was free to direct its attention to other matters.[118] One of the first was the appointment of a secretary and dispenser to relieve the matron of the task and from 13 applicants, Mr Edwin J. Nicholson was selected.[119] His salary of £200 was the same as that received by the chief dispenser at Perth Public Hospital. Although he lived out and therefore had no living expenses deducted as the nursing staff did, his salary was £100 more than the matron received.

The year 1897 had been trying and frustrating for most of those connected with the hospital. Beautiful as a home, The Knowle proved difficult for the limited staff to work as a hospital and its accommodation proved hopelessly inadequate for the town's needs by its second month of operation. If various staff members were disillusioned, it was not surprising. But there were small triumphs. In August 1897, the dentist Walter B. Jackson, who had been three years in Fremantle, offered his services to Hope at the hospital. As Hope frequently had dental operations to perform the offer was gladly accepted.[120] The importance of the work of the honorary dental surgeon was soon recognised by the hospital board at Perth who recommended the appointment of an honorary dentist there.[121] Henry Calvert Barnett, who had fought against insanitary conditions and fought for hospital accommodation at the port for so many years, lived long enough to see part of his dream fulfilled. While in 1897 the town was still dotted with cesspits and offended with its evil-smelling drains, there was at least a proper hospital to which the sick and injured could be taken. He died in Fremantle early in November 1897.[122]

The start of the New Year under new hospital control augured well but in the first months of 1898 a decision made by the board caused more upheaval. During the previous year Perth Public Hospital had benefited from the administration of Matron Hannah Gordon and the experienced sisters who came with her from Adelaide. Since 1896 it had also conducted a two-year training course for nurses. Perhaps in its legitimate desire to upgrade the standard of nursing at Fremantle, perhaps because of residual difficulties between Bessie Steele and her staff, perhaps due to conflict between the new board flexing its administrative muscles and the experienced matron comfortably powerful and settled in her position of authority over her nurses, the board proposed on 4 March 1898 that 'in the opinion of this Board, the present state of the nursing administration of the hospital demands reorganization, and the Board being of the opinion that the services of a more experienced Matron be obtained, Miss Steele be requested to resign that position'.[123]

118 CSO File 3502/97, Lovegrove to Under Secretary, 15 November 1897.
119 CSO File 3945/97, 20 December 1897.
120 CSO File 3029/97, 19 August 1897.
121 CSO File 3347/97, 30 October 1897.
122 *West Australian*, 4 November 1897.
123 CSO File 625/98, 4 March 1897.

Protesting her dismissal to Premier John Forrest, Steele wrote that she had been engaged by the government and dismissed by a managing committee; that she had served one year and nine months under Hope and Lovegrove to 'their entire satisfaction' and that both thought the committee's decision 'unjust and harsh'; that she had received no notice or salary in lieu of notice, and that she demanded a government inquiry.[124] Bessie Steele was a capable woman and a fine nurse, but she was no match against the combined force of the hospital's managers acting under the legality of the 1894 Act. The board paid her to 28 February and on 18 March she left the hospital. By May no action had been taken by the government and Bessie applied to them for her March salary. Colonial Secretary Randell privately thought that she had been 'somewhat hardly dealt with by the Board' but that nothing further could be done. Her letters sparked a flicker of concern in government circles when it was thought that 'she will sue us if she can'.[125] The problem was referred to the crown solicitor who agreed that although the matron's dismissal was a hardship it was quite lawful, but that it was customary to give a month's notice and sometimes more except in cases of misconduct of a gross nature. Under firm government prompting the board reluctantly agreed to pay the ex-matron. The salary was not sent by post as Nicholson suggested. In early July with her professional standing in question, her future undecided and a feeling of injustice barely concealed, Bessie Steele had to walk through the wide front door of the hospital in which she had invested so much of her concern and labour and time to collect her salary for March. In her place the board appointed Miss Jessie Warden of the Ovens District Hospital, Beechworth, Victoria.[126] There was much work yet to be done by the new administrative brooms but the foundations for the new hospital had been firmly cemented through adversity and hope.

[124]   *Ibid.*, Bessie Steele to John Forrest, 12 April 1898.
[125]   *Ibid.*, Colonial Secretary G. Randell to Crown Solicitor, 2 June 1898.
[126]   CSO File 914/98.

*. . . an institution belonging to the people and for
the people . . .*
Evening Mail, 21 August 1909.

In the first decade and a half of the new century, when the rush for gold changed to
a hopeful saunter, Fremantle's phenomenal growth of the 1890s checked, reversed,
stabilised, then once more increased, but not rapidly. Not until 1913 did the population regain its 1900 total of 20,000.[1] The newly built banks, offices, warehouses,
shops and other businesses, which had almost exploded into being following the
rush for gold, gradually lost the sharp self-consciousness of newcomers and with the
help of the sand which still buffeted the town, took on the softened, comfortable
aspect of belonging. The modern hotels—the P.&O., the Orient, Esplanade, the
National and the Fremantle[2]—and the boarding houses which had been quickly
erected in response to the need for accommodation, continued with a somewhat
reduced turnover. Stalls at the Fremantle Markets, which from 1898 sold everything
from fruit and vegetables to bric-à-brac, were still popular with townspeople, but
many also went to shops in the town. Others preferred the convenience of buying
from pedlars.

> The milkman called and one left out a billy. The butcher called and cut your joint on
> the back of the cart. The rabbit man called and sold you rabbits, a shilling a pair,
> skinned while you waited. The grocer delivered, always with some sweets for the kids
> with the weekend order.[3]

Chinese market gardeners with buckets balanced on poles across hardened shoulders
sold their goods door-to-door and invariably gave an exotic little jar of Chinese
ginger as a present at Christmas,[4] especially after 1900, when the drop in population
increased the competition for customers.

During this period, provisions for the hospital were purchased and delivered
under contract from different firms or individuals in the town, and sometimes the
arrangements left much to be desired. As the person responsible for stores, matrons,
frustrated at the late delivery or inferior quality of perishable provisions, sometimes
aired their discontent in reports to the board.

[1] Reece and Pascoe, *A Place of Consequence*, p. 57.
[2] *Ibid.*, p. 53.
[3] G. Clarke, *West Australian*, 11 November 1980.
[4] Recollections of C. E. Lundgren, cited in *West Australian*, 16 January 1980.

I have a great difficulty in getting poultry of decent quality from either of the fish mongers; and suggest that I may be allowed to get them from any private persons from whom the quality will be assured at the ruling prices. Mr Priestly (the hospital secretary and dispenser) can let me have a few ducks at present at four shillings each with your approval[5]

urged Matron Cameron in 1910. The supply of fish was often unsatisfactory: 'I have frequently had to complain about the quality and time our fish comes and on Friday last it came at twelve o'clock and was of such inferior quality that it had to be returned and tinned fish substituted as it was then too late to get any more'.[6] Sacks of potatoes were sometimes 'unfit for use', boxes of butter had to be returned and purchased elsewhere, good eggs were hard to get in summer, and conflict with the butcher was continuous: 'the butcher has been causing trouble this week'; 'the butcher supplied a bad load of tripe on Saturday last and did not supply any on Monday'; 'the butcher still continues to arrive late and often without the proper order'; 'major portion of meat supplied very bad quality for some weeks. Some totally unfit for human consumption.'[7] Storage facilities at the hospital were completely inadequate and one matron requested the purchase of proper lead-lined bins for stores, and '. . . that a cooler be made to store butter as it is close to the kitchen and as the weather gets warm it is very soft and a cooler would not cost much'.[8]

While some townspeople found entertainment browsing in shops, others, including league footballers, sported on the oval, often finding unwelcome evidence of the sheep which were used to crop the grass.[9] Some raced a bicycle around the cycle track at the oval's perimeter. More cheered their favourite teams to victory and wagered illegally on the outcome. Fremantle was a working-man's town and justly proud of its footballers, most of whom were wharfies who lugged bags of wheat and wheeled laden barrows on Saturday mornings before big games.[10] Men who daily balanced heavy loads on the backs of their necks and lumped them into ships holds were usually large in build and formidable opponents on the field. To the legions who supported them, the South Fremantle players often assumed the status of giants. Casualties from the game were inevitable but it was only a matter of minutes from the oval to the hospital casualty ward next door.

Occasionally sportsmen of another social class were injured, but they were treated at home. Cricketers and tennis players were rarely of the working class and they lived on Monument Hill and at Richmond Hill with views over the Swan, or in new houses on the northern side of Canning Road and around and along Preston Point Road. They played lawn bowls and croquet and the more athletically inclined were invited on hunts for kangaroo or to polo games. Fremantle's doctors were numbered among the town's élite and shared such activities. Doctor Owen Paget was known as

---

[5] Matron's Report Book, 25 January 1910.

[6] *Ibid.*, 6 September 1910.

[7] *Ibid.*, 8 and 22 February 1910, 3 May 1910, 28 June 1910, 28 March 1911, 18 July 1911.

[8] *Ibid.*, 5 October 1909, 29 March 1910 (lead-lined bins). In 1909 the government decided not to order stores from Chinese or Asiatics. In country areas this meant scarcity and high prices. See Public Health Dept File 1111/09, BL.

[9] Minutes of FMC, 27 October 1899. Council agreed to Councillor John's suggestion to graze out two or three hundred sheep on the oval to eat down the grass.

[10] F. W. Harrison, *Daily News*, 30 March 1978.

'Ah Good' due to his constant cry of approval at commendable play by his team at polo. His reckless rides on 'diminutive ponies with his legs nearly touching the ground' also earned him a certain notoriety. After one fall with his pony into an old saw pit 'it took a good part of the hunt to get him out full of prickles but none the worse'.[11] John M. Holmes was a surgeon from Fremantle Hospital taken by Lucius Manning, a member of one of Fremantle's oldest and respected families, on a different hunt.

> I took him wild horse hunting up Yanchep way, a rough game with hard living and hard long gallops over rough country to end with the throwing and roping of the brumby. He never complained about the conditions ... of the mosquitoes eating him at night and the sun burning his fair skin all day and the constant torment of bush flies, but he stuck it out for the ten days without a single complaint.[12]

Among the other doctors, Arthur White was also a keen horseman. It was a skill born of necessity, as most Fremantle roads were mere sand tracks and only passable by riding, and '... everyone rode that was able—the butcher, baker, doctors'.[13] Some, like Dr Hope, drove a sulky and bought their horse from the Mannings at Davilak, the principal horse-breeding establishment near Fremantle. Dr Thomas Anderson rode a bicycle, then graduated to a sulky driven by a coachman, before getting an Oldsmobile in 1905 in which to visit his patients.[14]

Perhaps the greatest impetus for change by the late 1890s was the opening of Charles Yelverton O'Connor's new deep-water harbour at the mouth of the river. The treacherous bar across the river mouth was blasted and the basin dredged, while two long, welcoming, stone moles, named by their geographic placement north and south, assured safe harbour to shipping from 1897. Four years later the massive coal-fired Royal Mail steamers from England joined vessels from other parts of the world and the eastern states in linking Fremantle on the 'highway of commerce and civilization from the Old World to the New'.[15] By 1910 only a small stand of masts and spars swung at harbour wharves where once there had been a thicket, testifying to the passing of an era.

Sailors from ships and lumpers from wharves still came to the hospital for medical treatment, and early in the century railway employees came too. Like police, the latter were entitled to free medical attention by the government medical officer for accidental injuries not contributed to by negligence in the course of their work. But they still had to pay maintenance if admitted to a ward. Barnett had a list of 108 railway employees who were entitled to treatment in 1888. In 1899 he was burdened with nearly 300.[16] By the turn of the century the railway workshops behind Victoria Quay were finally transferred to Midland Junction and the town lost hundreds of its families when they moved to new areas closer to Midland. On the tracks at Fre-

---

[11] Notes by Lucius Manning. Used by permission of Mrs J. H. Stubbe. For biographical information on Manning, see *West Australian*, 3 December 1975.

[12] *Ibid.*

[13] *Ibid.*

[14] C. W. Anderson, interviewed by M. Adams, June 1981—September 1983. O.H. 480, BL.

[15] Sir John Forrest at a postal conference 1895, cited in Ewers, *The Western Gateway*, p. 97.

[16] PHD File 310/99.

mantle, injuries still occurred and in the three years ending 31 December 1909, 13 railway workers from Fremantle or North Fremantle received work-related injuries and were taken to hospital.[17] Many of the railway workers who did not transfer to Midland became some of approximately 400 employees of the W.A. Fremantle Smelting Company Limited, situated south of South Beach between 1898 and 1920, working in a constant cycle of employment and unemployment as the company either shut down or worked full blast. Both working and living conditions for these men and their families were often deplorable. Those who lived in white-washed hessian huts were more comfortable than workers living in 'hotter than hell' corrugated-iron humpies in summer; others who camped in tents on the sand dunes, digging wells for water or getting it from the 'Works', shivered in winter.[18] Poverty, drink and an eight-hour shift seven days a week was an explosive combination and smelters often woke in hospital after evening fights. Workers on the roasting floors, or those near the furnace, sometimes suffered vomiting, sleeplessness, colic or anaemia from the poisonous sulphur fumes and had to be hospitalised. Many of the men paid a voluntary weekly subscription to insure themselves—a wise move considering that in 1904 Dr John Hicks alone was seeing between ten and 12 such patients, with as many as three new cases a day.[19] Accidents at building sites were still common. Often a victim of a street bashing was treated at the hospital. One youth brought to the casualty ward in 1903 required stitches after being attacked by 'three foreigners', one of whom slashed him with a razor.[20]

The wharves continued as the hub of activity in Fremantle. Silos were built to help move grain which poured from the south-west through the port, and livestock, timber, gold, manufactured goods, and even the paraphernalia of circuses was moved over the wharves. It seemed, as one old timer recalled, 'everything had to come into the wharf ... it didn't matter what it was, it had to come in from the wharf'.[21] Men too went over the wharves—to the Boer War and then the First World War. Alongside ships, horse-drawn lorries jostled to unload cargoes and the air was '... full of coal and sulphur dust then ... you couldn't walk along the wharf without tripping over big piles of cargo laying about'.[22] Seamen from the Orient, from India and many other parts of the world, could be seen cutting each other's hair and washing their clothes near their vessels, while Aborigines often sat and talked around the jetty at the end of Suffolk Street.[23] Some in the town eagerly scanned the horizon for the tell-tale smudge of smoke from steamers so that the ball on the flagstaff at the top of the hill near the Round House could be put up; as ships berthed, some opened a purse in anticipation of sales to be made, others groaned, knowing that departing ships would stock up on the town's fresh produce. 'There was not enough milk to meet demands. Whenever a ship came to port it would stock up on the milk, not leaving much for the people,' recalled one resident.[24]

17 A.N.347/1, Acc. No. 855, No. 44, 1910, BL.
18 S. Jones, Notes on Fremantle Smelting Works, Fremantle City Library, Ref. 128.3.
19 *WAVP*, Vol. 1, 2nd Session of 5th Parliament, 1905, pp. 496–8.
20 *West Australian*, 2 February 1903.
21 E. Ulrich, interviewed by Margaret Howroyd, 24 February 1984, FCL.
22 F. Harrison, interviewed by M. Howroyd, 8 February 1984, FCL.
23 W. E. Wray, interviewed by M. Howroyd, 9, 10 May 1984, FCL.
24 H. Wilkinson, interviewed by M. Scott and K. MacGill, April 1976, FCL.

Between 1897 and 1920 the experiences of Fremantle children varied. Many fished, crabbed with chaff bags, or helped around the house. Most swam and went to school. Some teased each other and the Chinese vegetable pedlar by turning his horse in the shaft. A few wagged school and all played the games of childhood—ball against the wall, hopscotch, marbles, kick the tin. Hoops were enjoyed and so were cubby houses. Some boys fought in gangs or threw sand under the lift-up flaps of pan lavatories when girls were inside. The police sergeant dispensed discipline—'a hit over the head, a boot in the tail and an order to go home and behave'.[25] At lunch time some boys went to the docks to sing or dance and play the mouth organ, for which lumpers sometimes threw them pennies. Other children were under greater constraint, especially girls. At St Joseph's Convent in 1908 'even when you had a bath, you had to put a garment on, even although you were in the bathroom on your own'.[26] Others endured social afternoons, when mothers exchanged calling cards and visits. Childhood accidents were common at home and school. The game of tip cat, in which a sharpened stick was hit into the air with a larger length, could cause a head injury, but other accidents 'just happened'. One child recalled:

> One dinner hour I was standing at the big door, which is still there I fancy at the Fremantle Boys' School, with my two fingers in the jamb of the door. The wind came and slammed the door and I was rushed off to the Fremantle Hospital and had stitches . . .[27]

Another child was exploring some houses under construction in Attfield Street:

> We climbed up a ladder onto the roof, and I decided to jump down. It was higher than I thought and I passed out after I landed. When my mother found out, I was taken to the doctor. Doctor Davy painted me all over with tincture of iodine (as they were want to do then) and I was told to rest in bed. I had been such a tomboy, and this seemed a terrible fate to me. As I didn't improve, the doctor decided to try to make a plaster of Paris jacket for me. It was in the middle of summer and I had to keep it on for five months. I had to lie on a firm cane lounge. Every Sunday, my father would lift me onto a table with my hair over the edge, and he would brush out all the knots.[28]

Women still dosed and nursed their families to cure or prevent illness. A linseed or mustard poultice could be made for 'a bad chest' and Bates' salve was a popular treatment for cuts and wounds. Senna tea on Sundays was often a standard family routine, while castor oil was administered to others. Sulphur and treacle were taken orally at every change of the season by the McGuffies and rhubarb was given to purify the blood.[29] At least one mother gave her family garlic and lemon juice to ward off bubonic plague. Some took asparagus to soothe an irritable heart. Others believed that a small piece of licorice slowly sucked would coat the stomach to treat dyspepsia and that home-made charcoal would absorb internal gases and give the sufferer relief. A cold in the head could be treated by sniffing fine castor sugar like

[25] L. Thomas, interviewed by M. Davis, 25 May 1984; E. McGuffie, interviewed by A. Reid, 8 September 1983, FCL.
[26] Ulrich, interview, FCL.
[27] M. Mundy, interviewed by L. Stevens, 12 September 1979, FCL.
[28] Wilkinson, interview, FCL.
[29] McGuffie, interview. See also Thomas, interview, FCL.

snuff, to dry the secretions and protect mucous membranes.[30] Among remedies from the chemist, Chamberlain's stomach and liver tablets could be bought, while Robur tea from the grocer promised to 'stimulate and yet soothe'. Men suffering debility and 'diseases of a special nature' resulting from indiscretions, overwork or other causes, could send for a free trial sample from the Boston Herbal Institute, sent from Perth in a plain paper wrapping.[31]

Fremantle spread geographically with the population increase of the 1890s. The élite gravitated to the north while workers generally lived in the south and to the east past Plympton. By 1895 North Fremantle was a municipality. East Fremantle followed in 1897, while the Melville Road Board was established in 1900. By the end of World War I, the Fremantle area had encroached two miles to the north, east and south, dimensions it retained right until the 1950s.[32] But 'South Fremantle was always the honest to goodness working men's place'.[33] From 1900 onward transport influenced this growth. At first horses continued as the principal means, with horse-drawn wool lorries rumbling along the streets beside horse-drawn buses, sulkies and individual riders. Railway travellers still passed hoardings near the station advertising Dingo flour, Pelaco shirts and Bushell's tea. By 1910 there were some bicycles and T-model Fords, 'but in those days ... with all the horses about it wasn't a matter of accidents with cars, it was whether a [rearing] horse was going to put his ... front feet through the top of the car ...[34] In 1905 two great innovations—electricity and trams—came to Fremantle through the Fremantle Tramways and Electrical Lighting Board owned by the Fremantle and East Fremantle councils. At first it seemed that the trams affected more people than electricity. Lines flashed out southwards from Fremantle down South Terrace, past popular South Beach to Douro Road; they stretched south-east to the new suburb of Beaconsfield; reached north-east along Marmion Street to Duke Street, North Palmyra, and were laid further north along Canning Road. In time, new lines extended along Fremantle Road and out to Point Walter and to Stock Road. It was a cheap, popular, and effective means of moving people, and even cheaper for the young boys who rode 'willy on the back of the trams' with head ducked below windows so that the conductor would not see them.[35]

Patients were brought to the hospital by cart or car and some arrived on foot. A North Fremantle resident remembered that early in the century people

> ... never had motor vehicles to convey patients to the Fremantle Hospital ... they only had—what do you call them—barrows like, you know, they pushed them away to the hospital and it had handles on with a canvas top on it and they used to push them from North Fremantle, walk on foot to the Fremantle Hospital ... I remember them going to one lady's place, a Mrs Tryson, and seeing her taken away.[36]

[30] *Morning Herald*, 14 November 1903.
[31] *Ibid.*, 23 October 1903.
[32] Ewers, *But Westward Look*, p. 101; Reece and Pascoe, *A Place of Consequence*, pp. 57–60.
[33] A. Parry, interviewed by L. Lauder and J. Brodsgaard, 5 February 1975, FCL.
[34] *Ibid.*
[35] F. Manns, interviewed by M. Howroyd, 9 December 1983, FCL. For tram routes, see Reece and Pascoe, *A Place of Consequence*, pp. 70–1.
[36] A. Williams, interviewed by M. Howroyd, 25 October 1983, FCL.

Due to the need for a better conveyance to take injured workers from the wharves to hospital, Frank Rowe, the Fremantle Lumpers' Union Secretary, organised the first ambulance van for the district in 1908. The well-sprung, especially designed horse-drawn cart could take three stretchers at once and was a great advance on the wheeled litter. In 1922 a new Ford motor ambulance improved the journey for Fremantle's injured. An applicant for a licence to drive a motor car had to be 18 and able to read a number plate from 25 feet. A policeman might instruct: 'drive it [car] down to the corner and I'll stand here and watch'. It was just as well that licences were easy to get. The town ambulance was kept in Bluett's livery stable and in an emergency 'anyone drove that was handy'.[37]

Industries expanded slowly. A foundry and a workshop for railway and harbour needs were set up by the Department of Public Works. It seemed to some that William Pearse's Tannery and Boot and Shoe Factory at North Fremantle employed everyone in the town at one time or another from 1895, and many worked at The W.A. Brush Factory at the corner of Drake and George Streets. There was work at William Mills' Biscuit and Cake Bakery from 1898. The tin shed bakery on South Terrace was impossibly hot in summer through sun and the heat from the ovens, but in heavy winter rain, floors flooded and workers, paddling around ankle-deep, had to find bricks to stand on to lift themselves out of the water.[38] William Watson expanded his stores into a thriving smallgoods factory with a piggery at Spearwood, and Charles Allen operated a cordial factory. The area where water and rail transport intersected was a fine place to conduct a business. Industrial accidents were not uncommon. One day at Pearse brothers' shoe factory, Clara Crowther absent-mindedly lent down on the 'little wheel side' instead of the 'safe side' of a machine, and her hair was whipped up into the unshielded belt. After that the girls had to wear mob-caps for safety. At another time the hot needle penetrated a girl's finger. Doctors operated successfully but it was found that the bone had been split and cracked.[39]

When they were not working, there was much to do in Fremantle and the hospital's off-duty nurses and other townspeople could enjoy open-air concerts or music hall shows. They marvelled at the new silent pictures and crowded into Vic's Pictures at the Town Hall to cheer and encourage their heroes: 'Look out, he's behind the door!' Later, at the Palladium, where children paid 'thruppence' to get in, the aisle seats were preferred because it 'was so darn hot with hundreds of kids jumping around like crazy'. Then the ushers would come by with big sprays of perfume and those in the aisles were covered with the cool freshness.[40] Full-length feature films at the Princess Theatre usually ran on six reels and the projectionist in his little sweat box was hard-pressed to maintain the continuity quickly enough for patrons. A reel placed on backwards or upside down was greeted with a slow hand-

[37] S. Gore, interviewed by G. Fowler, 3 October 1980, FCL. For ambulance, see *Fremantle Gazette*, 16 December 1977. Notes by S. Jones at FCL. Acc. No. 362.18. The ambulance service was run by volunteers between 1908 and 1929, after which the St John Ambulance Association took over.
[38] F. Thacker, interviewed by M. Howroyd, 22 November, 13 December 1983, FCL. For industrial development, see Reece and Pascoe, *A Place of Consequence*, pp. 55-8.
[39] C. Crowther, interviewed by M. Howroyd, 28 October 1983, FCL.
[40] A. Healy, interviewed by G. Fowler, 12 March 1983, FCL.

clap, and the 'One moment please' sign would be flashed on to the screen while the film was slid on correctly. Other signs requested 'Will ladies please remove their hats', 'We like dogs but not inside' or 'No smoking'.[41] Music teachers and music halls alike shared a lack of patronage as a result of the popular new entertainment.

Between 1897 and 1920 Fremantle was a small, bustling town with a very busy port. It was an intimate place where most settled residents knew each other by sight and usually by name. Twice during this period, townspeople saw their countrymen go to war and rejoiced with those who returned. These were particular periods when human life and health were thought about more than usual by the general population. High on the hill at Fremantle Hospital, however, life and death were constant concerns, both to those who sought help there and to those who attended them.

In its first eight months of office between November 1897 and July 1898 the board of Fremantle Hospital set to work with enthusiasm. Necessary guiding rules and regulations for the administration of the hospital were drafted, an office was arranged for the new secretary and dispenser, E. J. Nicholson, linoleum was laid down in the main corridors, and general furniture and equipment fitted. Surgeons were pleased when required instruments were obtained for the theatre. For the first time, fire-extinguishing appliances were fixed, a move which showed wisdom where open fires heated wards and sitting rooms, and fuel stoves and boilers cooked and heated water.

Admission to the hospital, unless due to accident or emergency, was through the recommendation of a doctor, a board member or a subscriber to the hospital. Those who paid £1 annually could recommend one in-door patient, for £5—three patients a year—and subscribers paying £10 a year could always have one of their recommended patients in the hospital. The really hard-up signed a declaration of their poverty and were not charged for treatment, but those able to pay were charged three shillings a day maintenance. It was a system which fostered and reinforced class distinction. Nonetheless there was no lack of patients. In the first six months, 432 were admitted to the hospital, 160 of whom had typhoid fever. In 12 months the number of admissions totalled 765 and the 68 beds were nearly always in use. Indeed when summer and typhoid came with vengeance in January, patients had to be turned away. The board visited the acting premier with a request for increased accommodation and The Knowle's first extension, a temporary, rectangular, galvanized-iron ward for 22 patients, was built from second-hand iron salvaged from Kalgoorlie.

Because of the increase in patients and the limited accommodation for nurses, a new nursing home was the next priority. But if their accommodation was inadequate at least the nurses under hospital board management and Matron Jessie Warden received training recognised outside the hospital. Each was engaged under legal agreement for a term of three years and following a successful pass in examinations would receive a certificate of competency.[42]

The board's enthusiasm for the local hospital was infectious and its members were conscious of their financial responsibilities under the Act of 1894. The people of Fremantle responded to encouragement to raise funds: over £80 came through con-

[41]   Gore, interview, FCL; Healey, interview, FCL.
[42]   Fremantle Hospital Annual Report, 1898, *WAVP*, Vol. 2, 1898.

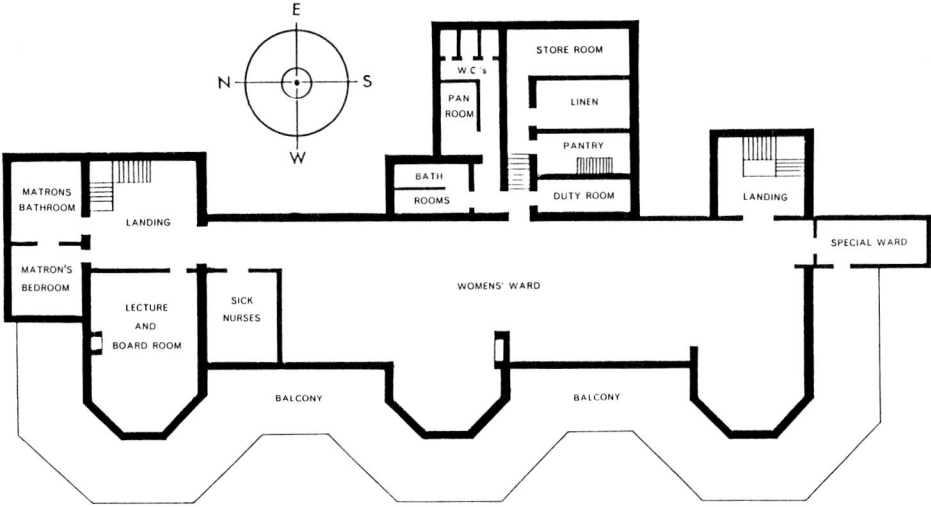

Fig. 11.   Map of Fremantle Public Hospital 1919—first floor of main building.

certs organized by the Fire Brigade, the Apollo Club and the Old English Fayre of Fremantle. Revenue from the Reverend Boas' lecture, invested since 1892, added another £24 and a cricket match between lawyers and doctors netted £4.14.1. Through some giving halfpennies and others pounds, the grand sum of £652.7.1 was raised in a hospital Saturday and Sunday appeal at the end of May. The board felt well-pleased with its efforts.[43]

In its second year of operation between mid-1898 and 1899, successful board management continued. There was a slight drop in admissions to the hospital, but the number of out-patients more than doubled in 12 months from 250 to 673. The total treated for typhoid was almost maintained at 157. Three people had measles, one scarlet fever, 13 were admitted with influenza and one patient was diagnosed as having whooping cough, while six suffered dysentery and 23 had venereal diseases. There was one hydatids case, 29 of rheumatism, 16 patients with cancer and 21 with phthisis or T.B. In a far cry from earlier years, only four patients had scurvy and five ophthalmia, but 20 were admitted due to the effects of alcohol. Perhaps the patient suffering opium or morphia poisoning was one of the local Chinese market gardeners. The soft glow of their pipes could be seen by those passing their houses at night. Only 68 of the total 661 patients were accident cases. Of these, 50 were treated for fractures or contusions, eleven for burns and seven for sunstroke. Two of three attempted suicide cases were saved. Just one patient was admitted suffering the effects of an abortion or miscarriage. Of 64 deaths, at least ten were admitted 'in a dying condition'. Doctors operated 51 times and only in seven cases were they unsuccessful.[44]

[43] *Ibid.*
[44] Fremantle Hospital Annual Report, 1899, *WAVP*, Vol. 2, 1899.

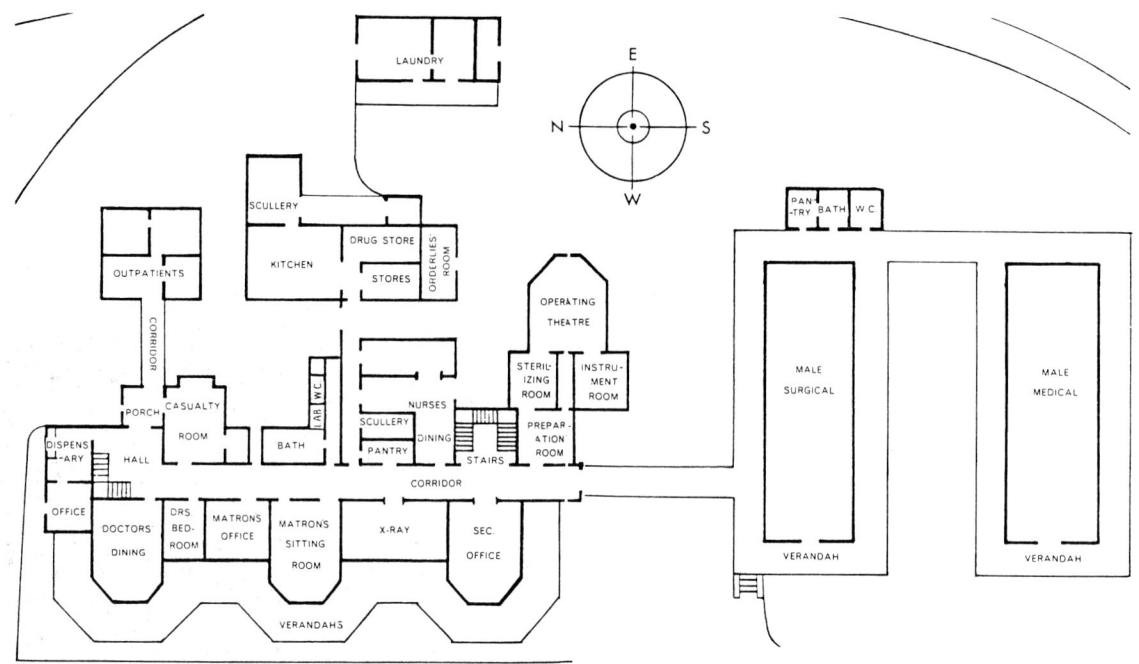

Plan courtesy Dr J. Stubbe

Fig. 12.   Map of Fremantle Public Hospital 1919—ground floor of main block.

The board was satisfied with its financial achievements between 1898 and 1899. 'By careful and systematic management' it saved over £700 of the government's £6,000 allotment to the hospital. In addition, patient fees totalled £112.4.3. and donations from the community totalled over £1,015. The new rectangular brick nurses' home built to the west of The Knowle, with seven double and five single bedrooms, a large sitting room, two bathrooms and a nine-feet-wide verandah all round, was—the board pointed out—'a monument of the generosity and support given to the hospital by the people of Fremantle' who had met the cost of over £1,000.[45] The interior of the hospital was completely renovated, the exterior land-scaped and an asphalt tennis court laid down for the resident medical and nursing staffs. It seemed that the only thing the hospital lacked was a pathological and bacteriological laboratory to bring it up to the 'most modern standard'.

Building at the hospital continued between mid-1899 and 1900. A porter's lodge was erected at the main Alma Street entrance to aid directly in the registration of patients and the indirect regulation of nurses' movements outside the hospital at night, and to the delight of Anderson and the honoraries, a pathological and bacteriological laboratory was fitted up for an outlay of £70. The board's previous year's parsimony was rewarded by a reduction of £1,000 in the government subsidy, and had it not been for the patients' contributions of just over £200, the hospital

[45] *Ibid.*

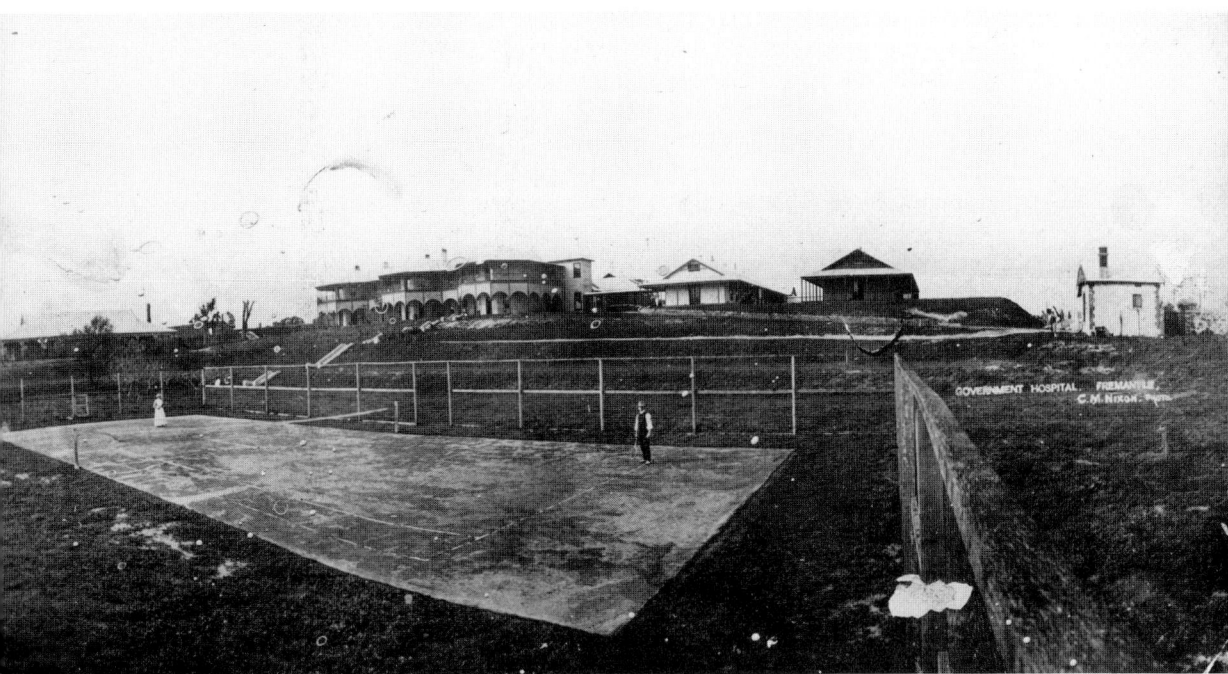

Photograph courtesy Fremantle Hospital

Plate 8. Fremantle Hospital at the turn of the century, looking east.

Buildings *(left to right)*: nurses' quarters, The Knowle, the laundry, two new wards and the Lodge.

> ... In the early days of the hospital, there was not any overall planning done at all. There was one honorary doctor who called it 'the hospital bitses' because there was just little bits added here and there.
>
> Matron Olive Jones

would not have had sufficient funds to cover its costs. This was the first year in which the board was really confronted with the problem of finances. It would be an ongoing battle of victories and defeats fought by many successive boards. Each carried a vision of high but costly standards of patient care but was bound by the necessity for immediate repairs and improvements. Between 1899 and 1900 the board also faced the problem of collecting outstanding patient fees, which by mid-1900 totalled over £1,900. The townspeople's new enthusiasm for practical support slowed, and the community raised only £645; this the board earmarked for an infectious diseases ward. Anxious to share the benefits of Rontgen's 1895 discovery of X-ray examination and no doubt because Perth Public Hospital had the facility, which constantly proved its worth, the board ordered a plant and some new surgical instruments and appliances for the hospital. Reluctantly the purchase of the X-ray equipment had to be deferred. In this year also, talk of their attraction to each other was confirmed when Anderson, the resident medical officer, courted and married

Matron Warden and set up in private practice. Their positions were taken by Patrick O'Meara and Alice Dixon respectively.[46]

The board was content with its administration and achievements on behalf of the hospital at the turn of the century. By mid-1901 an infectious diseases ward for eight patients had been built by the hospital, and an inebriates' ward for two patients was constructed by the government. Now infectious patients could be separated from the others, although the 65 typhoid cases during the year were still nursed in the wards. Sixteen inebriate patients were admitted that year. Men with reason dissolved in alcohol often disturbed the whole hospital with cowering, cursing and screaming and attacked staff and ward mates alike. Nurses were still responsible for the treatment of these men in the locked cells but the separate, secure rooms made it a little easier. Due to an order of the central Board of Health the mortuary attached to the hospital had to be destroyed and although the hospital was expected to use the public mortuary (and a gateway leading from the hospital to the 'morgue' and an ambulance trolley to run the bodies there were planned), the board protested and requested 'a small mortuary in a convenient position in the hospital grounds'. The government eventually agreed. A roadway from the front entrance gates to the hospital doors was laid, and an incinerator which had to be levelled to build the infectious diseases ward was re-erected further north. Public subscriptions dropped a little and 'maintenance fees outstanding' increased, but all in all it was good year for the board who spoke of a new operating theatre in their plans for the future.[47]

Their fourth year was yet another successful one and with confidence the board decided to demolish some old, unused cottages in the hospital grounds to make room for a new operating theatre. There was an increase of ward inpatients from 587 to 711, and of outpatients from 850 to 907, and although the public donated only £173 there was a slight increase in maintenance fees. The small laundry which, when all the beds were occupied, had to cope with the washing and drying for 75 patients, had to be replaced in 1902. As usual the board was thankful for the gratuitous service of the honorary medical staff on whose service the hospital depended.

Fremantle's town doctors were a close professional and social group in 1897. The private practitioners William Dermer, James Hope, William Birmingham, Arthur White, Owen Paget and the brilliant Henry Lotz, were joined by Richard Rendle and later by the erudite Thomas Davy, who joined the honorary staff of the hospital in 1898. The doctors met fortnightly at each other's houses and Dr Sidney Montgomery, the superintendent at the lunatic asylum, remarked that 'he had never before come across such an amicable number of doctors'.[48] While the core of honorary doctors practising in Fremantle changed little, the resident medical officers' tenure at the hospital was usually brief. Thomas Anderson, who was as good with a cricket bat as with his scalpel, joined the group when Rendle left in 1897 and, when he went into private practice in 1900, Patrick O'Meara filled the vacant position until November. In this month A. F. Deravin arrived at the hospital and served there before taking a well-earned holiday in September 1903. Meanwhile, Dr John Theodore Anderson had arrived as head of the lunatic asylum. Some of the doctors were

[46]   Third Annual Report of the Fremantle Public Hospital, 30 June 1900, WAVP, Vol. 2, no. 25, 1900.
[47]   Fremantle Public Hospital Annual Report, 1902, WAVP, Vol. 3, 1902.
[48]   Cited in Cohen, A History of Medicine, p. 110.

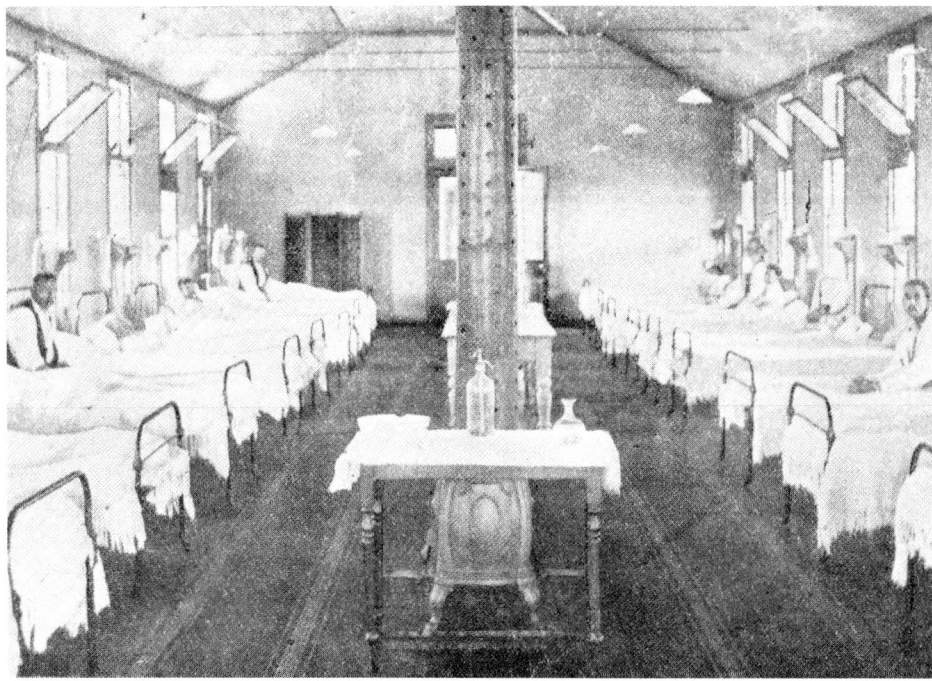

Photograph Courtesy the *Western Mail*

Plate 9.   The medical ward, Fremantle Hospital, 1908.

among the first to benefit as drivers of new motor vehicles, which didn't have to be caught and harnessed before setting out on a round or for an emergency call. Birmingham set the trend. Tom Anderson followed with a tiller-steered Oldsmobile and Thomas Davy, who never quite got the hang of the mechanical beast, carved out an almost legendary motoring career that included accidentally knocking a man down and, while attempting to pick him up to render first aid, running over him again.[49] Hope and White had already forged a medical partnership and it was not surprising when young Dr Alfred Martin arrived in Fremantle in July with a string of honours, credits and prizes from Cambridge University and St Thomas' Hospital, London, to his name, that he joined the esteemed and established Henry Lotz in his practice. Like Davy, Lotz was a skilled linguist and also invested heavily in surgical instruments which he reputably used efficiently, if deliberately, in his thoroughness. Such was his knowledge of anatomy that 'he didn't cut vessels and then suture them. He stopped short of cutting vessels.'[50] The first Board of Management to the hospital had a heavy medical bias with the appointment of Drs Hope, White, Wheeler and Birmingham.[51]

[49]   For an account of Davy's activities, see *Sunday Times*, 7 June 1908, reproduced as Appendix 2.
[50]   R. Barrington Knight, interviewed by C. Jeffery, 10 December 1986, FH.
[51]   *Government Gazette*, 12 November 1897, p. 2426.

Board membership continually changed over the years as some members resigned, others were not reappointed, or occasionally died in harness. The first to leave was Francis Connor, M.L.A., who found after some months that the time required for hospital affairs was too great in his busy schedule. He submitted his resignation to the hospital board in 1898, and the government encouraged the board to nominate a replacement. Three Fremantle 'Gentlemen' were suggested, but the minister asked for a single recommendation for the position. T. Smith was named by the hospital board and gazetted by the government on 10 June 1898.[52] Membership on the board was not taken lightly. There were government funds to administer and account for, and decisions to be made which would affect staff and patients in both the present and the future. Each board member was an influential man of superior status in the community and often joined with others in works of charity which were expected of one in his position. Board membership also conferred a certain power, and different interest groups were not slow to apply to the hospital for appointment. In 1898 T. Smith was nominated for consideration as a board member by the Sons of Temperance Society, G. Willis by the Protestant Alliance Society and W. E. Wray by the New Swan Lodge.

In 1899 Dr Louis Wheeler returned to England for a visit but decided to stay. When the board heard this, it requested the cancellation of his appointment as a board member and respectfully nominated Dr Lotz in his place. Lotz was pleased at the honour belatedly bestowed, and gratified when the government agreed to the board's nomination. Annual re-appointment to the board was not automatic and in 1899 Hospital Secretary Nicholson gently nudged the government on its tardiness in announcing the appointments for the year. A year later, when Chairman Lilly was asking about annual appointments, the government requested a list of attendances at meetings which was taken into consideration in 1901. The newly-introduced condition that three consecutive absences at meetings without permission would result in forfeiture of a seat was probably aimed at J. J. Higham, who had attended only one of the 12 monthly board meetings. In 1901, Elias Solomon resigned and a citizen named D. J. Doherty wrote to the colonial secretary suggesting the appointment of Captain Laurie, M.L.C., as he was 'a thoroughly representative man'. The government consulted the board, but as it preferred A. G. Leeds, the respected manager of Dalgety's, he was the man appointed.[53]

With its record of competent hospital management and the government's past acquiescence to its wishes in board appointments, the board felt confident in its efforts. However, 1903 was a period of testing. On grounds directly to the west of the hospital and fronting South Terrace, was a strip of land on which a two-storeyed house had been built at the Alma Street corner. The house which had been used by the Governor on occasion as a summer residence, was currently tenanted by Mrs Marmion. The hospital board had looked at this area in 1898 with thoughts of future expansion in mind, and realised that with its large, useful building, the property would suit them well. Colonial Secretary George Randell then assured the board that the site would eventually be granted to the hospital for its use. In 1903,

[52] CSO File 2763/97.
[53] *Ibid.*

when the board heard of the government's new plan to build a school for South Fremantle on the site, it protested vehemently. There would be noise from children and increased traffic to disturb patients and night nurses, and Marmion's House, as it had become known, would have served well as a ward for the incurables who were a quarter of the hospital's cases. Had not the council already surrendered to the Education Department a reserve at the corner of Mandurah and Douro roads for a school, queried the board. Although a deputation of the mayor, other members of the district and the hospital board met with the new Colonial Secretary, Walter Kingsmill, to ask him to vest the property in the hospital's board of management, they were not successful.[54]

Just a short time later, in June of 1903, Dr Thomas Davy resigned his honorary appointment at Fremantle Hospital to become the district medical officer for Perth, in charge of the city's various institutions.[55] At the Fremantle Hospital board meeting of 28 August 1903, when the board pondered the applicants to fill the vacant honorary position, young Dr Alfred E. Martin, who seemed 'the best man for the position' was preferred to the older and Australian- trained doctors Paget and Anderson.[56] His string of impeccable references ('a first rate surgeon . . . a good operator and thoroughly reliable in emergencies and on occasions of difficulty') from lecturers and surgeons at St Thomas' Hospital and the Children's Hospital, London, and his certificates and prizes and first-class honours for his achievements, spoke of his outstanding ability.[57] More on the board voted for the new arrival than the total voting for Paget and Anderson combined. Hospital rules were immediately altered so that an applicant of six months' residence in the state, rather than two years, could be appointed to the honorary staff, but to a board who could remove a matron in the hospital's best interests, this proved no barrier. Complacent in its wisdom and the government's acceptance of its past decisions, and outwardly a united group, the board directed Martin to commence work at the hospital and sat back to await the usual ratification of the appointment.[58]

In the context of hospital administration, Walter Kingsmill's tenure as colonial secretary had been fraught with problems of politics and power at Perth Public Hospital. He found that 'a great amount of friction and a great amount of scandal and many imputations of unfairness were made against gentlemen who had partners on the honorary medical staff, and who were practicing doctors and held seats upon the board of management'.[59] In 1902 the matter was brought up in the Legislative Assembly and veered off into a discussion of administration and hospital finance; but Kingsmill was still able to suggest and arrange the discharge of all local medical

---

54 *West Australian*, 2, 5 March 1903. See also *WAPD*, 11 November 1903, Vol. 24, p. 2026.
55 Like Dr Saw before him, who left the position in protest at his low wage of £250 a year, Davy found that travelling costs alone took 35 per cent of his income. His energetic, impartial condemnation of houses unfit to live in and regular visits to the government's institutions would stand to him as a monument in many memories after his untimely death in June 1908, PHD File 1043/08. See also Truthful Thomas, *Through the Spy-Glass*, p. 45
56 *Morning Herald*, 21 September 1903.
57 CSO File 3361/03.
58 *Ibid.*
59 *Ibid.* See also *Morning Herald*, 23 October 1903; *West Australian*, 23 October 1903; *WAPD*, 11 November 1903, Vol. 24, p. 2025.

practitioners from the Perth Public Hospital Board and the appointment of two out-side qualified doctors. Thomas Lovegrove, the principal medical officer, and Dr G. H. Blackburne, the chairman of the central board of health, proved to be com-paratively impartial medical advisors and were able to maintain a certain satisfying degree of government influence at the hospital.[60] To avoid a similar conflict in hos-pital administration, Kingsmill, with the approval of his colleagues, planned never again to appoint a privately practising doctor as both a hospital board member, and an honorary medical officer, nor to appoint the partner of a board member to the honorary staff in a public hospital. It was a policy, however, which was not announced publicly. The move was basically a sound one. One spoke for many in 1903 when he said, 'I never knew a place where there was so much jealousy among medical men as there is in Western Australia'.[61]

From 1897, honoraries at Fremantle Hospital treated public patients allocated to them at no cost but to their precious time. They also had the privilege of admitting certain of their own patients to the hospital. In 1901 this privilege was extended, and access to the hospital was granted to all Fremantle medical men. Despite this, an appointment to the honorary staff of a hospital was coveted: not only did it provide greater learning opportunities through access to a variety of medical cases and the opportunity for collaboration with other doctors, but it added to a doctor's standing in the community and enhanced his medical status for the prospective patients on whom his income depended. Because the number of honorary staff at Fremantle Hospital was smaller than at Perth Hospital, appointments were seen as more valuable and sought more avidly.[62] Professional envy was almost inevitable when two members of the one medical firm held board positions, as Hope and White did in 1903, or when partners served as honorary and board member respectively. As Birmingham pointed out, and Kingsmill was aware, 'a partner would naturally think more of his own partner than he would in a general way of other professional men. He would support and vote with his partner.'[63]

It was with shock that the board received Walter Kingsmill's letter of 9 September wondering if it was true that Alfred Martin was a partner of the present board member, Henry Lotz. The board bristled, and W. Bennett, the new secretary and dispenser, was directed to reply in strong terms to the official 'interrogation' and convey the board's 'utter astonishment that they should be asked to stoop to such an invidious position as to inquire into either of the professional gentlemen's privacy of practice'.[64] Actually the partnership was common knowledge, Martin having come with the express intention of joining Lotz, but the board believed that a principle

[60] See Bolton and Joske, *History of Royal Perth Hospital*, p. 69.
[61] *Morning Herald*, 21 September 1903.
[62] *West Australian*, 23 October 1903. So avidly were they sought, that when the board appointed young Thomas Anderson to the honorary medical staff in Lotz's absence overseas in 1900, the more senior men of the town—Drs A. Badock, W. Birmingham, T. Davy, W. Dermer, J. Hope, O. Paget, E. Tynan, H. Walter, and A. White—successfully petitioned the board against the appointment, CSO File 610/1900. Three years later, when Martin was voted to the position on the honourary staff, Paget and Anderson felt that their personal and professional status had been questioned. They visited a number of Fremantle members of parliament for reassuring references which they forwarded to the Colonial Secretary. See *Morning Herald*, 23 September 1903.
[63] *Morning Herald*, 7 November 1903.
[64] CSO File 3361/03, 12 September 1903.

was involved. So, too, did Kingsmill with his Perth experience behind him, and he tersely repeated his question.

At the board's next meeting the doctors monopolised the discussion. Birmingham supported the colonial secretary's stand, reminding the members of the intense bitterness at Perth Public Hospital when 'that institution practically passed into the hands of two or three firms' and he warned of drifting into the same situation.[65] Hope urged a civil reply to Kingsmill's query and Lotz confirmed that Martin was his partner. The answer was sent to the colonial secretary with another copy of Martin's glowing testimonials. But at that meeting in September another incident added to the board's discontent. On the resignation of Mr John, the board had recommended W. E. Moxon as its new member. In a surprisingly terse response the colonial secretary pointed out that under the 1894 Act the board could merely notify the government of a vacancy and not recommend an appointment. The rebuke, read at the meeting, rankled.

When Kingsmill's mild and reasonable letter was received later in the month, advising that Martin could not be confirmed as a member of the honorary staff because he was the partner of a board member, the board's simmering discontent was fuelled into anger. At a special board meeting convened to discuss the issue, hairline cracks of mistrust and animosity splintered into open schism as non-medical men spoke against medical, doctor spoke against doctor, and the whole board roundly condemned the government. Congdon expressed his long-held view that the board would one day find the medical staff outvoting the other members of the committee. Even though Moxon had just been appointed to the board, Smith thought that for some time the board had not been treated as it should have been by the colonial secretary, who had not generally acquiesced in the board's requests, and most supported his suggestion to reject Kingsmill's letter to show that they were not merely 'puppets and marionettes' of the colonial secretary.[66] Drs Birmingham and Lotz clashed over the medical merits of Anderson and Martin, while Smith—perhaps with the hospital's status in mind—supported Martin with his British training rather than Anderson who had trained in Melbourne and who 'came from a much inferior position than Dr Martin'.[67] By the end of the meeting, only Birmingham, the single medical representative on the board who was not committed in a partnership, firmly agreed with the colonial secretary that medical partners should not have a voice in controlling the hospital. For the others, the issue resolved into one of principle: if a government appointed a board, it should have confidence in its decisions. The board's recommendation to appoint Martin stood firm.

Chairman Lilly and Mr Hudson representing the board met the colonial secretary on 22 October. The issue of medical partnership was irrelevant, they claimed. The board wanted the best man for the position and the colonial secretary's attitude struck at the very root of the management of the hospital. Furthermore, they argued, the board felt that the government lacked confidence in its ability to administer the institution, and under Fremantle Hospital Rule 58, the board could nominate medical and other officers for appointment and could recommend their

[65] *Ibid.*, 23 September 1903.
[66] *Ibid.*, 14 October 1903.
[67] *Ibid.*

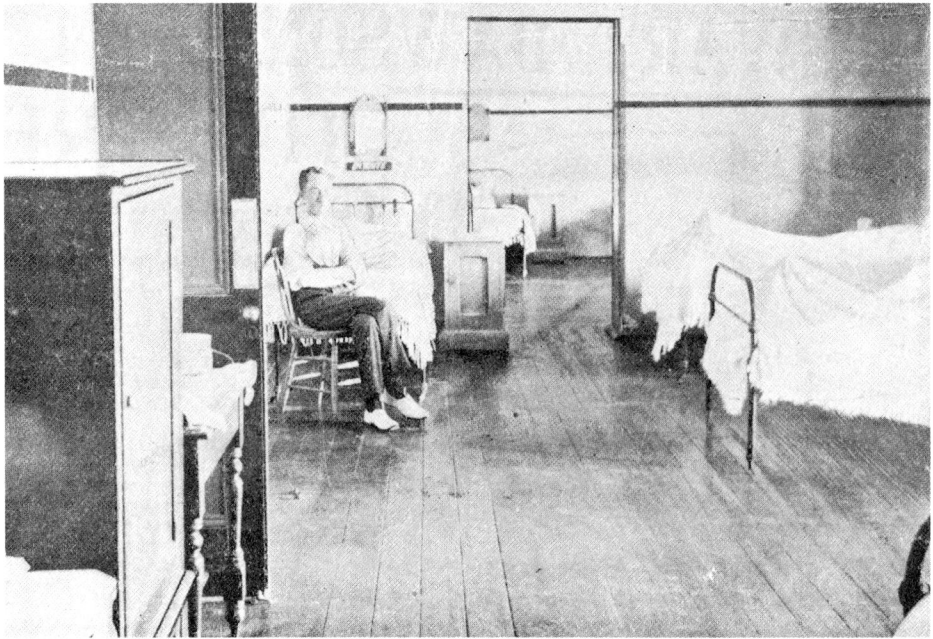

Photograph courtesy the *Western Mail*

Plate 10.   The surgical ward, Fremantle Hospital, 1908.

removal, subject to the approval of the Governor. Although Kingsmill assured the
two of his confidence in the board, expressed his regret at the situation, and explained his reasons for maintaining his decision, he promised to seek advice from the
Crown Solicitor to see whether the Government Act superseded the hospital rule. As
the answer did not arrive before the next monthly gathering of the board, the meeting was adjourned. When it came, it was inevitable that the judgement supported the
colonial secretary's stand. As Birmingham and Hope had reasoned—if the regulations clashed with the Act, the Act must be paramount—and so it proved.

    At the board's next meeting, feelings ran as high as the winter tides, and threats of
resignation were muttered from around the large table in the board room. James
Hope appealed for reason, but argument washed to and fro—against Birmingham
for his sustained opposition to partnerships on the honorary staff and his alleged
private correspondence with the colonial secretary; over Kingsmill for his lack of
confidence in the board and his policy which the board believed would lead to secret
medical partnerships; it eddied in talk of political influence and of board members
as being mere puppets manipulated by the colonial secretary. Only Drs White,
Hope, Birmingham and Mr Congdon were opposed to informing the colonial secretary that his reasons for declining to confirm Martin in the appointment were not
sufficient and that the board declined to make any further nominations.[68]

[68]   CSO File 3361/03; *West Australian*, 7 and 8 November 1903; *Morning Herald*, 7 November 1903.

Before Kingsmill could respond, seven indignant members of the Fremantle Hospital board decided to resign. Lotz was persuaded to reconsider his decision and, on 14 November, resignations were forwarded to the colonial secretary by Charles Hudson, Edward Duffield, Thomas Smith, Thomas Pearse, W. Moxon and the outspoken A. G. Leeds:

> ... It is with much regret that we now have to tender you our resignations as members of the Fremantle Hospital Board, consequent upon the Colonial Secretary refusing to make a certain appointment on the nomination of an absolute majority of the Board.
>
> This involves such a vital principle that we feel we have no option in the matter: furthermore, when a Minister thinks it necessary to differ from the Board of an Institution who are his advisors in a matter of local appointments, it is clear that they do not possess his confidence and therefore there is again no alternative to resignation ... Regarding the applicants for the present vacancy, it was impossible to select all three, and consequently two were bound to be disappointed, but the Board in a constitutional way by a majority, after careful scrutinizing each applicants credentials, selected Dr Martin as the gentleman, who, in their opinion, was the most fitted for the appointment on the ground that his experience in hospital work was of a higher class,—(vide the appointments held by him),—and more modern and up to date than that of the other two gentleman, and if a Minister is to overrule the deliberate advice of the Board of Management on such insufficient ground as that of 'partnership with another member of the staff', or through the representations previously referred to in the interests of disappointed applicants, then we are sure the hospital will suffer both in the class of men who will give up their time to serve on the Board and in the calibre of the professional gentlemen who will form the Medical Staff and minister to the necessities and alleviate the sufferings of the sick and injured poor ...'[69]

A few days before Christmas the remaining members of the board met to reconsider applications for the vacancy on the honorary staff and Thomas L. Anderson was returned as an honorary medical officer to the hospital where he had been a young resident.[70] It was a chastening experience for the board, which for a time, became cautious about the limits of its power in dealings with the government.

The years at the turn of the century brought other, different problems. With the increase in population from outside Western Australia came infectious diseases—smallpox, cholera and bubonic plague. From the port's earliest years successive Fremantle medical officers had carried out quarantine procedures, asking a ship's captain about the state of health of his passengers and crew. If an infectious case was aboard, a yellow flag would be run up the ship's mast and no one allowed to land. 'Constantly exposed as we are to the risk of contagion, it is only by exercising the most persistent care that we can hope to preserve the immunity we now enjoy,'[71] urged the *Inquirer* in 1874. At a local level, the Fremantle Board of Health in 1891 smugly wished to prevent the introduction into Fremantle of typhoid and other diseases which, if they were careless about, 'might be supposed to have been gener-

---

[69]   CSO File 3361/03.

[70]   *Ibid.* Young Anderson was appointed to the honorary medical staff just three years after the protests of more senior doctors in the town had resulted in his dismissal in 1900. See footnote 62.

[71]   *Inquirer*, 21 January 1874. For quarantine procedure, see *WAVP*, Vol. 1, 1874. Report upon the Quarantine Laws and Regulations.

ated here'.[72] Sometimes, however, a captain's answers to questions about health on his ship were untrue, and sometimes a party from a vessel came to shore before the ship was granted pratique. In heavy weather the quarantine officer often had to leap from the newly arrived and inspected ship onto the heaving, tiny deck of the pilot boat waiting to take him back to shore. 'No lefs [sic] than three times when boarding Vefsels [sic] as Health Officer ... I have been capsized in a boat,' announced Shipton in 1868, 'and but that I am a good swimmer must have been drowned.'[73] Western Australia did not escape the smallpox epidemics of 1880–85 and cholera in 1889, but bubonic plague between 1900 and 1906 struck harder. Each epidemic, however, served to tighten quarantine regulations.[74] Dr Frederick Ingoldby at the port of Albany was warned that he was 'at the gate of Australia and must keep guard'.[75] Such was also the position at Fremantle.

In 1900 the link between rats and bubonic plague was only just recognised. Under a consequent Central Board of Health regulation, each ship had to be held four feet away from a wharf by means of fenders coated with wet tar. All ropes, down which a rat might run, were replaced with wires which also had to be kept sticky with tar, and rat guards were required to be fitted to hawsers. Lights were set up to illuminate whole vessels and watchmen stationed to see that all precautions were taken. It had been easy for rats to get ashore at Fremantle where wharf bridged land, and for them to scamper into Cliff Street warehouses and into shanties where there was little sanitation or thought about cleanliness. In a massive cleanup, baits of oatmeal, sugar and strychnine, or phosphorus and arsenic mixed with wheat, were laid in the railway workshops, on the wharves and in warehouses, and a reward of sixpence for each rat caught was offered by the council. Ferrets, especially trained to hunt rats, were imported from W. Scarffe, a bird and animal dealer in Melbourne, and a keeper was paid to work, feed and house the hunters.[76] All cargoes arriving from plague areas were fumigated with sulphur for four hours under tarpaulins, or sprayed with a ten per cent solution of carbolic acid.[77]

Thomas Anderson quickly interested himself in the disease and was trained through the government in the treatment and prevention of the plague. His small son, from his narrow bed at night, could see the glow of the incubator, kept at 98.4 °F by a kerosene lamp, where his father's specimens were cultured.[78] People diagnosed as having bubonic plague were nursed at the Woodman's Point Quarantine Station. In 1906 a train called the 'Plague Special' was organised to run between Perth and Fremantle three times a day. Sufferers were loaded into a six-compartment coach behind a brake van and on arrival at Fremantle were transferred into a special ambulance for the journey to Woodman's Point. By 1908 special ramps were

[72] Minutes of FLBH, 24 July 1891.
[73] CSO File 617/1868. Letter to Colonial Secretary, 24 November 1868.
[74] See J. H. L. Cumpston, 'The Evolution of Public Health Administration in Australia', in *The Medical Journal of Australia*, 6 February 1932, pp. 194–8. A smallpox outbreak in 1893 claimed eleven lives out of 50 victims. Bolton and Joske, *The History of Royal Perth Hospital*, p. 51.
[75] CSO File 3278/89.
[76] CSO File 491/1900; PHD File 798/07 (ferrets); PHD File 882/07.
[77] CSO File 228/06.
[78] Anderson, interview, BL. Thomas Anderson was elected MD (Melbourne) in 1904 for his thesis on bubonic plague.

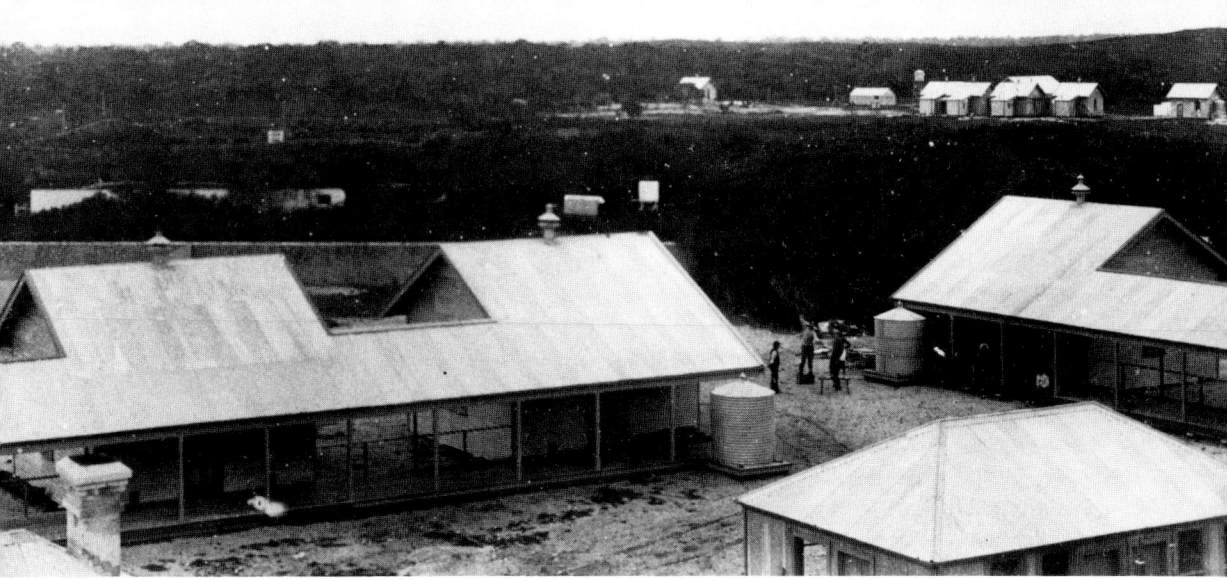

Photograph courtesy Battye Library

Plate 11. Quarantine Station Woodman's Point. On his return from seeing patients there, Thomas Anderson would often change his clothes in a back shed and burn the garments— even, to his wife's dismay, a new suit. He would then soak in a bath of 1:80 carbolic solution. Colin Anderson remembered trips to the Quarantine Station with his father, Dr Thomas Anderson:

> The corrugated iron wards ran at right angles to the road leading in. Smallpox cases were among those isolated there—men often from ships—with crusts all over their faces.
>
> Dr Colin Anderson

constructed so that the ambulance drove directly onto a flat rail car for the journey to Fremantle, and from the train, straight to the quarantine station.[79]

The first case of bubonic plague in Western Australia was that of a 19-year-old shunter working at the railway yards adjacent to the Fremantle wharf. On 5 April 1900, about 12 days after lumping some cargo from Sydney, he became ill and was admitted to the Fremantle Hospital where he died three days later. A routine post-mortem examination established the presence of plague. The ward in which the man had lain had to be closed and fumigated and the chairman of the board, Elias Solomon, announced, somewhat belatedly, that the hospital would not admit bubonic plague patients, or anyone suspected as having it. Another patient, however, was temporarily admitted in 1903 before being sent to Woodman's Point. It was not surprising that of the 77 cases of bubonic plague reported in Western Australia between

[79] PHD File 339/08.

1900 and 1906, 37 came from Fremantle, where ships carrying infection berthed and where rats scuttled freely through the limestone tunnels of Arthur Head and gorged on scraps thrown through the windows of workers' cabins on the wharves because there were no rubbish bins provided. The disposal of those who died as a result of bubonic plague initially posed perplexing problems of public health. The young shunter's body was placed in three coffins fitted one inside the other, which were flooded with carbolic acid and taken, hanging by chains, on a tug, far out past Rottnest for a sea burial. For some time no one would buy fish caught at Fremantle. The next body was burned on a pyre of two truckloads of railway sleepers at the beach near Woodman's Point. Dr Anderson had to pay the undertaker an extra ten shillings on the spot to help him wrap the body in carbolic soaked sheets and place it on top of the wood. Although gallons of tar were poured over it and the fire burned for over a day, the remaining pile of ashes with a human thigh bone protruding from the middle was an objectionable sight to those who saw it from the road. Only after their complaints were received was the old crematorium at Woodman's Point modified and extended so that it worked efficiently.[80]

The isolation of patients with a contagious disease was always a concern for the town's council. This was emphasised in 1897 when a young man named E. C. Elliott, working at the Jubilee Restaurant in South Terrace and without money or friends, was found to have scarlatina. With the hospital full of typhoid patients, there was nowhere but the police station to take the man, and he was placed in a small battered 'lean-to' which had once served as an artillery gun shed. The Fremantle gravedigger was appointed as an attendant and a constable was placed on duty outside, to keep intruders away. The gravedigger gave Elliott breakfast and left, and it was only after the hungry patient's clamouring appeals were heard that evening that he was given another meal. The government advised the town clerk that it was the council's responsibility to provide suitable places in which to locate infectious cases, but when three more cases of scarlet fever were reported, it granted the council use of the hospital at Woodman's Point Quarantine Station, provided that the attendant pitched a tent for himself to sleep in beside the wooden ward.[81] In 1903 Hope called for the building of an infectious diseases hospital at the port, to be maintained at municipal expense.[82] Although an infectious diseases ward was built at Fremantle Hospital, and the council and government haggled over who should pay the cost of treatment there, the infectious diseases branch of the Perth Public Hospital at West Subiaco remained the main centre for the treatment of infectious diseases in Perth. There was, however, a growing awareness about public health. Dr Blackburne was engaged full-time in 1907 investigating diphtheria among school children.[83] The need was due. In Fremantle, as in other areas in the metropolis, death was often the result

[80] See J. H. L. Cumpston, *The History of Plague in Australia 1900–1925*, Melbourne, H. J. Greene, 1926, pp. 35–9; CSO File 639/1900 (no plague cases by hospital); PHD File 882/07 (railway workers); *West Australian*, 2 March 1903 (patient 1903); PHD File 529/03, Medical Officer of Health's Annual Report 1902 to the Fremantle Local Board of Health and the Central Board of Health. Hope concluded that the public health of the town was in an unsatisfactory position; for disposal of bodies, see C. Anderson, interview, BL.

[81] CSO File 2745/97; *Inquirer*, 7 September 1897; Minutes of FLBH, 16 September 1897.

[82] PHD File 529/03.

[83] See PHD File 994/07; PHD File 1360/08.

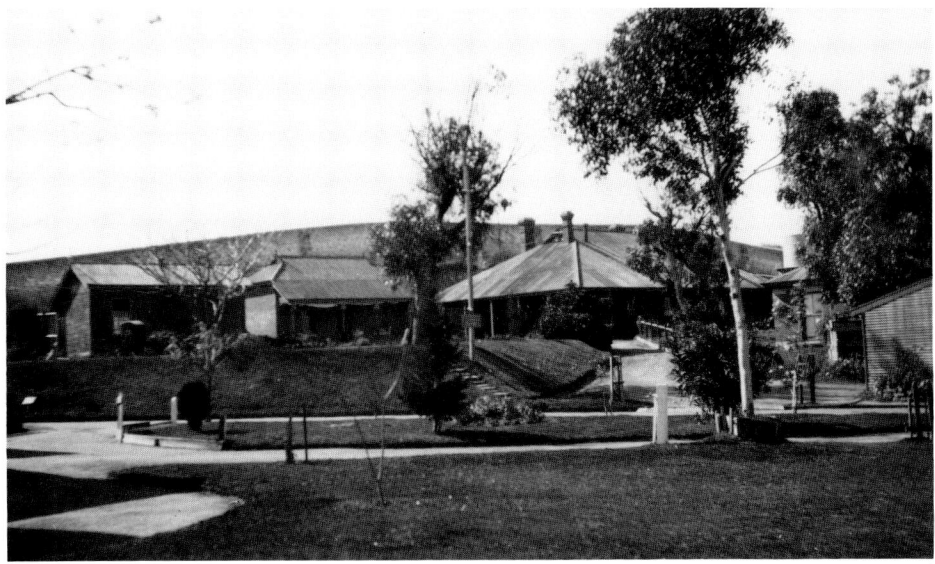

Photograph courtesy A. Orloff

Plate 12. *(Left to right):* The inebriates' ward, the old nurses' quarters known as Forrest ward, and the isolation ward.

> I think most people loved Freo. They liked the hospital. It was theirs. Even though it was a bit like a 'poorhouse'—it was theirs.
>
> Victoria Hobbs
> Nursing Sister, 1935

of the disease—five in a month not uncommon. In times of epidemic, such as in 1904, schools were disinfected weekly with formalin and sufferers nursed at home behind a sheet saturated with carbolic solution, strung up over the bedroom doorway to prevent cross-infection.[84]

As the place in town where people suffering the effects of alcohol were treated, the two-bed inebriates' ward at the hospital, although an asset, also posed difficulties. At times there was insufficient staff to nurse the patients there. One March night in 1906 when the hospital was filled to capacity, a man was arrested for drunkenness and lodged in the Fremantle lockup. He was joined by another who was riotously proclaiming himself of unsound mind, and when Dr Hope came to examine the men he ordered their removal to the public hospital. As there was no room available, the two were taken to the Gaol Hospital.[85] This action sparked conflict between the police, the gaol and ultimately the hospital. Although the inebriates' ward was obviously the more suitable place for these 'troublesome cases' unable to be admitted to an ordinary ward, the hospital board optimistically decided that the 'alcoholic cells' could only be used if the patients were attended by police. Three years later, in August 1909, a reporter was shown the ward by the chairman of the hospital board:

[84] PHD File 635/04.
[85] PHD File 500/1906.

'It is not fit work for any woman' stated the guide 'and, besides, it is positively dangerous for the nurses to have to handle such men ... You see here where a man the other
day smashed the locked door in with the bed, which he rent to pieces, and he afterwards
tore a hole in the galvanized fence, and got out. But in future a policeman is to attend
all such cases.'[86]

It was not a satisfactory arrangement to the small staff of police who repeatedly
offered to provide an off-duty attendant only if he were paid by the hospital.[87]
There the matter rested. By 1910 the inebriates' ward was also being used for cottage
cases and Matron Cameron suggested the provision of 'a bathroom, lavatory and
pantry adjoining; the present arrangements [there] being very unsatisfactory'.[88]

In 1907 there were further problems for the board. Edwin Nicholson left his position as dispenser and secretary in May 1903 after irregularities in the accounts were
discovered, and was replaced by William Bennett. Possibly the latter was better at
mixing solutions and powders than at keeping records. When an audit was about to
be undertaken in 1907 it was discovered that the books had not been written up since
1905. A 'deficiency in cash' was disclosed and when Elias Solomon, the chairman of
the hospital board, investigated, he found the irregularities '. . . due to negligence or
incompetence or both ... [but] no dishonest intent'.[89] In fact, when further enquiries were made, a surplus of £61 was revealed. Bennett explained that for some
considerable time he had been unaware as to how he stood with the maintenance
account, and concluding that something must be due to hospital funds, he had paid
in the amount he thought was short. The records were written up correctly, a new
system of bookkeeping similar to that at Perth Hospital was undertaken, and a
chastened but vindicated Bennett resigned. Out of 13 applicants for the position,
William Priestly was selected as the hospital's new secretary and dispenser in
November 1907.

It was a baptism of fire for the new employee in a time of economic constraint. In
1909 the cartoonist Ben Strange depicted Sir John Forrest lifting the Commonwealth
budget food cover off a lean portion of federal finances, with Western Australia
depicted as a cat hovering expectantly. 'Poor Pussy' was the caption.[90] The gross in-
debtedness per head of population was calculated at £76 in 1908, at nearly £80 by
1909.[91] As early as 1906 the under treasurer was urging the colonial Board of Health
to curtail its expenditure and to radically reduce the estimates for the following
year.[92] Constraints were not confined to the government. At Fremantle, the town
clerk's salary dipped, and those of the fishmarket inspector, the town hall caretaker,
the fireman and a labourer were reduced. Three council workers lost employment
and in all departments economies were practised.[93]

[86] *Morning Herald*, 18 August 1909. See also CSO File 4049/07.
[87] CSO File 4049/07.
[88] Matron's Report Book, 24 May 1910.
[89] Minutes of the House Committee, Fremantle Hospital, 26 July 1907. For Nicholson, see CSO File
      3945/97.
[90] *Western Mail*, 21 August 1909.
[91] *Ibid.*
[92] *Ibid.*, 14 August 1909. Reflections on 1906.
[93] PHD File 1051/1906.

By 1907 the full effects of economic recession were being felt at Fremantle Hospital. It was a heavy year for diphtheria cases with only one period of 24 hours when there were no patients in the 'isolated ward'. By 1908 the hospital was falling behind in its accounts despite 'a policy of stringent economy' and doing without 'things that are almost necessities'.[94] The board did rally subscribers to furnish its first children's ward more than six months before the new Children's Hospital was opened in Subiaco. Under Mrs Murphy's guidance, the ward was opened in 1908 with six cots and two bedsteads in one of the rooms on The Knowle's first floor. But not until late in 1909 was adequate mackintosh sheeting provided, and it was 1910 before a baby's bath and bassinette were bought. It was also difficult to find £250 each year to keep the ward open. Matron Dixon was summoned by the board to account for an excessive milk bill in May 1908: 'The extra milk was due to the number of patients on milk diet,' she explained—14 women had been ordered to have three pints daily and six to have one pint; in the male medical ward nine patients needed three pints of milk daily and 18 were having one pint each.[95] A suggestion to purchase or rent cows was made but not taken up.[96] Concern about milk was not unwarranted. Between 1909 and 1911 alone, seven vendors in Fremantle were convicted of selling adulterated milk.[97] Michael Healey, the vendor under contract to supply the hospital, had three convictions, one after the house committee's discovery that he was diluting hospital supplies. The vendor's reasoning that his cows supplied more water than milk on occasions was not believed, nor was his sworn statement that water from the milk cooler had 'eaten its way through one of the lead coils and assimilated with the milk' diluting it by 23.5% while he was absent in the potato patch. Magistrate Nicholas thundered:

> The ordinary cheat can be effectively punished, but the SNEAK (are you listening, Michael?) who would rob and cheat a patient lying on a sick-bed deserves to be held in utter contempt . . .[98]

Healey was fined the maximum penalty of £20—the cost of the hospital's milk account for a month.

The reduction in the financial vote for public hospitals hit Fremantle Hospital hard. In 1909, its subsidy was reduced from £6,000 to £4,000.[99] Three probationers had to be discharged; an orderly and the lodgekeeper, as well as two maids and laundresses also had to leave. The inebriates ward and the infectious diseases wards were closed. 'This will mean a menace to the health of the community and a great anxiety and expense to the municipality through its local Board of Health,' the *Evening Mail* warned.[100] The number of hospital patients was reduced to 42 and all were moved to The Knowle building. Many had to be wheeled onto the exposed verandahs but winter storms lashed so bitterly, that at the end of May the male medical ward along-

[94]   CSO File 400/08. See also PHD File 1281/07.
[95]   Matron's Report Book, 25 June 1908.
[96]   Minutes of BM, 5 February 1909.
[97]   AN 347/1, Acc. No. 855, 1911, p. 66, No. 128, BL.
[98]   Undated press article in FH Scrapbook, 1909.
[99]   Minutes of BM, 27 July 1909.
[100] *Evening Mail*, 3 August 1909.

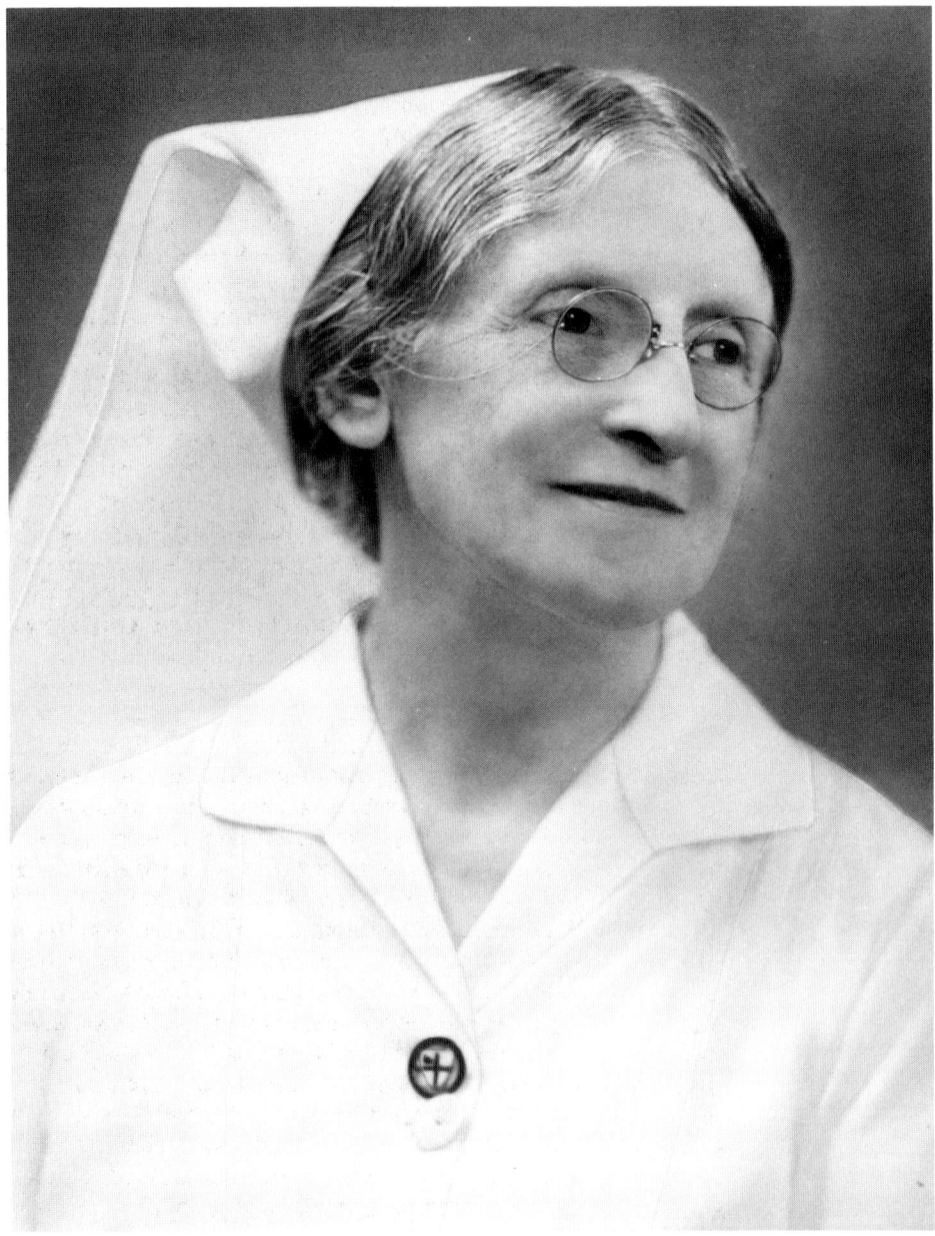

Photograph courtesy Fremantle Hospital

Plate 13.   Maida Balding, Matron of Fremantle Hospital 1914–1939.

Matron never—how will I put it—she always did what she had to do. She did it with grace and dignity and she—she was also reasonably tolerant.

Deputy Matron Mavis Fuller

side the Knowle was reopened. Despite Priestley's efforts to cut bed numbers and costs, patients kept coming—until the hospital held 59 instead of the planned 42 men, women and children. 'Will the people of Fremantle allow the work of the institution to languish for want of capital?' asked the *Daily News*.[101] Donations increased, but not by the needed thousands of pounds, although bequests from McKellar and Walter Padbury eased the position a little.

As a nurse trained at Melbourne Hospital between 1888 and 1890, Alice Dixon was welcomed as a senior nurse when she joined the staff of Fremantle Hospital in 1898 under Jessie Warden.[102] When the matron resigned, Miss Dixon was appointed to the position and for nine years, like matrons before and following her, she was responsible for the maintenance of hospital clothing, culinary requisites and stores; was required to 'inculcate' strict economy in the use of fuel and equipment, and was to see that 'order, cleanliness and punctuality prevailed throughout the establishment'.[103] When Dixon left in mid-1909, her position was advertised only in Western Australia. At a special meeting of the board, on which Drs Birmingham and Anderson were members, Dolinda Cameron was elected as matron. This was a period in which the honorary staff were testing the extent of their power. At the following board meeting, Dr Thomas Anderson moved on behalf of the honorary staff that Cameron's appointment be rescinded and her application with those of the eight other applicants be referred to the honorary medical staff for their consideration and report. The motion was lost by only one vote. While the honorary staff recommended the appointment of resident medical officers, the board selected the matrons of the hospital. When at the end of November 1911, Dolinda Cameron resigned, the position was again advertised in the Western Australian press. This time the board, which was little changed from that in 1909, agreed that if a qualified, capable Fremantle staff member applied, she should be appointed. The English-trained senior staff nurse, Margaret Brockbank, who had successfully filled the matron's position in emergencies, was appointed. On her resignation in February 1914—following press advertisements in New South Wales, Victoria and Adelaide, as well as in Western Australia—Maida Balding, who had trained at Perth Hospital between 1899 and 1902 before working at Coolgardie, was elected by the board to the position. The post of matron was not an easy one to fill and all matrons experienced frustrations with staff, suppliers, doctors and the board.

One aspect of a matron's duties was the lecturing of probationers. 'Nursing after operation of abdominal section', 'nursing special cases', 'general nursing', 'bandaging', 'attributes of a nurse and hospital etiquette' and 'poultice making' were among those delivered to all nurses. No matron attended board meetings but had to hand in her report book and await a summons if further explanation was required. Occasionally the board instructed the matron to arbitrate in disputes concerning her nurses. One patient complained of unkind treatment by staff, who observed that the woman could not lift her hands for anything when the nurses were in the ward but

---

101   *Daily News*, 18 August 1909.
102   Nurses had been taught at the Melbourne Hospital under guiding Nightingale principles with a trained nurse as Matron since late 1889. For training and division of nurses into four groups—sisters, nurses, probationers and pupils, see Inglis, *Hospital and Community*, pp. 96–101.
103   Rules and Regulations of the Fremantle Hospital, 1898.

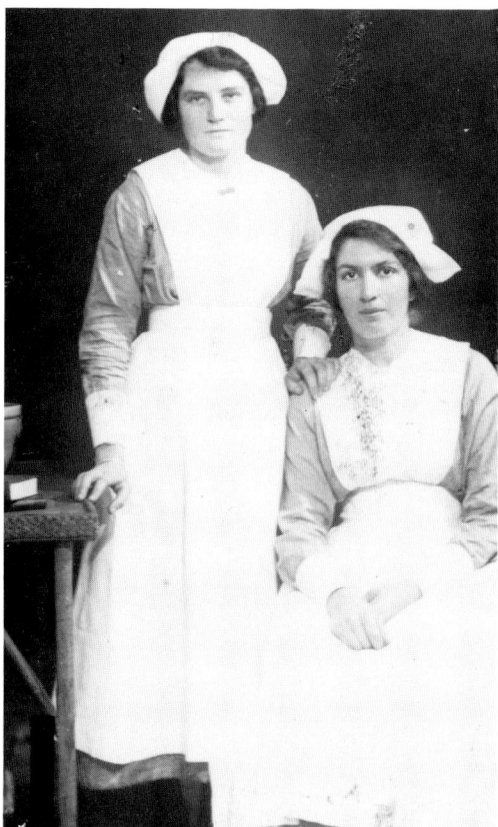

Plate 14.   Jean Kingswood (nee White)
[standing] was a ward-maid in the
Men's Medical Ward, c. 1918.

The ward-maids were under strict
supervision. At night bed checks
were made and each girl had to be
viewed personally.

Matron Olive Jones

Photograph courtesy Margaret McPherson

who 'could turn over and open her locker and help herself to fruit' when she thought she was unobserved.[104] The complaint was investigated by the matron and proven to be without foundation.

One of a matron's greatest problems could neither be avoided nor accurately predicted. Illness amongst the staff continually created havoc in her carefully organized schedule:

> I beg to report that Nurse Collins who went to the isolation ward to assist Nurse Breakel ... developed diphtheria. She was at once seen by the house surgeon and ordered to bed. No extra assistance was sent Nurse Breakel as the work being less she could manage by herself. Nurse Collins is progressing satisfactorily.[105]

Such reports were routine. It was not uncommon for other hospital workers, including the domestic staff for whom matron was responsible, to be warded after contact with an infectious patient. Evelyn Mason, a ward-maid, complained of feeling ill on

104   Matron's Report Book, 27 May 1904.
105   *Ibid.*, 16 August 1907.

a Wednesday in August 1907 and was sent to bed with typhoid. For three weeks her progress was favourable. Suddenly, on a Saturday, her condition deteriorated and by the following week she was dead. Coincidence perhaps, but that week three of her co-workers resigned.

The high turnover in domestic staff was another challenge to a matron's energies. They often found the work 'too hard' or 'too heavy', especially in the kitchen in hot weather; some left 'to marry' or 'to follow the family' or 'go on the 'fields'; some found work at a higher wage, a few suffered ill-health and others just didn't like the work. A few resented being told what to do. Housemaid Ethel Spencer in October 1903 'absolutely refused to do some work' that matron requested and was told 'either to do it or leave'.[106] She preferred the latter. One ward-maid left because she did not like one of the other maids who shared her bedroom and a laundress was replaced after 'returning to the hospital in a half intoxicated condition'. The cook, A. Peterson, resigned because she wanted a change. The assistant cook left also 'because A. Peterson is'.[107] Few stayed long enough to take their annual leave. It was not always easy to keep peace among the ever-changing domestic staff. Working in a kitchen over a wood stove, peeling, scouring, stirring, and lifting steaming-hot, heavy pots; boiling coppers full of objectionable linen in the stuffy laundry and spending hours over an iron were not conducive to harmony. Two laundresses walked out of the hospital when Matron Dixon assigned them the maids' personal washing to do. 'It will not entail much extra work on the laundresses,' thought matron, 'and will save bickering between them and the maids, if the maids are kept out of the laundry.'[108] Changes between different duties—laundry and kitchen, ward-maid and housemaid were common. When the doctors' and matron's house-maid left to go into business in 1908, the ward-maid on number two floor asked to take her place and a temporary ward-maid on the male medical ward requested a transfer to the number two floor. Ward-maids shared the responsibility of cleaning ward floors with the junior nurses and theirs was the task of polishing the floors after the nurse had swept it. 'If you dropped a spot of anything on that floor the ward-maid was on to you straight away . . . the ward-maids always growled at you,' remembered one nurse.[109]

Laundry workers were essential to the smooth functioning of the hospital, provid-ing clean, dry bedding and clothing for patients, and spotless, stiffly starched uni-forms for nurses. The tasks of washing and ironing were constant and heavy, and more than once in summer a laundress was reported as 'prostrated with the heat' and unable to work. On such occasions an extra laundress would be employed for five shillings a day. Not unnaturally, such bounty for labour irked the permanent laundresses who applied for a wage of £1 a week and Mrs Hunter threatened to resign if the increase was not paid. As the work was heavier in the laundry than it had ever been and few considered working anywhere for below £1 a week, the in-crease was granted.[110] Between 1911 and the beginning of war, N. McNally, Mrs

106   *Ibid.*, 2 October 1903.
107   *Ibid.*, 17 and 24 March 1905.
108   *Ibid.*, 3 January 1908.
109   Mrs E. Parker (née Eley), interviewed by J. Lancaster, 23 October 1986, FH.
110   Minutes of the House Committee, 26 March and 28 May 1909.

Petersen, Mrs Dixon, N. Regan and A. Regan were familiar faces over the tubs and irons.

By 1909 the laundry was in great need of renovation. The huge coppers had settled unevenly and the phenyl barrel was leaking where one of its hoops was missing and the wood was rotting. The ironing stand was broken through on one side where the hot iron stood on the stove, and the mangle wheel caught at the cover, making it difficult to turn. The drying room was also out of order and when washing was hung outside it flapped noisily against the windows of the operating theatre. The entire hospital was affected by the inadequacies, but in the children's ward, where the mackintoshes were so old they were useless, the position was intolerable. In November, when a new laundry was being built further from The Knowle, the male medical patients didn't really mind having to share their ward with laundry maids doing the ironing. The new laundry, however, closer to the isolation ward, was on rough ground with loose sand and it proved difficult for the staff to keep the clothes clean. Work there soon increased and two extra rope lines had to be installed to double the drying area for the loads of wet washing. Although the location changed, conditions did not, and the broken ironing stand made it difficult to get the irons heated. By early 1910 it was obvious that a third hand was needed in the laundry. Winter came. In the incompleted drying room the wash was slow to dry and wards experienced a continual linen shortage. Matron appealed to the board:

> The Public Works Department has not done anything further in the fixing of the drying room, and it is hardly to be wondered at, if people get ill, considering the damp clothing they are compelled to sleep in and also wear.[111]

Not until another three months had passed was the new blower installed and working. The board did try to help. In an effort to lighten the weight of wet washing, clothes baskets were fitted with wheels, but laundresses caught and tore their long skirts on the projecting fastenings, and guards had to be fitted to the wheels. Next, a portable laundry basket was tried, but proved too heavy to lift when loaded and matron recommended the fitting of a pivot wheel at the base to assist.

In the laundry the turnover of staff was particularly high. Some chose to leave, others were discharged as 'unsatisfactory', for 'using bad language' or for 'drunkenness'. The laundry remained a neglected area of hospital concern until 1915 when Mrs Carpenter and Mrs Murphy from the board visited the building and voiced their strong objection to conditions there. Together with the matron and Chairman Mills they formed a committee which met with the minister to inspect the area and a new laundry was promised when government funds were available.[112] Plans for a hospital laundry similar to that in Perth were drawn up in March 1916. By May of the following year, apart from new electric irons, the laundry was still in a 'deplorable' state. Once more the demand for clean, dry clothes could not be maintained throughout winter. Due to demands of war, 1917 was not a good year to build and equip a laundry, but so necessary was the work that by the end of September the main structure had taken shape under the direction of the Public Works Depart-

---

[111]   Minutes of BM, 21 June 1910.
[112]   *Ibid.*, 6 December 1915.

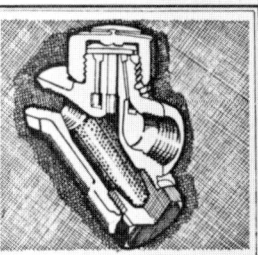
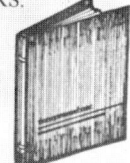
Fig. 13.   Spirax-Sarco Advertisement for steam valve.

ment. Machinery then proved difficult to get—a hydro-extractor, washing machine, some washing troughs, a soap boiler, wringer, radial horse mangle, disinfector and a motor to the drying horse. There was no ironing table, no folding table and no gas connected. The parts came slowly and irregularly. Twice the ships bringing a washing machine and centrifugal wringer were sunk by the enemy at sea. In April the hydro-extractor was 'hung up' in Singapore. Three months later, in 1918, it arrived and was installed. Then for the first time an engineer was required to monitor the steam power and equipment. A tall, gaunt young lad named Robert H. Benbow joined the staff on a month's trial.[113] He cut the fuel bills by covering the machinery posts with asbestos and overhauling the steam gauges, and arranged the construction of a coal and wood shed adjacent to the laundry. At the end of three months the laundry was working economically and well, handling 2,900 articles a week and fumigating others. Benbow stayed.

Women who nursed at the turn of the century were often viewed as more like Sarah Gamp of Dickens' novel, *The Life and Adventures of Martin Chuzzlewit*, than as Florence Nightingale. The dedication of Nightingale trained nurses, their strict discipline, both on and off duty, and their reputation for gentle, solicitous care to their patients, soon dispelled the reflection. However, at Perth Hospital in the mid-1890s, before a training course was organised, some nurses were 'affected with alcohol and morphia habits' and were described as 'rough and irresponsible',[114] which may have dissuaded some women against nursing as an occupation. Perhaps one young Fremantle woman entertaining more acceptable thoughts of training at the Children's Hospital, which was in keeping with a woman's accepted function, was so influenced:

> ... Well, I spoke to Doctor Birmingham, who was a great friend of ours. He was our family doctor. And in those days the doctors were very close to you ... he said it would be far better for me to go in to the general hospital. Well, of course, I didn't want to do that. So consequently I stayed at home.[115]

There were others who found that the compulsory accommodation, or the training received by a hospital nurse, which was becoming widely recognised, answered their personal needs; others had an esteemed relative who had been a nurse and generated enthusiasm for the occupation; some had always wanted to be a nurse ('my dolls were always sick').[116] The matron of the Home of Peace encouraged her nurses to train at Fremantle Hospital and many came with this nursing experience behind them. On the Legislative Assembly rolls of 1904 for Fremantle, 47 women were recorded as involved in the nursing profession—27 were specifically registered as 'hospital' nurses including those at the gaol; four were midwives and two were from the Sailor's Rest on the Esplanade.[117] Nursing was consistent with a woman's traditional role as comforter and nurturer, tied securely as it was to domestic work, and it was given status through need in war. By the 1920s it was a respected and respectable

[113]   Minutes of HC, 16 July 1918.
[114]   See Bolton and Joske, *History of Royal Perth Hospital*, p. 61.
[115]   E. Notley, interviewed by M. Howroyd, 13 April 1984, FCL.
[116]   Parker, interview.
[117]   Legislative Assembly Rolls, 1904, BL.

career for a young girl. Such was the regard, one nurse remembered that while walking in the town one evening with a fellow trainee, she was accidentally bumped by a sailor from one of the ships while coming around a corner. 'A man behind me saw this and knocked him to the ground.'[118] The chivalry was not greatly appreciated that night when the nurse found that the injured sailor was one of her patients and she dreaded his recognising her as the cause of his condition.

Many of the nurses who trained at Fremantle Hospital before World War I came from 'the east' or had family in New South Wales or Victoria and were perhaps enticed to travel for the higher Western Australian nursing wages.[119] In 1908 five out of the 12 trainees visited the Eastern States. Mary McDonald came from Castlemaine in Victoria to join her sister and brother-in-law in Western Australia following the death of her mother in 1899. She was accepted as a probationer at Fremantle Hospital in November 1902 by Alice Dixon. At the beginning of the following year Mary passed her junior exam. The only candidate to fail was allowed to sit a second paper, so that all the junior nurses—Brown, Collins, Cottell, McDonald, Bellamy and Marie continued together—nursing, learning, and sharing quarters and meals and off-duty hours. Each did three months night duty at a stretch with one night off a month, and occasionally one or the other was frightened at night when accosted by men lurking in unlit Alma Street. In May 1903, four nurses were isolated with diphtheria and another two with influenza, but it was a good year overall. During the week that Mary McDonald returned from her two weeks annual holiday in February 1905, Nurse Marie was isolated with the sore throat of diphtheria but recovered just before Nurse Bellamy was confined with the same illness. Then, in May, Nurse Marie reported sick with typhoid. It was a severe attack and it was not until the end of July that her condition improved, and it was August before she could get up. By early September she could be taken out onto the balcony of The Knowle, but still could not walk. A month later she was discharged and went to Melbourne to recover. She missed Nurses Cottell and McDonald getting their certificates in November 1905. Mary McDonald stayed on at the hospital and in March, when Nurse Marie returned to work and when the wards were glutted with the usual summer fevers, she reported a sore throat and joined Nurse McMahon in the nurses' sick room. Both battled the chill and fever of typhoid and a week later both were seriously ill. Despite careful nursing and prayers by her fellow probationers, Nurse McMahon died on a Tuesday morning and was buried the following Thursday afternoon. A week later Mary McDonald's condition had improved slightly, but not until the end of April was she was able to leave the hospital for sick leave. Four months after being warded she returned to work. In May two more nurses had typhoid. In August one nurse was confined with diphtheria and neuritis and one with measles, while another had typhoid. It seemed that the nurses' sick room was never empty. Nurse Bellamy, who had trained with Mary McDonald, left to join her sister in private nursing at Perth and at the end of October Nurse Marie completed her training, after making up for her seven months of illness during her three probationary

---

[118] M. Lund, interviewed by C. Jeffery, 2 December 1985, BL.
[119] In New South Wales it was reported that a matron, nurse and probationer nurse earned £67, £33.15.0. and £18.10.0. p.a. respectively, while in Western Australia the rates were £100, £55 and £27. *Morning Herald*, 18 September 1903.

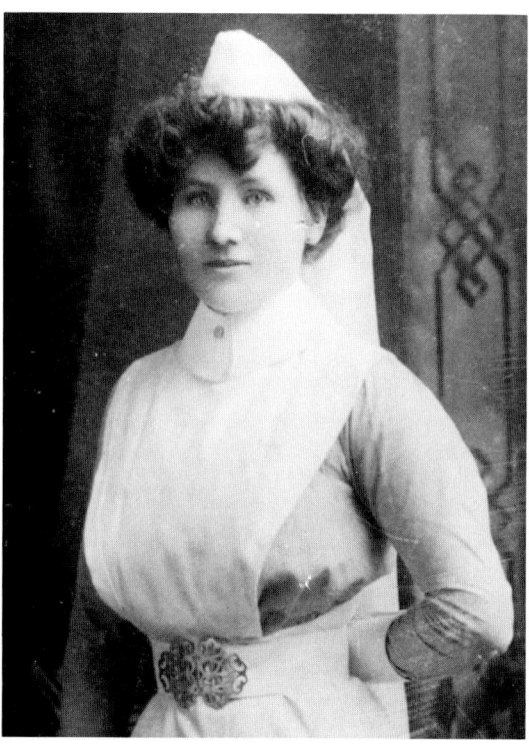

Plate 15. Sister Mary McDonald
trained at Fremantle Hospital
1902–1905.

Photograph courtesy Mrs D. Hesling

years. In February 1907, senior nurse Mary McDonald took her holidays. With plans underway for her wedding, Mary resigned in May and on 9 October 1907, was married by the Presbyterian minister in St Andrew's church, Perth, to Thomas Alfred Williams, a South Fremantle shopkeeper. It was a lavish celebration and for a year they were very happy. The couple were delighted when they found that Mary was going to have a child, but suddenly and copiously, on 26 March 1909, Mary haemorrhaged. Thomas took his wife to the hospital with which she was so familiar and Mary was admitted as a patient. Under an ether anaesthetic, Dr Lotz performed a laparotomy, but despite his skill and vast surgical experience, his limited nineteenth century knowledge and training were not enough to save Mary. Two days later she died from a ruptured ectopic pregnancy.[120]

Nursing skills were learned through a rigid system of apprenticeship. In the first decades of the new century trainees were placed on a month's trial before signing an agreement binding both the hospital and the probationer in a three-year training course. The honorary medical staff instructed in anatomy and physiology, medical nursing, surgical nursing and hygiene, while matron gave general nursing lectures and saw that invalid cookery lectures were given by herself or through the technical college. Time off from the ward to attend lectures was reluctantly given and it was

---

[120] Reconstructed from Matron's Report Books, and Fremantle Hospital Major Theatre Operation Record Book, Biographical notes on Mary McDonald courtesy of Mrs D. Hesling, Bindoon, W.A.

usual to attend lectures in off-duty time, often when a night nurse was supposed to be sleeping. Sometimes there was the invitation to attend a post-mortem for instruction:

> The morgue ... was a great big shed of a place, with a long slab of table which the bodies were put [on] and there were always two doctors there and they—any of the girls that wished to go up could go up and view. And seeing there was one from my own ward had died I was invited to go up which I did. And the doctor said, 'if any of you feel any queasiness get out, quick' ... nobody did. It was a liver complaint and they did a post-mortem. He explained ... it was one way of seeing all the functions of the body and it was really very interesting.[121]

But the real training came through the seniors. As one nurse explained 'we learnt more in the wards from the sisters than we did from any of the doctors', and 'the first year nurse had to watch everything that was done'.[122]

The decision in 1907 to form a Western Australian Branch of the Australian Trained Nurses' Association, which had been founded in New South Wales in 1899 and extended to Queensland and South Australia, formalised and standardised nursing education throughout most of Australia.[123] A basic education test was introduced prior to enrolment, while a suggested course of lectures directed the curriculum. An appointed board of examiners, including Alice Dixon while she was matron, tested nurses at the end of their training, and the successful were awarded certificates of membership and registration with the A.T.N.A. Some trainees dreaded the oral questioning by doctors, some feared the written tests, while others made clumsy by nervousness were anxious about the practical assessment. But registration with the A.T.N.A. conferred status and proof of competence when applying for a position. The examinations were sat 'three days running it was' in the Irwin Street University building.[124]

In previous years Fremantle probationers had attended cooking lectures given through the Education Department, each sharing the ten-guinea fee with anyone else that matron could talk into doing the course. In 1908 the board suggested that matron teach the course and although she demurred saying she was 'not a qualified teacher of cooking' and that the A.T.N.A. might not recognize the classes, the board paid ten shillings for cooking utensils and gave her the use of the hospital kitchen. Sister Sadlier, an Eastern States-trained registered A.T.N.A. sister working at Fremantle Hospital, acted as examiner and all who sat the examination passed. In the following year Matron Dixon declined the undertaking. 'I do not propose to do so this year as it is much too onerous a task. It is much better for the nurses to have a professional cook to instruct them.'[125] She provided Mrs Huxley, the recognized teacher for the A.T.N.A., and suggested that the six nurses each contribute to her fee of six guineas for their course in the hospital kitchen. The nurses objected to paying fees from their meagre wage and the board thought it prudent to reappoint

[121] Lund, interview.
[122] *Ibid.*
[123] See Hobbs, *But Westward Look*, p. 26.
[124] Lund, interview.
[125] Matron's Report Book, 14 May 1909.

FREMANTLE HOSPITAL.

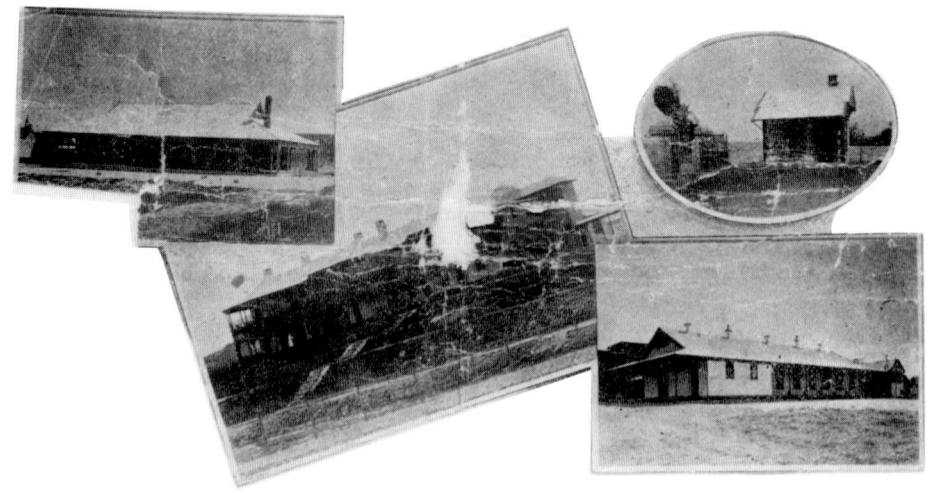

FOUNDED 1897.

Fremantle October 31ᵗ 1906

This is to Certify *that Nurse Josephine Marie resided in the* **Fremantle Hospital** *and received training as a Nurse for the term of three years, she has attended the prescribed course of Lectures, has passed the required examination, and is qualified to act as a skilled Nurse.*

Cravin Mtke Ct Rutell
House Surgeon.

DhCongdon
Chairman.

A.T. Dixon
Matron.

E Solomon
Vice-Chairman.

Fig. 14. Nurses' certificate 1906.

matron as instructor. Not until 1911 did nurses attend invalid cookery lectures at the technical school which were paid for by the hospital. However, two years later, the board again quibbled about costs, and Miss Mabel Yewers, 'a teacher of cooking', was employed at the hospital, and found the students' work 'very satisfactory, that of Misses McKay and Hornsby being excellent'.[126]

There was no gentle introduction to the profession of nursing. On arrival at the hospital a probationer would be allocated a bed to sleep on and a ward to work in and she soon learned the new diction and experience of 'bottle' (what do you want one for anyhow?), 'panroom', and 'sponges' not associated with the sea. Work started at 7 a.m. and continued until 12 noon. Some worked in the afternoon after the midday meal, others had a split shift and returned between 6 and 9 p.m. Night duty was worked between 9 p.m. and 7 a.m. In her first year the probationer was on duty at 7 a.m. when the night and day staff changed. Breakfast of porridge and bread and butter, sometimes with jam or honey, was served to patients and the dishes stacked for the wardsmaid to wash. 'Then we had to sweep the wards—the whole length. It was a nightmare at times really ... the wards were so long.'[127] Sponges had to be done 'one after another' behind heavy screens manhandled into position, and pan rounds completed after every meal and when necessary. Spittoons had to be emptied, lockers scrubbed, vulnerable pressure points attended to to prevent bed sores, infested heads treated with 'carbolic caps', patients' nails attended to and their hair done. Beds had to be made and covers centred with their large red cross right in the middle of the beds. 'I was just going off duty when one of the charge nurses came on and ripped them all off because they were not in the middle of the bed. So I had to go and do it all again. And I missed my train to Perth for which I was very annoyed,' remembered a nurse of 1919.[128] Barley water had to be boiled and the water strained and served to patients. 'It all took time.' While a second-year trainee didn't sweep and scrub she had to see that it was done. She made up trays, sterilized them in the big copper sterilizers, and lifted them out with a large pair of serrated forceps streaming steaming water. Urine samples had to be collected and tested for sugar and blood and for acidity or alkalinity in a screened-off section of the ward. Patients required medication and treatments, and some needed poultices. In her final year the nurse would supervise, and at times when there were insufficient charge nurses she would take control of the ward. Charge nurses supervised, wrote reports, did rounds with matron and honoraries, taught and assisted. Each day was demanding and the war period provided its own challenge. 'I was in charge of wards,' recalled a nurse thinking of her third year of training in 1919. Later:

> ... Because there were no sisters to be had, in the last three months I was in charge of the theatre and I had had practically no theatre training at all. Matron Balding said 'I'm giving you a senior nurse to help you instead of a junior', and she gave me my best friend, Mary Cooper, and the only thing that bothered me was we were both left

126 *Ibid.*
127 Lund, interview.
128 *Ibid.* All the social detail of nursing in this period is based on interviews of Lund and Parker. Their recollections give depth and insight into areas unobtainable from any other source.

handed. So we were an absolute nuisance to the surgeons because we had to do the assisting, and you always had to somehow keep your left hand free, to hand the scissors in case she [the other nurse] had to cut something, and the doctors were always swearing at you. We managed well, we had a tremendous lot of operations during that three months.[129]

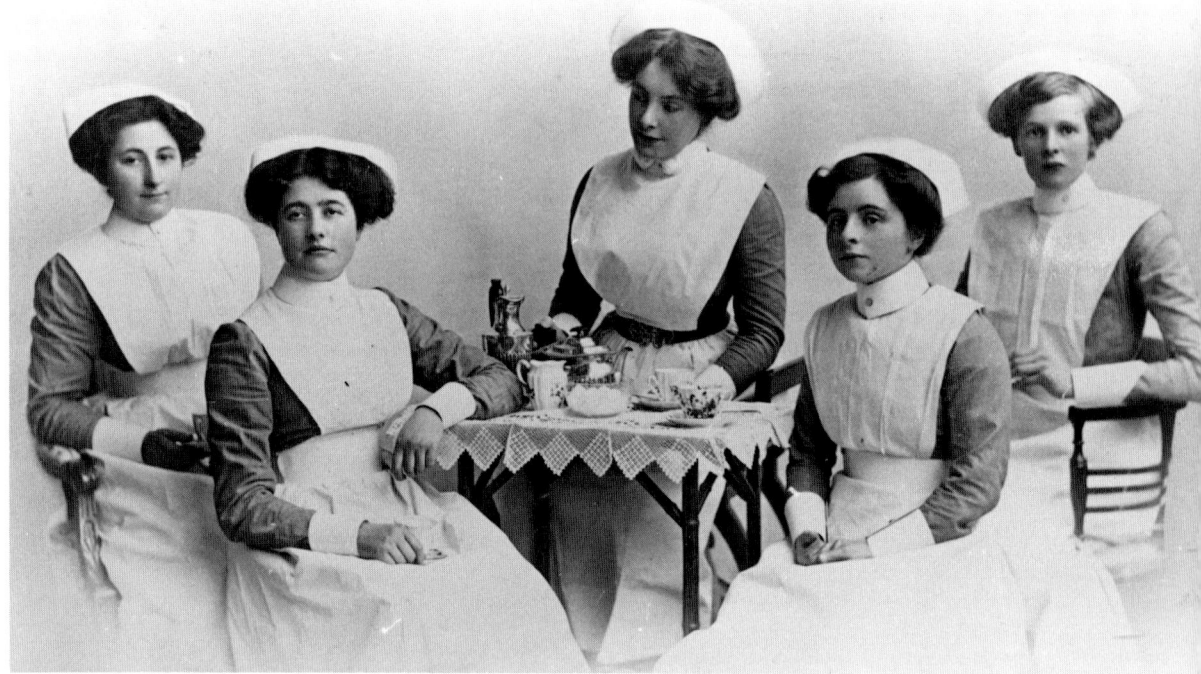

Photograph courtesy Dr G. Leyland

Plate 16.   Sister Agar pouring afternoon tea for the nursing staff, *c*. 1918.

Morning and afternoon teas were taken in the staff room but at midday a skeleton staff was left on the wards while the nurses lined up at the dining-room table and matron, at the head, carved the meat. Hospital food was not always satisfying. On a day off a nurse was entitled to breakfast in bed:

> You'd sleep in and the ward was supposed to send down your breakfast, which was an awful job because you wouldn't find anything to feed this wretched nurse on, that was off duty. Ordinary crockery was put on the tray. First you got a sketchy breakfast, porridge. There was always porridge of course. Porridge and bread and butter was all people lived on. We didn't get anything special. At our breakfast there was always a dish of chops on the table. They were always cold or burnt or greasy. We were always talking about those awful chops.[130]

129   Parker, interview.
130   *Ibid.*

A nurse's salary of four shillings and tenpence, seven shillings and sixpence and ten shillings in her first to third years respectively didn't go far, but sometimes at the Cannon Tea Rooms in Fremantle a friendly waitress would sell stale cake at half price. Whether off duty or on, '. . . we were always hungry'. One nurse recalled that

> You had to get morning tea in the ward you see, and of course there was nothing to eat so you would go across to the kitchen. I went across one morning . . . with another girl and when we got to the kitchen the cook had just taken a cake out of the oven. So she whispered to me, 'You get the jam, I'll get the cake—So I pestered the cook for some jam for our morning tea because you couldn't have butter and jam, you had butter or jam. And I looked around—my mate had gone—so had the cake. I saw her later on and I said, 'What did you do with the cake?' She said 'I have hidden it.' I said, 'Where have you hidden it?' She said, 'In your wardrobe.' Well nobody found it in my wardrobe so when we got off that night we had a party and ate the cake! Well the poor wretched cook, you know, she didn't stand a chance. She was always complaining about these dreadful nurses.[131]

Another source of food was matron's safe from which the back gauze wire could be cut and the contents rifled. Matron Balding said nothing but some years later she offered to show an ex-trainee one of the hospitals new acquisitions: refrigeration. Laughing, she said, 'You can't cut the back out of that'.[132]

Most nurses who trained at Fremantle Hospital between 1898 and 1920 were over 21 years but in times when new recruits were scarce, applicants as young as 18 were accepted. In 1914 a Miss M. Cannard, an 'over-aged applicant' was accepted as a probationer and the board decided to settle the maximum age of entry at 30. The nurse completed her three years' training with credit and only ten days' sick leave, unlike others, who left after illness or the common condition of flat feet. To decrease this dropout incidence, candidates applying for nursing training from 1918 underwent 'a thorough examination in bed'[133] by an honorary doctor as was done in other hospitals before they were accepted as probationers. Little wonder that foot problems were common among nurses—'you were on your feet for so long and we ran—we didn't walk,' recalled one. Dr Kerr, as medical examiner in 1919, despaired that 'there was not a good arch amongst the lot' of the probationers.[134]

Before she commenced training and each year thereafter, a new probationer was given 24 yards of print material to make her long, sweeping dresses and 12 yards for white aprons. In 1913 the lilac print for nurses' uniforms, ordered through the local Bon Marché store, was difficult to get and by 1916 nurses wore pink—well-starched and with a fine stripe like mattress ticking. Most made the uniforms themselves— with long sleeves and full, ankle-length skirts with two tucks in to let down in case they shrank. Detachable, stiffly-starched cuffs and close, stiff collars were fastened with studs. It was particularly uncomfortable in summer and although cuffs were removed for work and stowed behind an apron front, many nurses sponging a patient behind a screen took their collar off, too, for a moment of relief, invariably

[131]   *Ibid.*
[132]   *Ibid.*
[133]   Minutes of BM, 21 August 1918.
[134]   Lund, interview.

to be caught by someone looking over the top. The annual allocation of uniform material was a godsend to nurses on low wages, who frequently made their underclothing out of it. A change in uniform to a soft Peter Pan collar was attributed to the influence of a resident medical officer named Freddie Clark late in the 1920s.[135] White aprons had to be made to cover the uniform skirt, with straps crossing at the back. Black shoes with rubber heels for quiet walking, and black lisle stockings were worn. Staff nurses wore blue and Matron Balding's uniform was white, with which she wore a distinctive, English-style small cap trailing two tails about five inches wide down the back. A nurse's cap indicated her ranking in the hierarchical structure. First- and second-year probationers wore a basic cap—plain in front with five well-pressed pleats across the back—fastened onto their invariably long hair, which was swept up into a bun at the back. The third-year probationer had a beautiful single frill across the back of her cap. New patients quickly learned the ranking, and for nurses the difference in uniform reinforced the status that time, experience and learning gave them. 'You were always a little in awe of the ones that were very senior.'[136] Respect was necessary in a system where seniority made one a teacher of procedures that might either save a life or cause panic and faint-heartedness. Discipline of mind and in performance were integral in a nurses' training. The progress to staff nurse was marked by a change to a veil and sometimes by a ward's approbation. One graduate never forgot her reception: 'I was in charge of men's medical ward and I got a great clapping when I entered. It was really lovely of them.'[137]

The relationship between honorary medical staff and nurses was a distant one, although it privately seemed to nurses that they 'did the work, the doctors got the credit'.[138] Nevertheless they professed themselves 'very much in awe of the honorary doctors'. Newly graduated residents with minimal hospital experience were another matter and Dr Stubbe, who was firstly a junior resident, then an honorary medical doctor at the hospital for over 40 years, often said that the nursing staff taught him nursing.

Young women working and living together for three years, supporting each other, and sharing experiences relating to their work which would be difficult for an outsider to appreciate, grew close and often retained their contact throughout life. Being 'all hard up together' also helped.[139] Sometimes there would be a small gift of money or a cake from home, and then there would be a party in the quarters. Sometimes the nurses would organise a trip to the pictures—threepence on the ground floor and sixpence upstairs—or a trip by train to Perth. Often there was swimming off the rocks at South Fremantle in neck to knee bathers. Gentlemen friends were forbidden to enter the hospital grounds except for the annual dance, which was requested by nurses and held at their quarters. Nurses decorated and catered for it themselves, and a week before the event, probationers and their escorts gathered together with matron, who met the gentlemen and gave her tacit approval. One nurse's family supplied crayfish and everyone made something. A violinist and a

[135]   *Ibid.*
[136]   Parker, interview.
[137]   Lund, interview.
[138]   Parker, interview.
[139]   *Ibid.*

pianist provided the music. As staff numbers increased, the dance was held in the Town Hall but 'it was never quite the same'. The dominant memory, however, was that, 'we were really always too tired to do very much':

> Your main object was to sleep. But you see, as junior you had your time off very often in the mornings, ten till one or something, and you see you never got off on time because you hadn't finished your morning jobs. You had to be fully dressed in uniform for first dinner at one o'clock at which matron presided, so you didn't have much time to do anything and if it happened occasionally that you got off in the evening, well, then you had to go to a lecture.[140]

Days off for locals were usually spent at home, even though a train fare made a large hole in a weekly pay. A fellow trainee was often taken home, but the main occupation was still to 'sleep and eat'. Male friends had to be met in Alma Street outside the hospital grounds. Occasional evenings out were granted by a ward sister with matron's approval but it was a shared conspiracy that while the authorised late-comer handed her pass to the lodge keeper who opened the hospital gate at 10 p.m., others could pass below the window level, bent double, to avoid detection. If a nurse returned to the hospital outside the hour of curfew, the high wall surrounding the building could always be negotiated—'we had special places where we knew we could get over',[141] recalled one nurse. The knowledge passed on by a senior was not always medical.

Most Fremantle babies in the first years of the new century continued to be born at home under the direction of a midwife, although a woman could choose to be delivered at the Salvation Army Home. At first, few did, as it was recognised as a reception centre for wayward girls. Fremantle Hospital had no maternity ward, but occasionally an ill, pregnant woman, or one arriving at the point of giving birth, was not turned away. The practice of home birth was accepted both by prospective parents and the government; the former felt more comfortable with kin and community support, the latter considered the expense. Midwifery training was gained through direct experience and the shared knowledge of other midwives.

In 1909 there was a perceived lack of skilled maternity nurses and with the move to start a maternity hospital in Perth,[142] the government also moved to establish a midwifery training centre at Fremantle. The King Edward Memorial Hospital, which was built at Subiaco, was not opened until 14 July 1916, but the Fremantle centre was organised quickly. Midwifery training was placed unequivocally in the hands of male doctors. James Hope met with F. B. Allen, the director of technical education, and all the medical practitioners of Fremantle on 2 December 1909, to thrash out the rules and regulations. Applicants for training had to be aged between 24 and 45, and be of good moral character and physical fitness, with a certificate from a clergyman, a Justice of the Peace and a medical practitioner to prove it. The doctors wanted undisputed control of the centre and firmly decided against involv-

---

[140] *Ibid.*
[141] *Ibid.*
[142] P. Joske, unpublished history of King Edward Memorial Hospital; Bolton and Joske, *History of Royal Perth Hospital*, pp. 82–3.

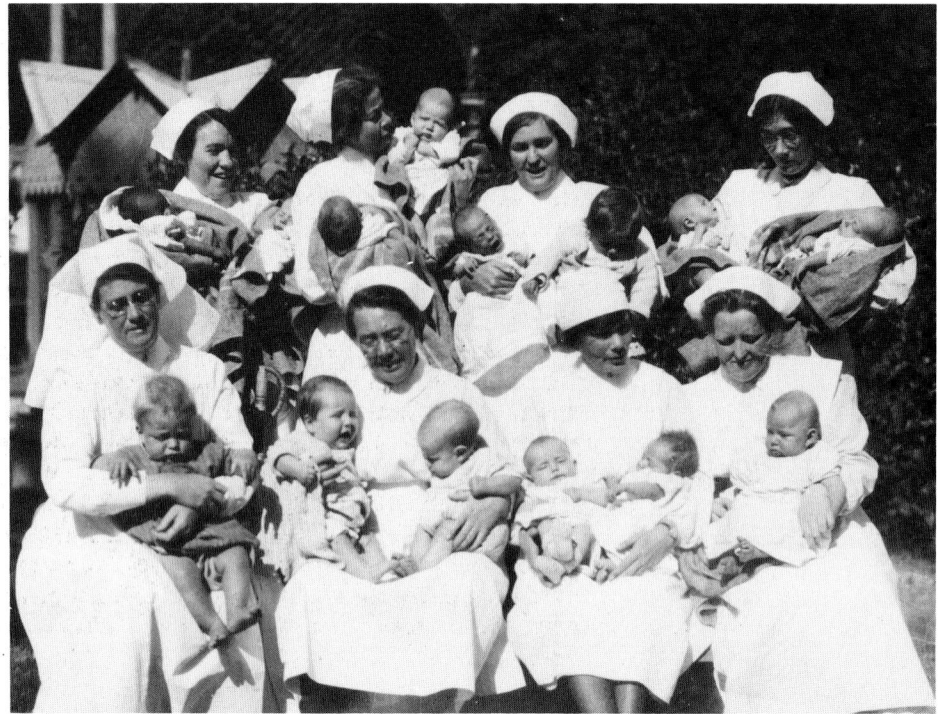

Photograph courtesy A. Orloff

Plate 17. Babies and nurses at the Salvation Army Hospital, Hillcrest, North Fremantle, 1920s.

On a couple of occasions Dr Dorothea Parker wanted to do a caesarean section and she brought the patient down from Hillcrest to the hospital ... There was one case that only had days to go and of course there was a fluttering upheaval in the women's medical ward when the baby was born. We kept the baby there until the mother was ready to take it home and everybody knitted and made baby clothes.

It was the 'in' thing for male babies to be circumcised, I don't know who the person was who said 'they shall be circumcised' but we used to do all the circumcisions at Fremantle.

Dr Stanley Barrington Knight

ing the technical school. Ten lectures would be given by two of their number in each of the six-month training periods held at the old lunatic asylum in Finnerty Street, which was being used as a home for old, sick or 'fallen' women. Practical instruction would take place at both the Salvation Army Home in North Fremantle and at the women's depot, where a minimum of 20 deliveries were to be observed of cases 'as are proper subjects for charity'.[143] The course included 'elementary female anatomy and physiology, the systems, mechanism, course of management of natural labour, haemorrhage, antiseptics in midwifery, the management of the puerperal

---

[143] PHD File 158/10. For brief history of the Salvation Army home, 'Hillcrest', see *Fremantle Gazette*, 18 August 1987.

state including the use of thermometer, catheter et cetera, the management and feeding of the newly born infant and the duties of the nurse with the regard to the seeking of medical aid'.[144] Jellet's *Short Practice of Midwifery for Nurses* and Merman's *First Lines in Midwifery* were recommended as text books. The fee for the class was set at ten guineas, one-fifth of which would go to the examiners and four-fifths to the instructors.

At the initial committee meetings held monthly at Fremantle Hospital under Dr David Williams, the resident medical officer at the women's home, it was reported that there were only two applicants, and eventually as the months passed, it was realized that the sum of ten guineas 'was prohibitive to the class of women desiring training'. On a decision to lower the fee to three guineas, with the government making up the rest of the doctors' fees, the school gained its first pupils and commenced in July 1910. Classes proved a great success and by the compulsory registration of midwives in 1911, 26 women had produced certificates by doctors as evidence that they had successfully conducted cases outside their training and were entitled to graduate as qualified midwives. Fifteen of the school's new graduates were among the 74 midwives registered in the Fremantle area.[145] Under the regulations of the Midwives Registration Board of 1911, training was extended to 12 months, so that pupils could gain more practical experience. Some difficulty was experienced with Salvation Army Staff Captain Gowden in his concern for their wayward sheep. He felt that unmarried girls expecting a child might not come for help if they became known by probationers. Drs White, Dermer and Williams were cautioned by the government to:

> Respect as far as possible their [the girls'] desire for secrecy, and when there is an opportunity of visiting this place for practical demonstration, the girls shall not be exposed to any curiosity to ascertain their identity by the probationers. I suggest that the girls when in labour in the presence of the probationers, should have a handkerchief or some light covering thrown over the face. As you know how necessary it is to have the use of this home, I should not [like] to have any possible excuse for them withdrawing it from our operations.[146]

The role of women as midwives and private nurses in community medical care was expanded in 1910 when North Fremantle council appointed Nurse Ryrie of Sydney as the North Fremantle District Nurse under the supervision of Dr Owen Paget. Hers was the task of teaching about cleanliness and adequate sanitary conditions, about the rearing of infants, and especially the need to keep their bottles clean. She was not to trespass on the doctors preserve by treating people who needed a physician's care. 'A trained nurse,' she assured 'would not do so; she knows the responsibility of her position.'[147] The Silver Chain nurses, with their newspaper-recruited club of children linked 'in a long chain of love, not to each other, but to all who come within their sphere of help and friendship' also made the community aware of their efforts to save life and relieve pain, especially among the 'suffering poor' and

[144]   PHD File 158/10.
[145]   See Register of Midwives in Hobbs, *But Westward Look*, pp. 209–29.
[146]   PHD File 158/10.
[147]   *Western Mail*, 2 July 1910.

less fortunate.[148] Nurse Thorup was the first Silver Chain nurse in the Fremantle district, and from 1913, she too visited the homes of the port's sick poor, counselling, nursing and cheering.

Although medical knowledge and practice had advanced by leaps and bounds by the turn of the twentieth century, there was yet much to learn. Early in the seventeenth century, William Harvey had shown that blood circulated through the body and although the microscope was in use and germs had been observed from the late 1600s it was not until Pasteur and Koch's work in the nineteenth century that it was proven that germs carried disease. Separately in Hungary and England, Semmelweis and Lister built on this knowledge to teach theories of antisepsis and the need for asepsis. Anaesthesia was used from the 1840s, and at Fremantle Hospital, the air always reeked of carbolic and chloroform. In 1897 William Rontgen's work on X-ray added an extra dimension to the usual diagnosis made by observation and palpation. Between 1898 and 1920 there was no insulin, no antibiotics, no intervenous therapy or sulphonamides. A doctor's ingenuity and a nurse's skill often directed a patient's healing. The house surgeon Freddie Clark once operated on a ten-year-old girl and

> . . . opened up her leg from one tuberosity on the knee to right down—and it was full of pus so they had to rig up a kind of drainage system and she had to have an anaesthetic for the first two or three dressings. And then Doctor Clark said, 'This will never do!' so he got to work and he got a hat rack from somewhere, and he got one of those winchester bottles, drilled a hole in it and a cork and he fixed up a drip system and that was the first time I ever saw a drip system put in—a continuous drip which was not painful—and we watched that child. I specialled that little girl. She was a marvellous case and a lovely little girl and you could see . . . I called sister over to say, 'Do you see what I see?' and there was little pink dots all down where the marrow was forming and it was really . . . we just about clapped our hands to see it, but she was in for a long, long time . . . and that girl walked out, thoroughly healed. No penicillin.'[149]

War surgery, although horrific, added new dimensions to medical knowledge and by the end of the war, blood transfusions were occasionally performed at Fremantle Hospital, 'but not directly'. Instead, a donor's blood was collected into a bowl and a nurse stood with aching arms, stirring and stirring, to prevent the blood clotting until it was transferred into the recipient.[150] Notwithstanding war, poultices were still standard treatment—linseed, mustard or antiphlogistine—the former made by spreading and folding up a putty-like mixture of linseed meal and boiling water on old linen ('a poultice properly mixed should leave the sides of the bowl perfectly

[148] *Ibid.*, 4 September 1909. The club commenced in 1905. See also *Western Mail*, 21 August 1909. 'I will try and collect some money for the poor, little sick children', wrote Nurse Cherry, the visiting nurse, in her weekly column, *Western Mail*, 14 August 1909. A week later she recorded, 'The difficulty is to find funds to tide patients who are seriously ill over their poverty and illness. This aspect of the work takes as much time and attention as does the work of actual nursing'. *Western Mail*, 21 August 1809. N. Stewart, *Little But Great. Saga of the Silver Chain (1905-1965)*, 1965, pp. 44-6.

[149] Lund, interview.

[150] *Ibid.* The existence of the four blood groups was discovered in 1907 by J. Jansky in Prague. Not until 1914 was sodium citrate recognized and used as a safe anticoagulant. See G. Williams, *The Age of Miracles—Medicine and Surgery in the Nineteenth Century*, 1981, p. 127.

clean') and bandaging it firmly onto the patient's chest or the required area. But it invariably seemed that one 'either had the linseed too hot, or too cold, or too thin, or too thick. If it was too thin it trickled down under the binder and into the bed. It was always wrong.'[151] Pneumonics had linseed poultices applied four-hourly day and night, while antiphlogistine was more commonly used for boils or areas showing pus. Foments of flannel or towelling dipped in hot water, wrung out and applied hot to the patient, were frequently ordered.

The board had planned and plotted for an X-ray unit for diagnostic use and cancer therapy from its earliest days, but it was not able to realise its ambition until 1907. In this year, when he went to England, Dr Thomas Anderson was entrusted with £120 of precious hospital funds to purchase 'the most useful and uptodate X-ray apparatus'. The £14.5.0 extra that was needed, Anderson paid out of his own pocket. The doctor returned in November 1907, a month after the steamship *Echunga*, with its precious medical cargo which was so eagerly awaited, but it was the end of January before the apparatus was delivered and installed in the out-patients' department. Perth Hospital loaned a part which had been omitted in packing and by February, private patients sent to the hospital by medical men for X-ray examination were paying between one shilling and sixpence and 21 shillings for the privilege. The dangers of X-ray were not fully appreciated and in the doctors' initial enthusiasm during the eleven months between April 1908 and April 1909 (no figures available for July), 450 X-rays were taken of hospital patients and 55 of private cases. By 1913 the number had dropped to 165 hospital and 28 private cases, while in 1918 only 75 hospital and three private patients were X-rayed. In 1917 the X-ray department and laboratory fittings were moved in the first of a series of moves over the years, to the old surgical ward in The Knowle, where a new laboratory was installed which extended the whole length of the room. So dependent had the honorary staff become on the apparatus, that when it was out of use in 1917 the doctors were reported as 'greatly handicapped thereby' and moves were made for its speedy restoration. The whole of the surgical ward was then taken over and used as an unsatisfactory dark room for developing the negatives on glass slides, but it was September 1919 before tenders were placed for a proper dark room. In July 1919, following his return from war, Mr W. S. Priestly commenced duty as radiographer and dispenser, and in this month he screened one hand, one foot, one hip, one elbow and one skull case. It was the first of many such working months.

A young junior house surgeon writing in 1906 from England to inquire about professional prospects in W.A., was rightly told by Lovegrove that 'vacancies occur fairly often in the service'.[152] Hospitals quickly engaged young doctors graduating from medical schools in Sydney and Melbourne and were delighted to employ young British-trained doctors on their staffs. Theatre work was one aspect of a doctor's training and surgery performed at Fremantle Hospital between 1898 and 1920 was

---

[151] Parker, interview. See also Nurse J. Brown's own lecture notes 1897–1898, Fulwood Hospital, Preston, Victoria—held at FH ... 'however careful you are' [when making a poultice], warns the instructor, Superintendent Nurse Back, 'you will make some mess and the kitchen where there is usually a large fire, always appears to be the best place, and if you are quick and have everything nice and hot you can always take it to the patient even hotter than they can bear to have it on.'

[152] PHD File 143/1906.

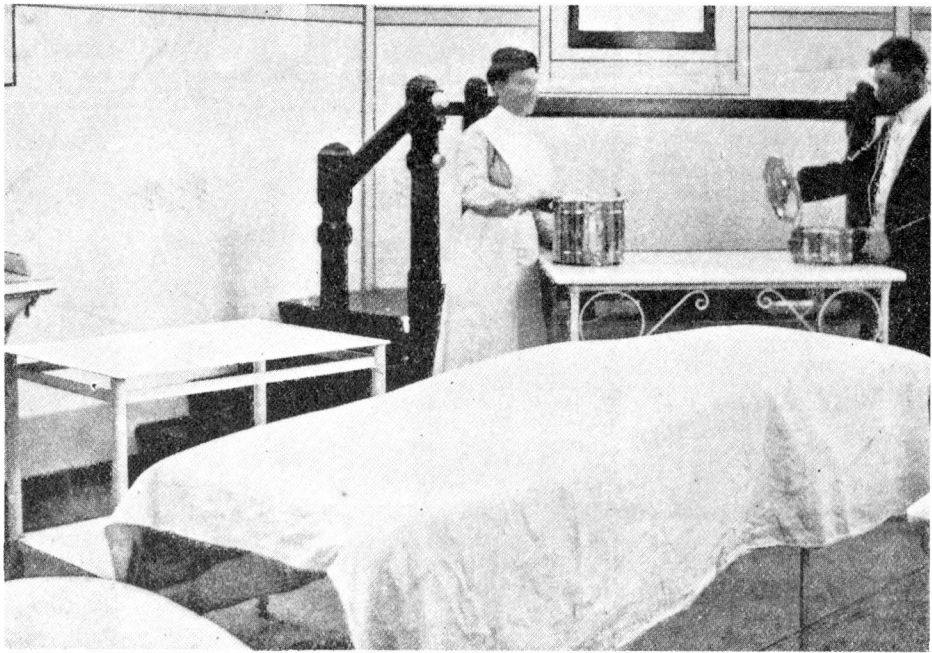

Photograph courtesy *Western Mail*

Plate 18.   The operating theatre, 1908.

Matron Balding told me that the theatre was designed to a plan by Dr Lotz who had been overseas and came back with this idea of having a platform a few feet out from the inner wall. The idea was that they would have a platform so that medical students or other people could observe the operation.

Matron Olive Jones

diverse and instructive. Some was diagnostic and at other times corrective. The long period of routine amputation was passing; a doctor in 1908 noted that 'today surgery is conservative, save if possible instead of lop off'.[153] Some surgery was major. A laparotomy for intestinal obstructions, ectopic pregnancies, peritonitis or a ruptured liver; trephining for cerebral tumours or a fractured skull were not uncommon. Breast cancer was scheduled for operation, a fractured patella wired, a haemorrhage removed by ligature and hysterectomies done. A thiersch graft was performed on an ulcerated leg, a hair lip repair attempted, and cataracts removed. Two men were shot in big toes within a week. One was cured, the other died in the rigor of tetanus. Tracheotomies for diphtheria cases were performed frequently and this operation also saved the life of a four-year-old after her larynx was badly scalded. Bones were set and an occasional amputation was still carried out. Tendons were divided to relieve a club foot and varicose veins removed. It was not unusual for a woman aged between 15 and 17 to come to the hospital to have a sewing needle

[153] PHD File 2044/1909. Report of Phillip Nutting to Principal Medical Officer, 24 October 1908.

removed from her hand or knee.[154] The nursing staff were treated when necessary: one received treatment for a floating kidney, and another for a septic thumb which became a septic hand within three months. A nurse had deformed toes straightened in 1914, whilst a senior who had been a charge sister for seven years by 1909 needed a hernia operation.

Henry Lotz was a brilliant surgeon, and leading doctors in Britain and Europe often sought his opinion on their research.[155] His decision to practise from Cantonment Street benefited both the people of Fremantle and the hospital's other honorary medical staff who consulted with Lotz over difficult diagnoses and treatments. John Thomas Smith was such a case. Diagnosed by a doctor on the goldfields as having blood poisoning in the brain, he was sent to the coast for a change of air. On the morning of 31 May 1903, Smith boarded the train at Perth but when it arrived at Fremantle railway station, he was found lying insensible in the carriage and was taken to Fremantle Hospital. Although in a torpor, when he was sharply pinched Smith responded in protesting slurred monosyllables. The man was not drunk or suffering narcotic poisoning and the honorary staff were perplexed at his condition. Henry Lotz, however, diagnosed 'a brain disorder' and scheduled immediate surgery to save the man's life. Deliberately he cut and removed a portion of skull behind Smith's left ear and immediately found three large abscesses, one extending an inch and a half into the brain. Lotz removed all three abscesses, operated on the man's inner ear, which had been diseased for over ten years, set drains in position and closed the wound. It was one of the first operations of its kind ever performed successfully and the press joined with townspeople who spoke of Lotz' skill: 'Several like operations have been performed in Sydney, but always with fatal results ...'[156] After nearly four months in hospital John Thomas Smith was discharged as fully recovered. The following month, through the press, he thanked the doctor and the sisters and nurses of the ward who had restored him to 'perfect health'.[157]

The death rate under surgery at Fremantle Hospital or within a few days after it, was not considered excessively high. There were eight deaths from 198 operations in 1909 and two deaths in 171 operations during 1910. But a man crushed by a train, or a patient with an intestinal obstruction, or one with a ruptured liver after being thrown out of a trap, or even one with a perforated typhoid ulcer, was a challenge to most doctors of the first two decades. With the arrival of Edward Thomas Brennan, a 1909 graduate from Melbourne, as senior resident medical officer in 1911, children between the ages six and 13 were diagnosed as having 'P.N.G' (Post Nasal Glands). They were operated on in blocks of between two and nine in number, one following another. The operation was soon known as 'T's and A's' (Tonsils and Adenoids). Brennan's example was followed by Anderson and to a lesser extent by Dr Barker. Young patients were less enthusiastic about this sudden interest in their sore throats.[158]

154   Fremantle Hospital Major Theatre Operation Record Book, 11 September 1908-3 November 1916.
155   R. Barrington Knight, interviewed by C. Jeffery, 10 December 1986.
156   *Morning Herald*, 21 September 1903.
157   *Ibid.*, 10 October 1903.
158   Fremantle Hospital Major Theatre Operation Record Book, 11 September 1908-3 November 1916. It
       is interesting to note that an appendectomy was first performed on 24 August 1883 at Guy's Hospital, London. *West Australian*, 19 January 1939.

Chloroform and ether, sometimes straight chloroform, occasionally ether, or a local anaesthetic were used in operations. Restrictions in war years brought changes; ether and cocaine were principally used in 1914 and only in a few instances was chloroform given. A hernia was done under a local anaesthetic and on 6 January 1915, novocaine was used for one patient. In 1915 chloroform was reintroduced as the most-used anaesthetic. Holding a gauze mask over a patient's nose with one hand and feeling the throb of pulse under the jaw with an extended finger, the anaesthetist, would slowly drizzle anaesthetic onto the mask—just enough to avoid patient reflexes and maintain good colour. A patient's colour, breathing, and pupils were the guide to his or her condition. The work required observation and skill. Although a doctor knew he had to watch for respiratory failure, the danger in using chloroform was as yet unappreciated. Post-operative vomiting was common and often tested the catgut stitches. Occasionally no anaesthetic was given for a thiersch graft on an ulcerated leg or for a patient with cardiac disease.[159]

Only one Aborigine appears to have been operated on. Registered only as 'person' he was diagnosed in June 1910 as having chronic osteomyelitis and his leg was incised and drained. His femur was scraped in August and again in January 1911.[160] Most patients registered with distinctly Anglo-Saxon names, but settlers and seamen from distant countries with names such as Bozonich, Edstrom, Sanmiguel, Siro, Schultz, Zuponovitch and Amid Bin Cassin were also patients. In unfamiliar hospital surroundings, sometimes unable to communicate with doctors, nurses and other patients, frequently fearful about their condition, these immigrants and sailors often felt great alienation. One sick sailor admitted from the visiting Dutch ship *Koningin Regents* in 1910, had the companionship of crewmen from three visiting warships when they visited him. Although ailing for some time, his not unexpected death was a blow to fellow sailors, who saw to his burial with Naval ceremony. Fremantle undertakers A. E. Davies & Co. had the coffin loaded onto a gun carriage led by dark shining horses and three squads marched through Fremantle streets to the cemetery on Carrington Street with the body of their crew mate. The coffin, draped in the Netherlands tricolour with the sailor's uniform cap on top, the four kettle drummers and two accompanying fifers, the ship's officers, and government and town council mourners, added to the ceremonial gravity of the morning, and small boys talked for weeks about three traditional bursts of shot fired outside the cemetery gate, beside the grave and then into the grave.[161]

In 1908, ten full years after the appointment of a board of management at the hospital, only Solomon, Hope and Birmingham were still involved in directing the business of the institution. Another set of the Fremantle respected joined the ranks, including jovial Fred Instone a noted plumber, and W. Mills, who owned the local thriving cake and biscuit factory. Hope left in 1909 to become the Principal Medical Officer, a position which was changed to Commissioner of Public Health in 1911,

---

[159] Fremantle Hospital Major Theatre Operation Record Book, 1908–1916. See also Anderson, interview.

[160] It is possible that three different Aborigines, each designated as 'person', may have been admitted at different times, each requiring similar treatment. There were few Aborigines left at this time in Fremantle. In 1897, only thirty-two were registered as eligible to receive the government's gesture of a free blanket each year.

[161] *West Australian*, 12 November 1910. This issue is marked 13 November in error.

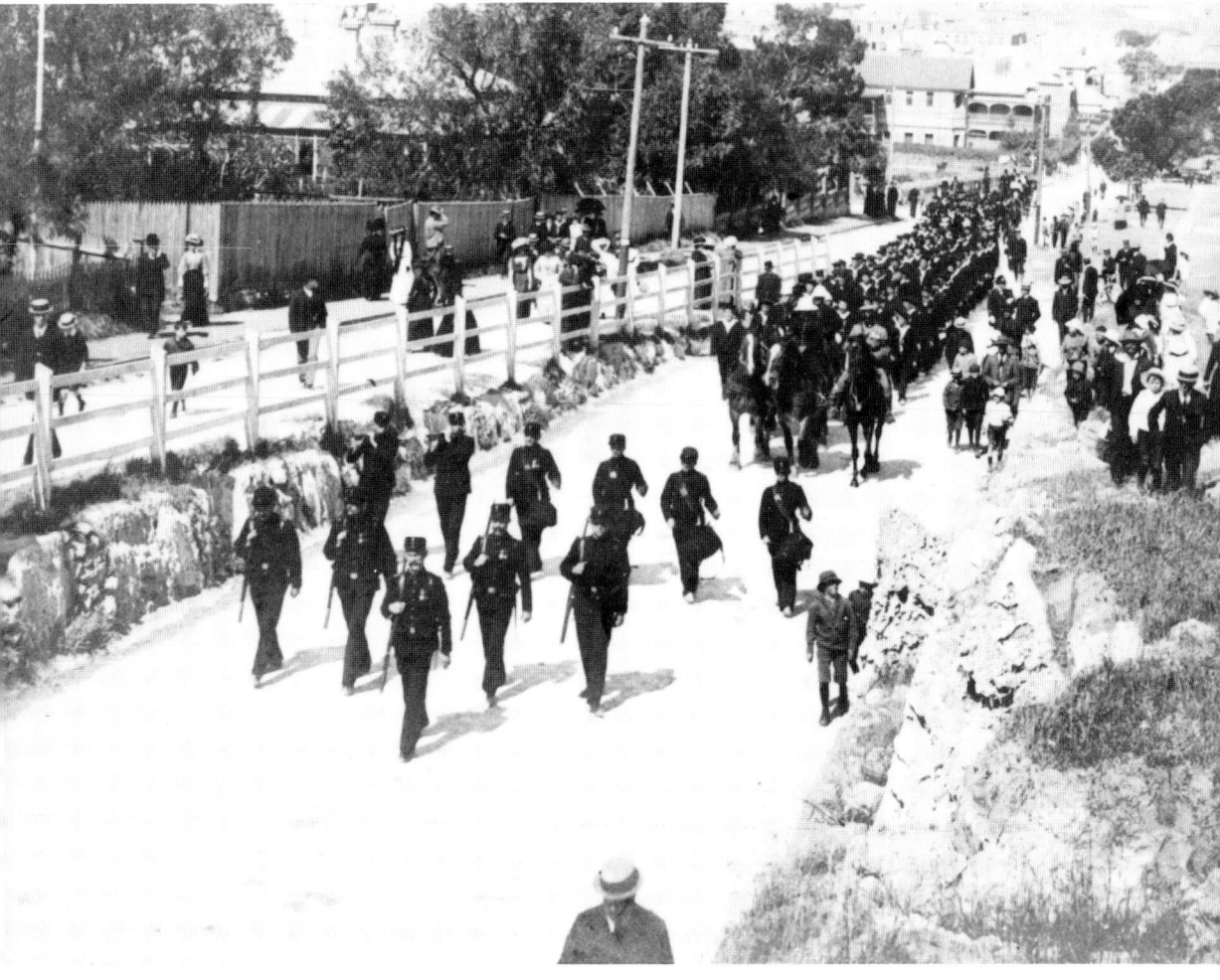

Photograph courtesy of West Australian Newspapers

Plate 19. In 1920 a Dutch sailor from the *Koningen Regentes* died in Fremantle Hospital. His funeral procession marched up High Street to the Carrington Street cemetery.

Despite the early hour the streets were lined with people ... In place of the band were four drummers and two fifers, who to the slow beat of the kettle drums played an old Dutch funeral march.

West Australian, 12 November 1910

and from this time, the number of medical men on the board was usually one but occasionally two. In 1911 Mrs W. A. Murphy was the first woman appointed to the board and Jean Beadle of the Fremantle Labour Women's Association joined her in the following year. When she resigned a few months later in July, her place at the board table was taken by Mrs A. K. Carpenter. By the second decade of the century, more local council representatives and fewer state politicians were on the board. Frank Rowe's appointment as the lumpers' representative in 1911 was a wise move. Energetic, conscientious, and down to earth, it was he who agitated for fire equipment, for work on the lift when the machinery lay rusting and open to the weather, and for basic maintenance that others did not see. In November 1912 the board decided to change the system whereby patients were admitted to wards through the patronage of subscribers to the hospital. At times, those recommended by subscribers were not the genuinely needy, and the board took upon itself the issue of orders for all treatments. The notice on the board at the gate was altered to read:

FREMANTLE PUBLIC HOSPITAL

for treatment of Indigent cases only

Persons desirous of Hospital treatment must obtain an order from a member of the Board of Management. The addresses of whom can be obtained from the gatekeeper. No order is necessary for accident or emergency cases which are attended to at any time.

Visiting days: — Wednesdays and Sundays between 2 p.m. and 4 p.m.

Two Visitors only.[162]

The change stressed the families of board members. William Wray remembered that when his father was on the board their family rarely had a meal in peace. Questions about an applicant's health and ability to pay had to be asked, and it seemed that prospective patients always came when the family sat down to eat. Harold Watson reflected that although the family had survived the period of his father's involvement in government and on the hospital board, it had been a big strain.[163]

In 1914 questions of an international nature were asked, and answered in blood. For four years the wharves at Fremantle, echoed to heavy military boots as soldiers from Western Australia joined ships and men from the eastern states with whom they would fight in a war which it was said would end all wars. For four years Fremantle people gathered on the wharf to farewell them, and one cornetist after another played 'Now is the Hour When We Must Say Goodbye'. For four years the lists of those who would never return was scanned with dread, and many, many families in Fremantle and throughout the country mourned. Some soldiers returned supported by an attendant, some limped and many on stretchers had suffered shocking wounds, the like of which were rarely seen in times of peace. Once again the old immigration depot on South Terrace which had been used as an emergency hospital in 1896 under K. Borough, housed the casualties of a greater emergency as the No. 8 General Australian Military Hospital.[164] In the group of scattered corrugated-iron and wooden buildings around the central courtyard of the A.G.H., or Base Hospital

---

[162] Minutes of BM, 26 November 1912.
[163] Wray, interview, FCL; H. A. Watson, interviewed by M. Howroyd, 7 and 8 May 1984, FCL.
[164] The building would later be used at various times as the headquarters of the Fremantle City Band, the Police Boys' Club, the Unemployment Relief Depot, The Labour Bureau, Police Quarters, St John Ambulance, Police Athletic Club, Infant Health Centre, Fremantle Benevolent Society. See index card, BL.

as it was called, men were treated mostly for gunshot wounds and shock. Those who were able, ate in the downstairs dining room and here pyjamas and dressing gowns were as common a uniform as the traditional khaki. Others preferred to lower coins down to the street on a piece of string so that a passer-by could get them fish and chips from the shop opposite.[165] On the first floor, officers were granted the privilege of a separate entrance to their ward and in all rooms and verandahs of the buildings, beds were crammed together for men who needed them. Trained sisters, doctors and volunteer wardworkers from the St John's Ambulance Brigade and the Red Cross joined with others to nurse the wounded. The work was long and continuous as hospital ships kept coming. Experiences were unforgettable to nurses, visitors and patients alike:

> ... and there were stairs up and we had one man in our ward and he had a leg operation, and he used to go up and down those stairs on his seat one at a time ... they managed exceptionally well. They helped one another so much and waited on one another ...[166]

Another recalled that as a paper boy he:

> ... would go down to the *Daily News* office and get a parcel of newspapers—and take the *Daily News* around to the patients in the wards. Oh, and they were smashed up terrible some of them too. Oh ... no legs, no arms. Yes, they went through a lot those poor souls ...[167]

The horror was too much for one patient who went into the flower garden one night and took his life.[168] As a patient, Albert Facey recalled his cardiac treatment after other external wounds had healed:

> A plaster about six inches square was placed over my heart. It had a drawing effect and caused a blister to form the full size of the plaster, and when the blister had drawn the fluid out about half to three-quarters of an inch, the nursing sister would put a kidney-shaped bowl underneath and tap it. About half a pint of fluid would run out into the bowl—it was the colour of muddy water. The sore that was left was dressed and bandaged until it healed properly, and then they would put another plaster on and I had to go through the same routine again.'[169]

In the town fishing was abandoned until daylight, and a search light beamed out from the mole to Rottnest and Garden Islands to check for enemy craft. Some young men wearing their heavy military boots were taught how to dance by the town's young ladies, and at East Fremantle Town Hall—in a reluctant response to the regretted imbalance of the sexes due to war—freak balls were sometimes held and no males were allowed to attend. White feathers were sent or delivered to those considered too cowardly to join up. Although between two and five soldiers might

---

[165] Notes by N. J. Foster, held at FCL.
[166] Lund, interview.
[167] Wray, interview.
[168] Lund, interview.
[169] A. B. Facey, *A Fortunate Life*, 1981, p. 283.

be brought directly to Fremantle Public Hospital each month for treatment in the early years of fighting, the impact of war was felt more in the depletion of staff and commodities, and in the continuing battle for funds.[170]

The board entered 1914 with a deficit and the position worsened. The welcome addition of Marmion's Cottage in 1913, after more than a decade of board-badgering and government refusal, caused some additional financial stress and routine maintenance and replacement was a continual drain on precious hospital funds. The new quarters were used to house the secretary and the domestics, and at times some nurses, but the rambling, isolated house made supervision of the staff living there, difficult at night. Early in 1914 the United Friendly Societies planned an Easter fund raising for the hospital, but so desperate was the financial plight that the board could not wait and wrote in February to the minister for public works explaining that it was impossible to carry on without either an increase in funds or the closure of some of the wards. Board members did their best. They went to West's Theatre company's 'Hospital Picture Night' to support the hospital cause and acknowledged a sweep that was organised to help raise funds. Contribution boxes were ordered to be placed in conspicuous places about the hospital with written notices inviting patients to contribute, even if they couldn't pay full charges, and six collection boxes were distributed throughout the town in places such as the Terminus Hotel and travellers' and workers' clubs. The financial status of patients was scrutinised even more carefully, even though the usual finding was 'not financially sound', and the hours of the gatekeeper who collected the out-patients' fees were reviewed and extended. During the year a masquerade concert was held on the hospital's behalf and £50 was gained from North Fremantle's 'Hospital Saturday' and their evening concert in December.

Goods donated to the hospital certainly helped—including fruit and vegetables from gardeners at Jandakot and 371 fresh eggs from an egg collection at a Caladonian hall dance. The occasional donation from either an individual or a company such as the Liberal Gathering Committee, the Fremantle United Friendly Societies or 'the sugar company' were welcome. During these difficult years, costs were saved by an increased use of prison labour from the other side of the high stone wall. A necessary incinerator was constructed by prisoners from materials supplied by the Public Works Department. The suggestion to work some vacant hospital ground with prison labour to provide a vegetable garden was allowed to slide, but in 1916 the prisoners' preparation of Forrest ward for male medical patients cost the hospital £20 compared to the £55 quoted by an outside contractor. Prisoners then renovated and painted the vacated medical ward and repainted the isolation ward, inside and out—including the cots, bedsteads and fittings—'. . . making an excellent job of it' with 'really good workmanship'.[171]

But the constant accounts for provisions and salaries and other costly urgent items outweighed the income. A new hot-water service, surgical instruments, a wheelchair, an urn for boiling water, a new laundry and a new mangle for the laundry were

---

[170] See H. Fletcher, interviewed by L. Stevens, 17 and 24 November, 2 December 1981, FCL; M. Foster, interviewed by G. Fowler, 27 March 1983, FCL; S. M. Kingsbury, interviewed by M. Howroyd, 12 March 1984, FCL.

[171] Minutes of BM, 16 May 1917.

needed. Fred Instone gave a fair deal on sterilizers for the theatre at £3.10.0 and on the 25 extra beds that had been needed for years and which were finally bought from a bequest left to the hospital by Walter Padbury. Patients painted the white screen frames ready for the 36 yards of sheeting bought to provide for their necessary moments of privacy. Nor could the purchase of blankets, sheets, draw sheets, pillowcases and towels be put off any longer. These, however, were charged to the Medical Department. The financial position was grim. The hospital workers' union, seeking a reduction in hours for orderlies, was told that, 'owing to the condition of funds and general arrangements' their claim was impossible.[172]

In May 1914 the accounts were £146 over the subsidy and the milk account of nearly £112 could not be paid. In the following month the colonial secretary paid this bill from the hospital subsidy and forwarded the remaining amount to the hospital. The board was outraged at the action, and considered that it should have been given the opportunity to pass the amount in the usual way. Chairman Mills stewed over the slight, and the following month, when the hospital was £258 in debt, he resigned from the board. His absence affected neither the deficit nor the board's determination to reduce it under Mr McLaren. It found in September, however, that there was no item where economy could be further exercised. So grave was the situation by October, that the board considered handing the administration of the hospital to the government. Earlier pleas for a special grant or a subsidy increase had been met with a shake of the official head; this time a boost of £471.1.1. and a promise to increase the subsidy by £500 eased the situation, but the accounts were still £73 in arrears. Mills was restored to the board and elected to the house committee with the 1915 appointments and Dr Campbell was voted as chairman, but the financial position remained serious. However, in light of war demands, hospital needs paled. The colonial secretary called for a reduction in hospital expenses and staff salaries in April 1915, but in a united decision the board and the entire staff rejected the notion. The board pointed out the increased number of patients—from 60 in-patients, 16 operations, 217 new out-patients and 784 reattendances in March 1914, to 65 in-patients 34 operations, 173 new out-patients and 869 reattendances in March 1915—and the waiting list for beds which grew daily: 'Our staff at present is undermanned and overworked and in no case overpaid, and we can see no way of making alteration',[173] they countered. By the end of September 1916 the hospital's deficit totalled £700.

The board's decision in February to close the infectious diseases ward, merely caused the unsympathetic government to call for general reductions in the board's spending rather than to close a ward. Real help, however, came through the community. The Lumpers' Union had always supported the hospital and had been its first contributor at the Point Street building in 1896, with a donation of £10. That hot February in 1915, when five guineas were collected by sympathetic troops for refreshments to cool the lumpers working on their boat, the lumpers decided to donate the sum to the hospital. While donations had always fallen short of that hoped for by the government, like the lumpers, many Fremantle people consistently supported their hospital. In October and November of 1916 alone, £2.2.0. was

172   *Ibid.*, 3 March 1914.
173   *Ibid.*, 6 April 1915.

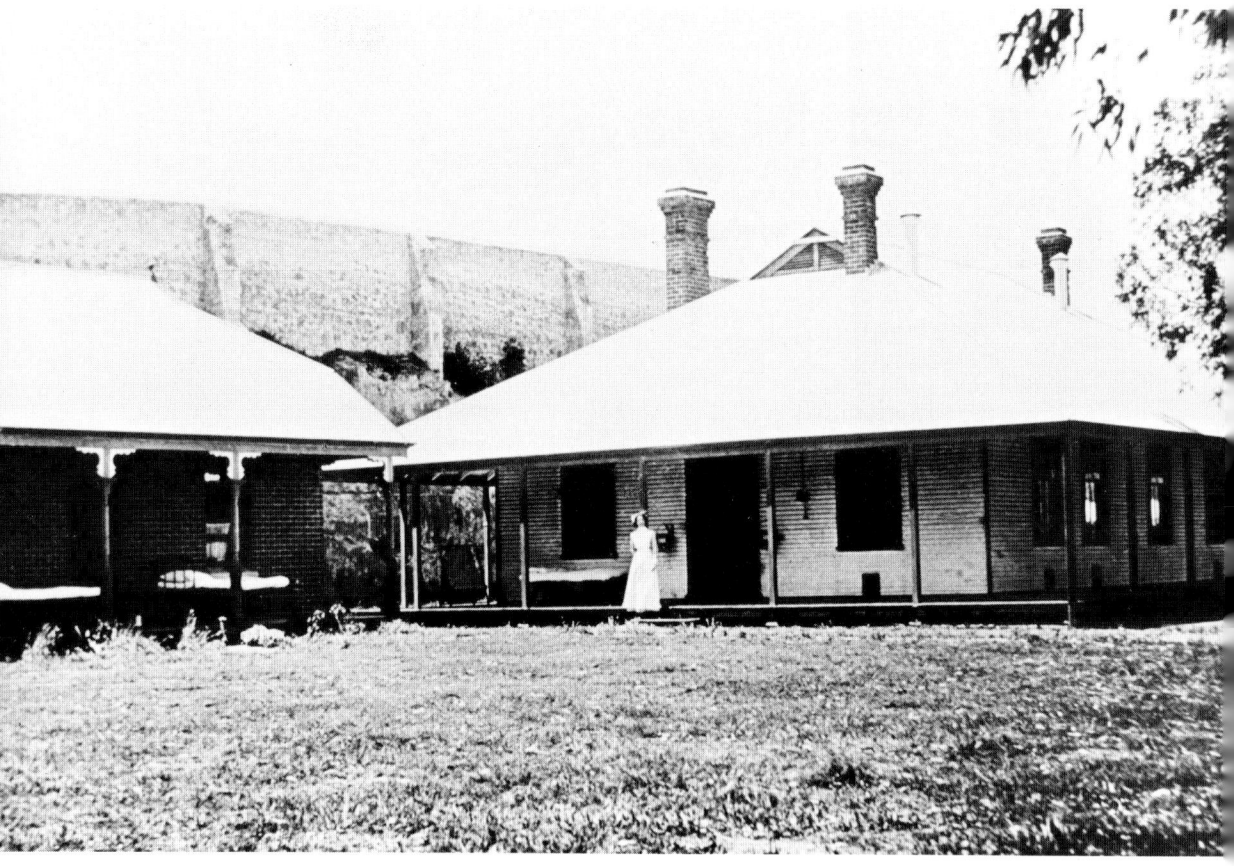

Photograph courtesy Fremantle Hospital

Plate 20.   Nurses' quarters and isolation ward, with the Fremantle prison wall in the background.

received from M. Riley, £1.0.0. from Mrs Chester, £2.6.4. from the Tramways Board and R. Salter offered part of the proceeds from the East Fremantle Childrens' Fancy Dress Ball. The grand sum of £18.15.0. was raised by the Economic (Fremantle) Girls' Football Club and £1.12.10. came from the collection boxes. Although appreciated, these monthly donations by individuals and organisations were not enough for the hospital's needs.

In early 1917, however, the committee of the Owners' and Trainers' Association decided to organise a horseracing carnival at Bicton for the hospital. The 24 March proved a wonderful day. Prominent racing men came from Perth for the event, and many racegoers paid five shillings to enter the enclosure and gain the chance to win the racehorse Harry Lauder. The jockey E. Bowden who held the winning ticket, number 650, redonated the horse for sale and raised another £8. A committee of Fremantle ladies made a collection and everyone cheered the running of the six races—the Doctors' Plate, the Nurses' Purse, the Hospital Handicap, the Orderlies' Trotting Handicap, the Benefit Handicap and the Patients' Handicap, each with a purse of 20 sovereigns.[174] At the end of the afternoon £819.6.9 had been collected for the hospital. Not only had it been an enjoyable day, but contributors received the private satisfaction of giving and some perhaps the satisfaction of public approbation when their names appeared in print in the *West Australian* and the *Daily News*.

To the hospital's satisfaction and relief they were only £136 overdrawn for the financial year in 1917. While government assistance to the hospital was restricted during the war, the help of Fremantle people continued, although the 40 wooden collection boxes in various hotels reluctantly had to be changed to sturdier ones of metal ordered from Cumpston's Store. In July 1917 an Ugly Women's Carnival raised the magnificent sum of £750 to supplement smaller donations from individuals and companies such as the National Bank, the Union Bank of Australasia, Fremantle Tramway and Electric Light Board, Fremantle Workers' Club and Mills and Ware employees, Fisherbeard, F. H. Faulding and Co. and the North Fremantle Amateur Dramatic Society. The Barmaids' and Barmens' Union, the Melbourne Steamship Company, the Federated Seamen's Union of Australasia also gave. A little revenue was made by increasing hospital charges to the shipping companies who paid three guineas a week for the treatment of their sailors and it was pleasing in June when patient fees reached a record of £243. One man paid his account with three blocks of land. In January 1918, for the first time in six years, the books showed a credit balance.

In the last year of the war and despite the sharp sword of refusal that seemed poised always ready to trim plans for extensions and improvements in the name of 'insufficient funds', it was apparent that something would have to be done about a new nurses' home when the military commandeered Marmion's Cottage. The 25 new Bon Marché beds bought for the nurses when the old ones threatened to fall apart in 1916, were only a palliative measure of comfort. Matron pointed out that conditions were trying at the nurses' home, with 23 probationers sharing only eleven bedrooms. On warm nights a large number of nurses slept outside. By 1917 hospital authorities feared that they were liable for prosecution under the *Health Act* with nurses having to sleep on the verandah due to overcrowding, and Matron Balding despaired.[175] A new wind-screen of trellis work, fixed to shield nurses sleeping in bays on the verandah was helpful in fine weather but proved useless in winter storms when an umbrella of ingenuity was of greater protection. An enterprising nurse recalled:

> One girl and I slept together in the bed one night when it was raining and blowing and we slept on my bed—and her mattress (they were the good old horsehair mattresses) we stood up against the bed to keep the rain off us.[176]

The quarters which had seemed so fine early in the century were positively inade-

[174] *West Australian*, 25 March 1917.
[175] Minutes of BM, 11 July 1917; Matron's Report Book, 11 July 1917.
[176] Parker, interview.

quate by 1918 and plans to extend the old building were condemned by the house surgeon who inspected the nurses' quarters:

> I find that the circumstances under which they are housed are most unhealthy and must needs cause very great inconvenience and annoyance. There is no element of comfort. During inclement weather the conditions are such in several cases three nurses were obliged to sleep in a room which in itself is not capable of containing three beds. The proposed addition as per plan would be inadequate for the comfort and convenience of the staff.'[177]

Premier Hal Colebatch, visited the hospital one Sunday night and reaffirmed his support for a new nurses' quarters. Many meetings later the government finally decided to build a new, rectangular, two-storey home to accommodate 30 nurses and to use the vacated home for the smaller number of domestic staff. The contract price of £3,928 was viewed with complacency. 'It is gratifying to know that the new building will cost less than the estimated cost of patching up the old quarters.'[178] In August the footings were dug. In September the lower-storeyed framework was completed. By November, when the town rocked with celebrations of peace, the roof was almost on and the board was fighting to have a 'lavatory basin' supplied to each bedroom.

> The board still desire that if possible this work should be carried out. The suggestion that same may prove unhealthy should not be allowed to prevent the carrying out of work of such importance to the convenience of the nurse, and we are satisfied that the abovementioned risk is infinitesimal ... all up to date buildings such as hotels et cetera are fitted with basins as suggested in our previous request.[179]

With its deficit in mind, the board launched an appeal for £2,500 for hospital expenses and the fitting up of the nurses' home. In February 1919, the new home was completed with its box room erected off the verandah to leave more sheltered space for relaxation, and the jarrah woodwork oiled ready for polishing. A good reliable supply of hot water was laid on from the laundry. The new quarters stood unfurnished in splendid isolation while funds were raised for fittings. Twenty-three promises of £20 each were made by townspeople towards suites of furniture and it was hoped that prisoners might fill the ground around the home and lay out the grounds to cut costs. Before everything was ordered and in place the military took over Marmion's Cottage and the nurses moved into 'The Home'. In the quickly-renovated old quarters, each maid was provided with her own room in which was a wardrobe and a wash stand and duchess. The old laundry was divided into three bedrooms and a sitting room with a verandah on three sides for the orderlies. In its move to Marmion's Cottage, the military indirectly served the hospital well.

In no way did the war affect Fremantle Hospital more than through the insatiable demand for its staff. The board worried as resident and honorary doctor alike left to serve his country and the hospital prepared to lose its matron. The drain was under-

---

[177]   Minutes of BM, 15 May 1918.
[178]   *Ibid.*, 21 August 1918.
[179]   *Ibid.*, 18 December 1918.

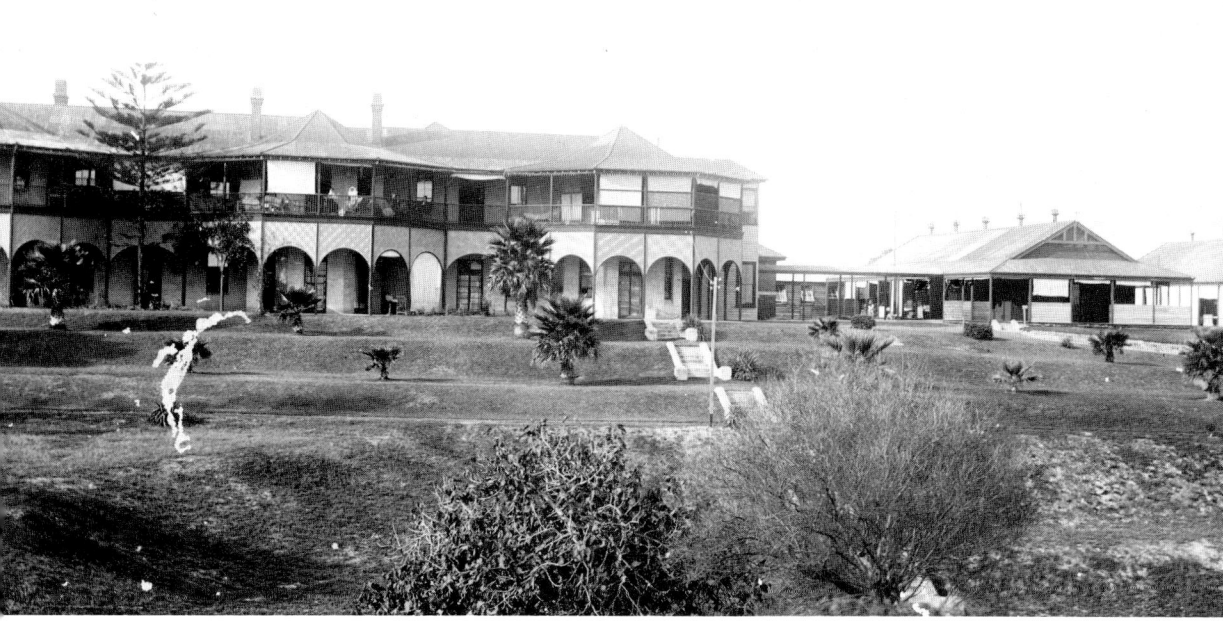

Photograph courtesy Fremantle Hospital

Plate 21.   The Knowle, c. 1920s.

> ... there were big verandahs all the way round. We had patients out there during some of the finer months, you know ... when it was nice and when they were able to be wheeled out.

> Margery Lund
> Nursing Staff

way by October 1914, when Dr Sawers, the senior resident medical officer, departed, leaving Dr Yuille as the only resident doctor. Young Dr Parer was recruited to the hospital later in the month, but both doctors soon resigned—Yuille to go with the military in December and Parer in March, the month in which Anderson from the honorary staff also left. Another resident doctor was quickly engaged. His frequent absences which left the hospital with no medical attendant, frustrated the other staff, especially in emergencies, and the board often heard reports of its medical officer's lack of attention to his patients. After his resignation was called for in September 1915, the hospital vied with the military for a surgeon and for nearly three months it had no resident doctor. At the end of the June 1915 meeting, the board lost its chairman when Dr Campbell resigned because of 'military duties now cast upon him'.[180] White and Anderson had already sought leave from the

180   *Ibid.*, 21 June 1915.

honorary staff until the end of the war and in July 1915 Dr Lotz left his honorary position to take that of honorary consultant. The new honoraries, J. S. Landon and W. E. Blackall, received a baptism of fire as they joined with the old honorary staff—Birmingham, Parer, Blaxland and Dermer, helping to hold the medical services at the hospital together. Sometimes they were assisted by doctors passing through Fremantle on their way to the front, but the night sister, sometimes with matron's help, had to cope with emergencies at night. The board offered a £75 incentive to a doctor who would work 12 months at the hospital, and were relieved in January 1916, when Phillip Nutting from Busselton was loaned to the hospital by the State Medical Department.

The first weeks under Nutting passed uneventfully as staff and doctor felt their way in the mutual relationship that was necessary to best benefit a patient. Nutting performed only one operation at the hospital but acted as anaesthetist many times. If a deterioration in relations in the theatre was reflected in the keeping of the hospital operations book there was not always harmony when a patient needed it most. The total number of patients admitted in the six months prior to Nutting's coming was 364, just 28 more than the number admitted after his arrival, and there were only five more operations performed while Nutting worked at the hospital, than in the previous six months. The average number of deaths after surgery was almost constant.[181] However, when an unprecedented total of nine patients died following operations in June, tempers may have frayed. Neither was Matron Balding's temper the best after Nutting started to intrude on her area of administration. Not only did the doctor enter the nurses' dining room at 6.30 a.m. to disturb the morning meal, but he went to the kitchen daily at dawn to supersede her instructions to the cook.[182] Small wonder this challenge to matron's efficiency was resented.

Phillip Nutting had a tendency to alienate certain of his contemporaries and when he took a dislike to someone it was not done in secret.[183] His dissatisfaction with one of the sisters was expressed in rudeness to her in the wards and in front of patients and staff. When matron took him to task the doctor extended the disrespect to her. So awkward and unseemly was the situation and so adamant matron's complaint, that a special board meeting was called to which the protagonists were invited. On the afternoon of the scheduled meeting, 26 July 1916, Nutting received news that his eldest son had been so badly wounded at the front in France that little hope was held for his recovery. The worried father asked secretary Priestly to give his apologies to the meeting, but no message was relayed to the board. Mills, as chairman, concluded for all present that 'the whole trouble is that Dr Nutting has acted in a most ungentlemanly way to matron and nurses and nothing could justify such conduct from one in his position'.[184] Since he had not availed himself of the opportunity to attend

---

[181] Calculated from Fremantle Hospital Major Theatre Operation Record Book. The average number of deaths during and following surgery increased from 6 to 6.1 in the six-month period after Nutting's arrival.

[182] Minutes of HC, 21 August 1916.

[183] After coming to Western Australia from St Kilda in Melbourne, Nutting had worked in harsh conditions at the isolated prospecting field of Blackrange for 15 months from 1905, and later at Wagin. His health, not the best, was undermined by his conflict with townspeople wherever he lived. See PHD File 2044/1909.

[184] Minutes of BM, 26 July 1916.

the meeting as matron had done, Nutting was informed that the board had unanimously come to the conclusion that matron was in the right and that his resignation
was expected. Nutting, however, refused to resign, and appealed to the colonial
secretary:

> ... As I have received no explanation as to the reasons which actuated the Board in
> taking this step, and as I am prepared to uphold my conduct to the fullest extent, I must
> ask you, as my chief, to make the fullest inquiry in the matter . . .[185]

Once again the government and the board faced each other over a principle. Why,
demanded the colonial secretary, had Nutting been asked to resign? The board had
investigated the matter, replied Mills and decided that Dr Nutting's services to the
hospital should cease forthwith. Perhaps, he suggested, further friction could be
avoided if Nutting was recalled and transferred. But the doctor continued to reject
the idea of resignation and the board united in this challenge to its authority.

On 9 August, with the authority of Section 12 of *The Hospitals Act* of 1894
behind him, the colonial secretary drew the board's attention to the fact that while it
had administrative authority over funds, the board could only nominate persons for
appointments and dismissals subject to the Governor's approval. The echoes rever-
berated back to 1903. On Wednesday, 16 August, with 'a state of unrest amongst the
whole staff' at the hospital, the house committee went to Perth to explain to the
colonial secretary how urgent the position had become. By the time of the special
board meeting on the following Monday, there had been no official reply. Priestly
rang the colonial secretary only to find that he was out of town and nothing had
been done in the matter. It was an anxious and unsettling time for those involved.
Matron Maida Balding was invited into the meeting and assured of the board's support and an urgent telegram was sent to the colonial secretary:

> Extremely surprised at no reply to our personal interview 16th. Hospital in state of
> chaos. Position intolerable. Special meeting today adjourned until 4 on Wednesday
> afternoon. Your decision requested.[186]

Patients and others wrote to the colonial secretary of Nutting's 'attention and
great kindness to those under his care'[187] and the colonial secretary replied in time
for the special hospital board meeting on 23 August: 'I am requested that your
board will hold a full inquiry, and that the witnesses including Nutting be examined
on oath.'[188] Full power of discretion was to remain with the board members who
would be appointed as a legal commission. The board, however, was not agreeable.
Had it not already made a full inquiry into the matter? Chairman Mills maintained
that although no objection could be taken to the professional qualifications of Nutting, the issue was that as matron and the nursing staff could not agree with the
doctor, Nutting should be recalled. Declining to accept responsibility for any trouble
if Nutting was retained, the board went ahead and arranged for the passage from

---

[185]   *West Australian*, 25 August 1916.
[186]   Minutes of BM, 21 August 1916.
[187]   *West Australian*, 19 October 1916.
[188]   Minutes of BM, 23 August 1916.

Sydney of Dr Marshall as their new medical officer. The members even thought about resigning. In Mills' 15 years on the board, the minister's confirmation of an appointment had never been withheld, but he professed, that as he did not want the matron and part of her staff to follow his lead and resign, he would stay: 'To see that justice was done to those of the staff who were unable to help themselves'.[189] The press delighted in the affray and began to speak of the power of the government as '... only a matter of the impression of a rubber stamp'.[190] The government bristled and determined to protect its officer. For his part, Nutting explained to the press that although he regretted fighting three members of the opposite sex, he was compelled to defend his name and hitherto untarnished reputation. The conflict had come about as a result of his reproof, merely offered in an effort at reformation necessary at the hospital.[191] By the end of August the board was calling for an independent inquiry into the hospital conflict. At the out-patients department and in the wards, the honorary medical staff worked overtime.

Between 3 and 4 o'clock on the morning of 29 August, Nutting collapsed in the corridor outside his sitting room. Dr Blaxland stayed with him until 9 a.m. and two of the senior sisters, Skinner and Larity, and two orderlies under matron's direction were ordered to attend to him. Dr Webster, who was Nutting's medical advisor, in consultation with W. E. Atkinson and Dr Anderson, then organised two male attendants to care for the doctor. It was no time to hold an inquiry. Nutting was pleased, however, when his brother arrived from Sydney and visited him each day. Nevertheless the board remained unmoved in its opposition to the doctor. On 4 September it agreed that while Nutting's serious illness was regrettable, his services had already been dispensed with and he could not be granted sick leave. Futhermore, that as Dr Marshall was arriving in a few day's time the resident medical officer's quarters were needed for his use. Marshall was appalled to arrive in the midst of such chaos on the 11 September. His stay in the nurses' sick bay and the board room which was hastily cleaned and converted for his use was brief. A little over a week later he resigned to take up a military appointment. Neilson Hancock, the medical agent, held no hope of obtaining another doctor from Sydney and once more the board faced the daunting prospect of finding a medical officer in time of war.

Despite Nutting's serious illness, it was not he who died, but Chairman Mills, on 7 October. A cab and a wreath were sent as a gesture of the board's regret, and most members attended the funeral of the man who had worked for so long for the hospital. As the need for a resident medical officer was great, the board was anxious to settle the matter of Nutting, and offered to expunge from the minutes the resolution dismissing the doctor, provided the colonial secretary would gazette his recall to the Medical Department. If no settlement had been made by the following board meeting, however, they threatened, they would have a full statement ready to release to the press. At the end of October and after yet another board deputation to the colonial secretary, word was received from Premier Frank Wilson claiming to be generally indignant and surprised that his earlier agreement to recall Nutting had not been carried out. This time action was rapid and the following day, Nutting—a man as

189   *West Australian*, 25 August 1916.
190   *Daily News*, 24 August 1916.
191   *Ibid.*, 25 August 1916.

determined as his great grandfather Captain William Bligh[192]—was ordered to leave the hospital. He would practice medicine at Mandurah and at Gingin as a valued medical officer before spending three years in retirement near the sea at Cottesloe, in ill-health. No one from Fremantle Hospital was mentioned as being present at his funeral 15 years later in 1931.

For a month the hospital had no resident. So serious was the position that the board promised a fee of a guinea to any doctor willing to give anaesthetics for operations performed in the hospital by the honoraries Birmingham, Landon, Parer, Blackall and Blaxland. On 1 December 1916, the hospital recruited young Dr Arnold, fresh from Melbourne University, who lived and worked at the hospital for six months before donning a military uniform. Of the honorary staff, Blaxland left in March 1917 and Charles Douglas Kerr from Meekatharra was temporarily appointed in his place. Dr Blackall was replaced by Dr East when he was called to military duty and Drs Paget and Tregonning also temporarily joined the honorary staff. Birmingham left on 16 January 1918 after 'long and continued valuable services'[193] to the hospital. The next to leave was Owen Paget in 1918. It was a period of much upheaval.

The need for doctors to treat the thousands who fell at Gallipoli, Flanders and in France did not waver. Twelve thousand of the 32,000 West Australians who fought, came home with awful, visible, physical proof of their involvement. Six thousand did not return.[194] Others lived an internal hell that often could not be shared with those at home. It seemed that every family lost someone. Many of the men and women who joined the military or service groups such as the Red Cross or the V.A.D.'s left their work at Fremantle Hospital to do so—gardeners, office boys, orderlies and occasionally domestic staff. In October 1916, secretary Priestly followed his wife, a nursing sister already a year at the front, and Mr H. Arliss Robinson was appointed secretary and dispenser at £5 a week with board and lodging. Domestic staff at the hospital worked where the need was greatest. Housemaids acted as cook or laundry maid. Staff combined positions or just filled in. A German patient, Otto Bigeleki, was sent to assist in the kitchen for a few days and even the male gardener, J. Kirby, worked as a kitchen-maid for a while in 1916. The turnover of domestic staff was high. Some maids became ill, others proved unsatisfactory in their positions, a few left to marry and one or two were dismissed after being found under the influence of alcohol. In 1916 the board heard with relief that cook Sampson had commenced on 14 December, and 'the members of the Domestic Staff resumed their usual duties'.[195] When Sampson left in May the new cook worked just 13 days, the next cook only three weeks, and Mrs Murphy of the board was told it had 'long been a difficulty to secure and keep a cook'.[196] Sometimes a cook left after a day. At these times Matron Maida Balding would step in: 'She'd roll up her sleeves and go in and do the cooking for the whole hospital.'[197] The work was always heavy

192 *West Australian*, 22 January 1931.
193 Minutes of BM, 16 January 1918.
194 See Crowley and de Garis, *A Short History*, p. 67.
195 Minutes of BM, 10 January 1916.
196 *Ibid.*, 12 June 1916.
197 Lund, interview.

and hot in summer and new kitchen-maids had to be trained each few weeks. After eleven years at the hospital, N. McNally was transferred from the laundry to the position of cook and finding the kitchen work 'too arduous'[198] she left in 1918. The age group of orderlies increased, as most men between 18 and 44 were away at the war. They received £1.2.6. a week and a white half coat as uniform from August 1916. Despite the fact that 'great inconvenience had been caused by inability to obtain efficient orderlies' a second ranking orderly was immediately dismissed in 1918 'for being insolent to matron and general insubordination'.[199] Some of the orderlies who worked were only filling in time until their call to the military. There was still talk of matron being called up, but the dearth of doctors was constant.

The Fremantle Hospital Board worked diligently for the institution entrusted to its administration but most of the members were conservative in outlook. In 1903, when the Perth Hospital Board broke new ground in appointing Dr Ethel Ambrose to the resident medical staff, their contemporaries in Fremantle possibly sided with the Perth honorary medical staff who protested at the move. While a nurse was expected to insert an enema or catheter, and sponge or dress the different sections of her male patients' anatomy in the performance of her duties, it was considered different for a lady doctor. It was also expected that while women would unhesitatingly unburden themselves to a male doctor, that a man would never make a confidant of a lady. 'It is unfair to ask her to so absolutely unsex herself,' reasoned one of the Perth honorary medical officers, and 'unfair to the patients that they should be compelled to continue their suffering because they are precluded from confiding in their medical attendant.'[200] So desperate was the board at Fremantle, however, that when Arnold left his position as resident medical officer in June 1917, the members contemplated engaging a female doctor. Debate was brisk but as the secretary concluded, 'the idea of engaging a lady as house surgeon was discussed as unworkable'.[201] Douglas Kerr filled the position until Milton L. Coutts arrived on 1 January 1918 for a six-month term. After that the hospital was for three months without a resident medical officer. One applicant for the vacant position was Dr Hilda Kershaw. Exceptional times demanded exceptional measures. It was not an easy decision and it generated great discussion, but at length the board decided to appoint a woman as Fremantle Hospital's resident medical officer. Her arrival was delayed by a strike on the transcontinental railway and she did not arrive until 24 October 1918. When she left the hospital 12 months later, the board gave her a special letter of genuine appreciation.

The war affected all areas of hospital administration. The cost and scarcity of groceries, butter, meat and drugs inevitably unbalanced carefully calculated estimates. The cost of some drugs increased by over 100 per cent. In October 1913 the drug bill for a daily average of 58 patients totalled £16.4.4. but by October 1917 it was £64.1.0 for 50 patients.[202] While all departments suffered dislocation, none affected the hospital's operation more than the depletion and rotation in trained

[198]   Minutes of BM, 17 July 1918.
[199]   Ibid., 20 February 1918.
[200]   West Australian, 15 August 1903; Bolton and Joske, History of Royal Perth Hospital, p. 70.
[201]   Minutes of BM, 11 July 1917.
[202]   West Australian, 9 January 1917.

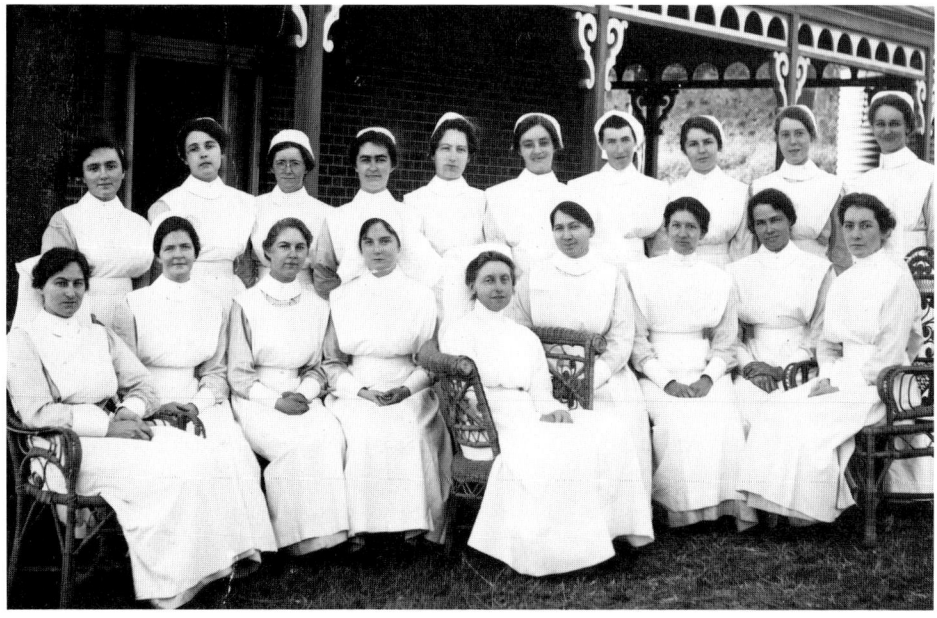

Photograph courtesy Fremantle Hospital

Plate 22.   Due to war, a very junior nursing staff, 1917.

Back row (left to right): Nurses Bell, Leo, Elphick, Kiernan, Donnelly, Livermore, Grono, Evans, Jouning, Mercer.
Front row: Nurses Leeds, Taylor, Draper, Doherty, Matron Balding, Nurses Cannard, Cowcher, O'Shanassy and Sister Agar.

> Miss Sharpe—Charge Nurse—commenced duty 25th, left for Military May 1st; Charge Nurse Jeffrey left hospital for military duty May 9th; Charge Nurse Larsen on day duty April 22nd; Staff Nurse Reidy taking night charge duty from annual leave April 29th; Probationer Draper off duty sick since April 25th discharged from ward May 12th and is on leave for one week; Probationer Grono off duty sick since May 14th; Probationer Leeds off duty with injury to head May 2nd to 7th; Probationer Cannard completes her training May 31st and is entitled to her certificate.
>
> Matron's Report to Board,
> 16 May 1917.

nursing staff. By 1916 it was—as one nurse remembered—'embarrassing, it was almost impossible to get trained staff. They'd come in and matron would be thrilled to think she had got a staff and then one by one they would go off to the base hospital—the call-up.'[203] In June 1914 the nursing staff comprised the matron, three charge nurses, three staff nurses and 16 pupils. The exodus was well underway by May 1915 when Nurse Walsh and newly-graduated Staff Nurse Scanlan were given leave to serve abroad. Until this time nurses just left and joined up. In June, Sister Parker left for the military after working only three weeks at Fremantle Hospital and in July she was joined by Sisters Carson, Baillie and Cronin. As a result of press

[203]   Parker, interview.

advertising (later as far as Sydney and Adelaide) and an invitation to graduating Fremantle Hospital nurses to stay as staff nurses, the level of trained staff was almost maintained. Despite the departure of Staff Nurse Cowcher in November 1915, there were four charge nurses, two staff nurses and 17 pupil nurses at the hospital in that month.[204] Staff Nurse Croham, then Charge Nurse Edsall and Sister Irene Kiernan were specifically recorded as leaving for military service in 1915 but others also left the hospital and joined the services soon after.[205] With the involvement of Australian troops in France and at Gallipoli and with the first use of military tanks in 1916, the need for military nurses increased and it became extremely difficult for the hospital to recruit trained staff. 'Charge nurses have again been advertised for,' reported matron in 1917, 'and every effort has been made to replace sisters who have resigned'.[206] Other hospitals were similarly affected and Fremantle Hospital lost one of its valued charge nurses when Sister Howard was appointed matron at Meekatharra Hospital in March 1917. A new charge nurse was recruited in her place commencing on 25 April but left for military service just six days later. Within a few days Charge Nurse Jeffrey joined her. Sometimes military nurses, between movements or when demobilised, worked for a few days or weeks at Fremantle Hospital to help out. Sometimes they came for some peace: 'Two sisters from Military Hospital slept here Jan. 28 and 29 on account of noise of building. They brought their own beds', reported the secretary in 1916.[207] By May 1917 the staff was greatly reduced, with only two charge nurses, one staff nurse, seven third-year probationers, four second-year probationers and eight in their first year of training. Of these, two were off sick and one on holidays, leaving 22 on duty. A month later there was only one charge nurse and one staff nurse. With so few senior nurses, the system of nurse training—whereby a senior instructed and supervised and the junior nurse under her listened and learned—broke down, and no one was more aware of the fact than Matron Balding:

> I should like to point out how junior my nursing staff is at present with a view of endeavouring to get some trained staff. I have six nurses under three months, five under one year, four under two years (two of which are off staff sick) and six third year nurses, three of which must fill charge nurse positions—this makes work very difficult and training inefficient.[208]

Matron not only worked alongside the nurses as her help was needed, urged the sometimes reluctant honoraries to diligence in their lectures to nurses, and gave lessons on general nursing herself, but also took opportunities to further a probationer's training:

> She taught you things. She'd come round when you were on night duty, she always

---

[204] In June 1914 the nursing staff comprised the matron, three charge nurses, three staff nurses and 16 pupils.

[205] For a list of nurses from Fremantle Hospital known to have served in World War I, see Appendix 3. By 1918 between 25 and 30 nurses had left the hospital to take up military duties, see undated press article, FH scrapbook.

[206] Minutes of BM, 21 March 1917.

[207] *Ibid.*, 7 February 1916.

[208] Minutes of HC, 5 September 1917, FH.

visited to every one of the nurses. She'd come along one evening and she'd say 'has so and so had his ten o'clock sponge yet?'—that would be a typhoid. 'No, not yet, I was just going to do it'. 'Well I'll come back in ten minutes and help you,' and she'd come back and that night *she* would sponge that patient with your assistance, and tell you why she did this, that and the other and the exact way to do it to reduce the temperature. She'd sponge that patient from head to toe, never missed an inch. She helped them back to bed, then she'd go on her way, thoroughly pleased with herself. A few nights later she'd turn up again and ask you some question about somebody with typhoid and that night you would sponge the patient and she would assist you and see what you came up with. Anything you did wrong she would put you right.[209]

Due to the pressure of work, matron's lessons could not always be given and she reported in 1918: 'my own lectures suspended pro tem until domestic arrangements are more satisfactory'.[210] It was difficult for nurses to study when they were overworked. One nurse who twice failed her junior exam had to be given some study leave before she passed, and in 1918 the seniors all did so poorly in the medical examination that Dr Kerr deferred the paper for two months and gave extra lectures before they sat again. Significantly, in October 1917 all the senior nurses with their sound earlier training behind them, passed their medical theory examination but three of the new juniors failed theirs. By February 1919 matron despaired:

> The nursing standard is the best possible under present conditions, it is most essential that each ward has a trained Nurse of some experience for practical instruction and supervision of pupil Nurses, which has not been systematically obtainable lately, trained staff being most difficult to secure. I would also suggest a small library of nursing text books up-to-date, to assist the Nurses in their studies.[211]

When one nurse recalled that 'there was no sisters available, no sisters at all' she was almost right.[212] Towards the end of 1917 there were two—one in charge of theatre, the other as the night superintendent. The six third-year students were in charge of the wards, doing all the supervising, instructing, and helping where necessary. When they graduated, five stayed on as staff nurses, but there were no third-year nurses left at the hospital. Staff Nurse Quealey, Staff Nurse Seldon, and Charge Nurse Ryan donned military uniforms in the first half of 1918; by the end of the year, Charge Nurses Minister and Scanlan had also left the hospital. In 1919 the entire trained staff was temporary. Illness and accident continually reduced staff numbers and in May alone various nurses were suffering scarlet fever, acute rheumatism, tonsillitis, influenza and enteric fever. The number of nurses required to staff the hospital each 24 hours was 27: six for women's ward (22 adult beds and seven cots), four each in the medical and surgical wards (22 beds in each), two for theatre and casualty work, seven for night duty, two in isolation with its 13 beds, one for holidays and one for emergency or when someone was sick.[213] Although the number on duty was sometimes as low as 21, it was usually 23 and sometimes there

[209] Parker, interview.
[210] Minutes of BM, 21 August 1918.
[211] *Ibid.*, 19 February 1919.
[212] Lund, interview. From 19 May 1919, senior nurses were referred to as 'sisters'.
[213] Minutes of BM, 15 January 1919.

was only one trained nurse on the staff apart from matron. It was a heavy responsibility for these young women, especially when there was no resident medical officer at a time of emergency. One remembered acting as night superintendent for the whole hospital and having to report to matron 'every morning at nine o'clock in her office. And we had to know the temperatures of any of the people. We used to write them on our cuffs and on our hands . . . we had to make that report.'[214]

Holidays had to be postponed or forfeited, days off were irregular and their allocation rarely known in advance: '. . . sometimes we were told at 6 o'clock in the morning that you had that day off . . . the night sister used to have to come around and call us up . . . and so we got a bit tired of that of course'. In the end the nurses approached Matron Balding:

> We were lucky to get a day off when matron could give us one, and that was a bone of contention . . . Nurse Bishop went to matron and said she was going to call a committee meeting to say that they wanted to know when their days off were the night before, and also they wanted to know when the holidays fell due, so that they could make arrangements to do something outside the hospital . . . so she went to matron and told matron that she was going to call a committee meeting. 'Well,' she said, 'I had heard rumours of it nurse but I was hoping you'd come and tell me about it.' 'Well,' she said, 'We couldn't do it without you.' So that was held in the secretary's office.[215]

For a short while, time off was more organised.

Fremantle resounded with joy at the armistice of November 1918 and the excitement continued for months as the men came home. The returning troopships would hoot as they drew close to land, the steam locomotives whistling in reply could be heard out at Spearwood, and small ferries jammed with people churned circles around the ships, whose decks were lined with smiling, tearful, laughing and relieved faces under the well-known slouch hats.[216] The *Melbourne Argus* boasted of the expeditious manner in which disembarkations were conducted in Melbourne. The record there was 360 men in two hours. But at Fremantle, 833 men left the *Konigin Luise* and were 'finalised' in two hours and five minutes. From the *Oxfordshire*, 470 men were put through at Fremantle in one and three-quarter hours.[217] The streets of the town were often thronged with men in khaki, jostling and whooping, home from the battle fronts, and there were always crowds outside the embarkation shed to greet loved ones. On one weekend alone, six transport ships berthed. At the hospital, matron sighed with relief as the nurses gradually came back.

The relief was short-lived, for it seemed that an unseen enemy stalked the soldiers to their homeland to taunt the population there. The virulent pandemic influenza of 1918–1919 cut a swathe through Europe, Britain, Africa, Asia, the Americas and down to New Zealand.[218] Its natural sea barrier coupled with a stringent maritime

[214] Lund, interview.
[215] *Ibid.*
[216] Gore and Healey, interviews, FCL.
[217] *Western Mail*, 14 August 1919.
[218] See H. McQueen, 'The "Spanish" Influenza Pandemic in Australia, 1912–19', in J. Roe (ed.), *Social Policy in Australia: Some Perspectives 1901–1975*, Stanmore, Cassell Australia, 1976, pp. 131–47; J. H. L. Cumpston, *Influenza and Maritime Quarantine in Australia*, Melbourne, Albert J. Mullett, 1919.

quarantine defence, lessened the impact in Australia. Influenza was no stranger to Australian populations and Western Australians shared the experience many times—including during epidemics in 1860, between 1891 and 1893, and in 1899. At Fremantle in winter the local board of health would routinely hear that 'influenza is still prevalent' or that the town was in good health 'although as usual at this time of the year a good deal of influenza prevails amongst the juvenile portion of the community', or perhaps that there were 'no fatalities from the influenza epidemic, but many chest complications'.[219] At Fremantle more than at inland cities, people on the shore were aware of the closeness of the 'Spanish Flu' as they watched at least 32 trading and troop ships ordered into quarantine. When the *Boonah*, transporting over 900 soldiers, came from Durban in South Africa and berthed in Fremantle on 11 December 1918, it carried 300 cases of influenza of whom 150 were landed at Fremantle Quarantine Station that night. Eighty-six were unloaded the following day. By the end of January, 22 of the 496 reported ill had died, including four of the eight local nurses at the quarantine station.[220]

The strict maritime quarantine procedures coincided with a seamen's strike early in 1919, cutting the availability of butter and other perishable goods to Western Australia. On the S.S. *Dimboola*, bringing such cargo from the Eastern States in May 1919, several cases of pneumonic influenza developed, but before the ship had completed the requisite period of quarantine, shipping agents and local traders wanted the goods unloaded. The long-serving lumpers, and the volunteer 'loyalist workers' union' funded and organised by employers in 1917 when lumpers were striking, at first agreed not to unload the ship until it was declared free from infection. The scab labour, however, bowed to their employers' wishes. The Western Australian government supported the unloading, and the two interest groups— lumpers and those under the cloak of legality—exploded in violent confrontation on the wharves.[221] Hospital treatment was not needed for Premier Hal Colebatch and his party, who were pelted with missiles as their launch passed under the railway and traffic bridges on Sunday, 4 May 1919; but it was required for others among the police and the three- to four-thousand-strong crowd which quickly congregated to support the lumpers. In the fracas, seven lumpers were wounded by bayonets or police rifle butts, and 26 of the policemen assailed with nuts and bolts, stones and other missiles, also needed medical attention. The following day a group of police were attacked with iron pickets torn from St John's Church fence. On the Wednesday, a lumper named Tom Edwards died from a head injury sustained on 'Bloody Sunday'.[222] Although the community, which was linked in location and interest to the wharves, rallied in support of the lumpers, and although many of the hospital patients on 4 May would have preferred to have been at the wharf hurling bed pans instead of using them in the ward, the official hospital attitude to the lumpers was ambivalent. In its own battle for financial survival, able-bodied unemployed lumpers and their families must have often seemed subversive to a balanced hospital

[219] See *West Australian*, 18 December 1896; Minutes FLBH, 24 October 1888, 26 June 1890; Cumpston, *Influenza*, pp. 139–40.
[220] Cumpston, *Influenza and Maritime Quarantine*, pp. 139–40.
[221] See B. K. de Garis, 'An Incident at Fremantle', *Labour History*, 10, 1966, pp. 32–7.
[222] *Sunday Times*, 11 May 1919.

budget. Frustration was not always contained and a woman was moved to write to *The Truth*:

> My little girl was ordered to the hospital and admitted on Christmas Eve. Today I went to bring her home and the nurse took me around to the secretary to get her discharge. After asking my husband's full name and occupation and learning he was a lumper the secretary's lips seemed to drop and he asked me if I had brought the money to pay for my child's keep. I told him that I did not have it but would pay it as soon as I could as my husband had done very little since the trouble on the wharves started. Then he told me that I knew my girl was being discharged today and I ought to have brought something off the account and that it was my husband's fault for being out on strike. I told him I did not know whose fault it was but I did not want to hear any arguments about it but he said he had to send a report in as to when he could get the money and started off again about the 'lumpers had ruined the port' etc, but I told him that I could not help it and that I did not want charity and would pay it when I got it and I thought the lumpers had been pretty good contributors towards the upkeep of the hospital. He asked me when I could pay it and I told him that I did not know. Perhaps in a month, six months or twelve months ... I think my only fault was in being a LUMPER'S WIFE.[223]

The secretary's concern with finances was temporary distracted in the latter half of 1919. The influenza virus found its land legs in Victoria in June and strode with ever-increasing confidence to New South Wales and then into other states. In Kalgoorlie the transcontinental train was impounded, quarantined and the service terminated in an effort to discourage the invasion, but the action did not stop the assault. Accommodation for influenza sufferers at Perth metropolitan hospitals proved hopelessly inadequate and patients overflowed into the old military camp on Blackboy Hill and out to the infectious diseases branch at Subiaco. By June the 'Spanish Flu' was reported in Fremantle and by July it was rife. On 1 August the Fremantle Hospital was placed under quarantine regulations.

The decision to open the hospital to influenza patients was not made lightly. With the number of cases in the town increasing, the house committee—Len Bolton, Harry Woodhouse, William Watson and Mrs W. H. Carpenter—met at the end of July to discuss the situation and to decide whether the hospital's resident should be allowed to help the private medical practitioners in their efforts to cope with the increasing number of cases. The doctors had given their time and expertise to the hospital as honoraries, and the hospital decided that Hilda Kershaw should be permitted to help the Fremantle doctors in this time of need. On the following day, 30 July, the greater question of direct hospital involvement in the epidemic was discussed at a board meeting so hastily convened that only Mrs H. E. Bolton was able to attend with the house committee, and it was decided that Dr Atkinson's suggestion to use the hospital as a centre for emergency treatment should be endorsed. Rather than have the hospital's resident out working in the town it was agreed 'that our resident can better serve the interests of the sick in the Fremantle district by having them under her care in this institution'.[224] Most existing hospital patients were quickly discharged and the remaining cases who were too sick to be nursed at

---

[223] *The Truth*, 12 January 1918.
[224] Special Meeting of the BM, 30 July 1919.

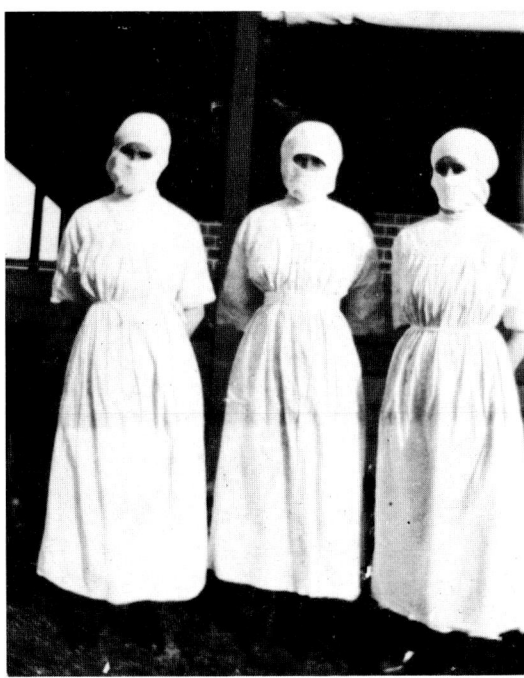

Plate 23. Nursing during the Spanish 'Flu, 1919.

We had some very sad cases ... Some went off their heads and some kept their heads ... One man jumped from one bed onto the next one ...

Margery Lund
Nursing Staff

Photograph courtesy Mrs Lund

home were warded—male and female carefully segregated ('they just put a partition across, that's all'),[225] medical and surgical together—in the women's ward which had been made into one large Nightingale ward early in 1918, when all the separate dividing walls had been knocked out. By the following day the men's medical and surgical wards had been prepared for influenza patients—one for men, the other for women. The isolation ward and the old nurses' quarters were quarantined for sick nurses and domestic staff, and the upper storey of the new nurses' home was reserved for the staff nursing influenza patients.

Between 1 and 19 August, 104 influenza patients were admitted and 33 died. Other sick men, women and children were brought to the hospital but no room could be found for them. By 18 August, accommodation for patients was increased when the South Terrace School, adjacent to the hospital, was used as an auxiliary hospital. The staff employed to nurse there was housed in the domestics' quarters and the domestics were transferred to the nurses' cold, open verandah. Extra nurses, orderlies, and domestic staffs were engaged. The laundry workers washed and dried copious quantities of bedding and linen, and the dispenser prepared medicines for patients in both centres. The out-patients' department continued a reduced service. 'It was,' as one nurse recalled, 'a very, very busy time for everybody'.[226]

Nurses volunteered to work with influenza patients. 'Notices were put up and ... of course everyone volunteered—because of the pay. You see, we were only getting

[225] Lund, interview.
[226] *Ibid.*

such a small pay and for the influenza epidemic we were going to be paid £3 a week
...',[227] explained a nurse. The parents of another nurse, who had recently lost a son,
did not want their daughter exposed to the virus, but she went ahead anyway: 'I
didn't tell them; so they were none the wiser'.[228] Despite the protective gowns and
masks they wore, it was not long before the staff joined patients in illness; it seemed
they went 'one after another'[229]—domestics and orderlies and nurses, the office boy
and then the lodge-keeper. Of the 15 nurses who staffed the influenza wards in the
first two weeks, ten were subsequently hospitalised in the isolation ward, which was
hurriedly prepared for them. At the end of two weeks matron had organised the
three wards under 13 nurses, three wardsmaids and two housemaids. No trained
nurses could be found to work at the hospital, but three new probationer nurses
were taken on, all of whom came down with influenza in an inauspicious beginning
to their nursing careers, as did two housemaids, the doctor's housemaid and the
cook. After their recovery, nurses were given a few days off and then they were back
in the wards. By the end of the first fortnight of the crisis, a temporary dining room,
30 by 15 feet, had been knocked together just outside the kitchen to help feed the
small army of staff at the hospital and the school.

Matron reported to the board that work in the wards was long and 'strenuous'.[230]
Many patients suffered the chill and high temperature of fever, the cough and sore
throat, aches in the head and all through the joints and muscles, the vomiting and
'pea soup' diarrhoea. Only the most urgent cases were admitted to the hospital and
these required constant nursing—four-hourly sponges to reduce temperatures,
aspirin, and cough mixtures. 'You had so much to do you couldn't do half the treatment,' remembered one nurse.[231] Four hourly mouth washes were ordered, sensitive
pressure points on backs and heels had to be rubbed to avoid bed sores—the
measure of a nurses proficiency and especially difficult when 'they used to walk their
feet up and down in the beds'.[232] One nurse recalled working

> seven weeks night duty, twelve hours a night without any night off ... and people died
> like flies ... The men would walk in at night and said they didn't feel well, they thought
> they had the 'flu. And they'd be carried out before morning—it was awful'.[233]

Another recalled of her patients, 'some went off their heads, and some kept their
heads ... some got very restless, some were very quiet'.[234] All had different tem-
peraments, and the high temperatures caused some erratic behaviour:

> ... one poor woman got out in the nude, running round the lawns in the front and
> everybody chasing after her. We had some very sad cases and one man jumped from
> one bed on to the next one and oh ... We couldn't handle the very heavy cases.'[235]

[227]   Parker, interview.
[228]   Lund, interview.
[229]   Parker, interview.
[230]   Minutes of BM, 20 August 1919.
[231]   Parker, interview.
[232]   Lund, interview.
[233]   Parker, interview.
[234]   Lund, interview.
[235]   *Ibid.*

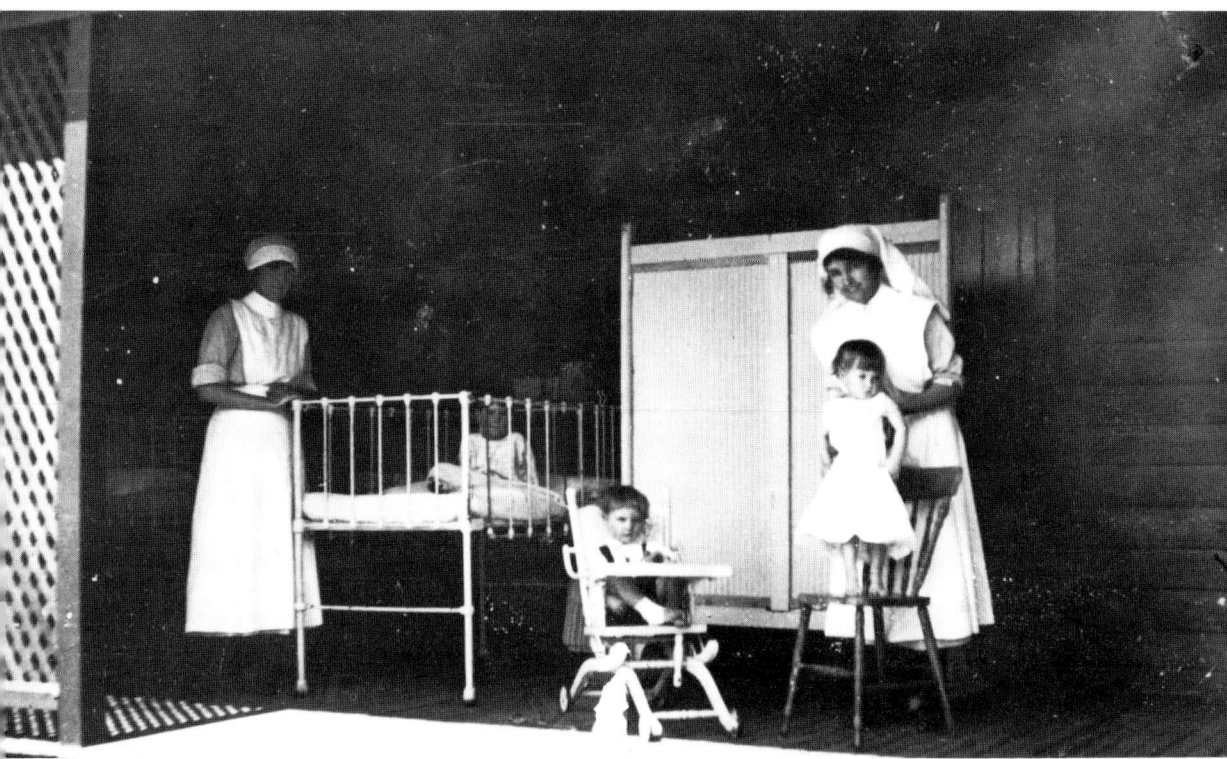

Photograph courtesy Battye Library

Plate 24.   Children's Ward, *c.* 1920, with Sister Leo and Nurse Arnold.

During the weeks of the shocking flu, Maida Balding joined her girls. 'She also then rolled up her sleeves and went to work—in the wards and went around doing mouths all day. She worked with us, cleansing, cleaning mouths, mouth washes, glycerine and lemon juice.'[236]

Some in the town helped in the best way they could, sending lemons and oranges to the hospital. Mr Watson of the board provided extra milk through his small-goods business, which was appreciated when supplies were low. In the midst of the dying in a quarantine ward, a baby was born on 5 August. Churchmen, particularly the Roman Catholic priests, often visited in the wards, comforting and administering. By mid-September most of the nursing staff who had been taken sick were back in the wards. There were 14 nurses available to tend the 29 influenza patients, nine for the 21 patients in the general ward, two were on holidays, one was sick and one was on sick leave. Although there were never less than 24 influenza patients until 7 October, the worst was over.[237] It was reported that in the metropolitan area, from

[236]   *Ibid.*
[237]   See Appendix 4.

the beginning of the outbreak to the end of August, 2,041 cases of influenza had been reported with 185 deaths.[238] At Fremantle, by 15 October the auxiliary ward at the school had closed, the hospital's domestic staff were back in their quarters and the quarantine staff had been reduced to six. By 5 November, payment of the special quarantine nursing rate had ceased.

For her excellent work as the hospital's house surgeon, tall, dark-haired and somewhat severe-looking Hilda Kershaw received a commendation from the board. Although she had shown that her worth as a surgeon, as an anaesthetist and as a medical attendant in an emergency of an unparalleled dimension was not curtailed by her gender, the opening of Fremantle Hospital to 'lady doctors' was a gesture born of desperation in wartime and was not repeated for many years. Her successor was one of the young junior resident medical officers from Perth Hospital, Dr J. H. Stubbe.[239]

There was much cleaning up to do after the epidemic. The men's medical and surgical wards were scrubbed and renovated. In the isolation ward, the old 'lino' was pulled up and the floorboards polished to show the beautiful grain of the timber. The dining room, so quickly erected in the first weeks of the epidemic, was eyed covetously as a children's ward by the board. Permission for this use was granted, but only provisionally, in case of a second outbreak. The experiences of war and epidemic were forgotten by none, but put behind them as Fremantle launched into the 1920s under the Nationalist-Country Party government of James Mitchell. Sister Irene Keirnan returned as a senior sister in November 1919, after war service during which she had been with Lord Forrest when he died unexpectedly while on a troop ship going to London. Others too came back, relieving the shortage of nursing sisters, and re-establishing the efficient nurse-training system of practical apprenticeship to experienced skilled senior nurses. Honorary doctors returned to their work, as did honorary masseuses Mrs Shepherd and Miss McBean, and although it was gradual, there was an increase in the theoretical teaching given by honorary doctors and the matron to the new probationer nurses. The knowledge gained from treating war casualties refined some medical procedures, such as plastic surgery, and expanded the text of some nursing books to include a chapter on war wounds, with graphic illustrations of men with a face or a limb half shot away.[240] In the wards in 1919, patients received their Christmas cheer as customary, while the church bells tolled the faithful to prayers of thanksgiving. But somehow things were never quite the same again.

[238] *Western Mail*, 4 September 1919. Statement by Huelin, Secretary to the Commissioner for Public Health. For weekly figures of influenza reports and deaths in the metropolitan area, see *Western Mail*, 4, 11, 18, 25 September 1919; 2, 9, 16 October 1919.

[239] For some of his impressions and experiences as a junior resident doctor, see Stubbe, *Medical Background*, pp. xix-xxvi.

[240] See E. W. Groves and J. M. Fortescue-Brickdale, *Text-Book for Nurses. Anatomy, Physiology, Surgery and Medicine*, Third ed., 1925, pp. 410-25.

Chapter V

I hope that a bright future may be in store for the Hospital.
Dr F. J. Clark, SRMO
8 December 1923.

It wasn't just the short skirts and shorter hair that women wore, or their employ-ment in previously predominantly male domains such as factories, shops and offices. It wasn't just the motor cars manoeuvring side by side with the horse-drawn drays that still transferred wool and other loads from warehouses, although the new motor buses certainly moved more people more easily than horse-drawn vehicles. When Charlie Spicer's Char-a-banc service started with two old 1914 Bluebird Ford buses which had to be cranked by hand, Fremantle people could travel between Perth and Fremantle for half a crown return;[1] the consequent preference to shop at Perth rather than locally affected Fremantle's large firms only for a time. In the late 1920s, when women rarely drove themselves, let alone others, Marion Bell really raised eyebrows and words of condemnation when she became Fremantle's first woman taxi driver. However, young Amy Healey was probably not the only young lady to be glad of Marion's chosen profession. At almost twelve o'clock one night—two hours late home and stranded because she had spent her bus fare—Amy asked the taxi driver for a lift and promised payment at another time. Not only was the lift given but Marion Bell went in and set things right with Amy's worried mother.[2]

It wasn't just in private households, where some had not returned from war, that there was an obvious difference. Many of these families came together and sug-gested building a commemorative obelisk on the cleaned-up Monument Hill site, high above the town, overlooking the port where soldiers had embarked. It wasn't just the big bands playing at dances, for which the girls dyed their dress a different colour each week. Nor was it the new talking pictures which introduced an outside world to the known and familiar territory of Fremantle. After the war there was a different way of looking at things.

It was time to take a deep breath and to work for the future. Wheat farmers between 1920 and 1929 extended and consolidated inland areas under crop. James Mitchell encouraged dairy farming in the timber areas of the south-west, and sheep were often run alongside wheat. Roads and railways were laid to reach far into pro-

---

[1] Wray, interview, FCL. See also Reece and Pascoe, *A Place of Consequence*, pp. 92–3.
[2] Healey, interview, FCL. Amy had been taught to dance by her mother, who ran the Kelly's School of Dancing. As an eight- or nine-year-old she had danced at the lumpers' picnics at South Fremantle beach and, later, in the chorus line during interval at the Princess Theatre, and at many fund-raising charity concerts.

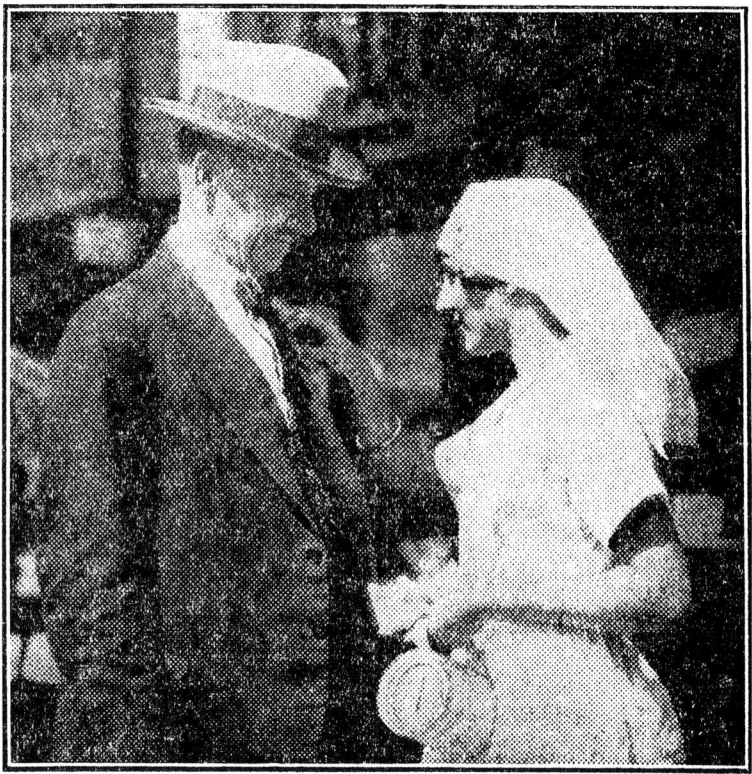

Photograph courtesy A. Orloff

Plate 25. For decades, donations were collected for Fremantle Hospital as shown in this newspaper photograph in 1928. A staff member of the late 1940s recalled:

If we were trying to raise money we would say 'Would you give a donation'. There would be raffles, either legal or illegal. Then they ran a popular nurse competition.

Sister Bette Needle
Nursing Staff

ductive areas. In towns, optimism and growth were reflected in new buildings, and motor transport extended the suburban sprawl. A 44-hour week in industry and a state basic wage were introduced.[3] At Fremantle the wharves were always busy with produce going out and immigrants from the United Kingdom coming in. Many of the 43,700 who were assisted were granted pocket-sized blocks of farming land alongside grants settled by returned soldiers. Poverty, heart-break and toil were the lot of many, but overall the increase from the earth was bountiful.[4] After the crisis of war it verily seemed that there was a season for all things and that this was a blessed time for growth.

[3] See Crowley and de Garis, *A Short History*, p. 108.
[4] *Ibid.*, p. 101.

The individual cycle of human lives—birth, life and death, health, injury and illness—and the natural increase of population in Fremantle, supplemented in waves by the arrival of immigrants, meant a continual need for improvements and maintenance at the hospital. The ebullience resulting from the state's development was not extended to hospital expenditure and the board continually lived its own challenging cycle of hospital maintenance, improvement and expansion within the rigid confines of a minimal £5,000-a-year subsidy from the state government. In 1919, the costs associated with the influenza epidemic plunged the hospital account into deficit, a position from which it rarely recovered in the following decade. In February of 1920 the accounts could not be paid, although the March subsidy had already been received. 'From these figures you will gather that the financial state is bad,' observed the secretary.[5] A board deputation organised to appeal to the minister for an increase of £750 was only partially successful, and it was May before the special grant of £500 was approved and July before it was received. Donations such as £100 from the W.A. Turf Club, £5 from the lumpers, £19.13.2. received through the domestic staff's euchre party, or the proceeds from Mr Wray's Easter self-denial, failed to lift the figures into the black. In August alone, salaries amounted to over £313, gas more than £42, drugs topped £10, meat and milk cost £64 and £43 respectively, while dressings and bandages amounted to over £12. There was insufficient to pay the latter three accounts and the expenditure was an ominous monthly average of £487 above the subsidy.

The notion to appoint a hospital collector was not new to Western Australia. In 1906 the usual commission paid for the work in country areas was ten per cent, but there had been some objection to solicitors doing that character of work 'which one can scarcely expect gentlemen of that profession to do'.[6] The Fremantle Hospital board's decision to appoint a 'lady collector' was made in 1908 and Mrs Fordham was paid 21 shillings a week, with a five per cent commission on all the subscriptions, donations and fees that she could collect. Mrs Inkpen followed her three months later, travelling by tram to different debtors' homes and prospective donors' residences. Debtors of likely means were reported to the board, who could then take them to court. Of four names submitted to the board in March 1909, one was considered by Dr Birmingham to be unable to pay, one was thought to be insolvent, and another had his account promptly written off. Just one man was threatened with legal action and he could manage to pay only half of his fee for hospitalisation before it too had to be written off. In December 1920, Mrs McMonagle was appointed as a house-to-house collector at 35 shillings weekly with ten shillings for expenses. She collected over £34 in her first three weeks. Sometimes, especially near Christmas, the monthly total was nearly £50 and the collector was soon granted a pay increase to £2 with 12 shillings and sixpence weekly for expenses. The Fremantle Tramways Department also gave her a free pass for travel by tram. But the hospital finances needed a greater lift than a collector could give.

In 1921 the secretary was directed to write to the Ugly Men's Association and the United Friendly Societies at Cottesloe for aid, and in September, with a massive debt of £2,000 and the government's hospital bill before the House, by which it was

5   Minutes of BM, 17 March 1920.
6   PHD File 32/1906.

hoped hospital funding would be restructured, it was decided to call a meeting with Perth Public Hospital and the Children's Hospital to discuss the implications. No action resulted from the combined conference, but it helped the Fremantle board shape its own views.[7] The board strongly rejected any move to raise funds through a tax based on the rateable value of property and preferred instead a more equitable, centralised state supertax on per capita income. In parliament, Frank Broun's plan to transfer responsibility for hospital administration to local governments made the council at Fremantle gulp, but after a perceptive and penetrating Royal Commission presenting evidence for and against the bill, and much discussion both in and out of the house, the *Hospitals' Bill* of 1921 was rejected by the Legislative Council.[8] It was a disappointment to many. For nearly 30 years since the passing of the *Hospitals Act* of 1894, under which only Perth and Fremantle were administered as public hospitals, no hospital legislation had been considered, and the act was outdated and ineffectual. The government hospitals were no better off. At none of the 48 hospitals in the state which were managed by the Medical Department or assisted by it, did a committee have the statutory authority to sign as much as a contract for supplies. The defeat of the bill effectively dashed hopes of improving administration and raising more much-needed finance for hospitals for years.

The colonial secretary subsequently pointed out that government funds for hospitals had been:

> ... cut down to the finest possible point, with the result that everytning but sheer necessities has had to be eliminated, and various subterfuges have had to be adopted ... secondhand furniture, bedding, and bed clothes have been utilized to the fullest ... Those in control of the expenses of hospitals have had to examine very closely practically every penny spent, and no expenditure which could be avoided or which could be postponed has been undertaken.[9]

Of this the board at Fremantle was well aware. Townspeople also were concerned about the situation and both businesses and associations such as the Western Australian Turf Club, W.A. Brushware, the banks, some of the steamship companies, newspapers, lodges, and private individuals including Drs Blackall and Tregonning, rallied to support their hospital. One of the hospital's greatest financial strengths in these years of the second decade of the century was the Fremantle Ugly Men's Association, which gave £260 in August 1921. Formed in 1917 as the brainchild of a group of leading citizens to raise funds for those in need as a result of war, it conducted a competition through penny votes to find the ugliest man in Perth. Based on the same principles and with the same philanthropic ends in view, a parallel Ugly Women's Association was formed. These organisations continued to raise funds for charitable concerns long after the war ended, and the Fremantle branch established a giant fairground opposite the railway station, strung with lights, where chocolate wheels spun, merry-go-rounds whirled, and concerts, dances, mild gambling competitions, stalls and sideshows could be enjoyed. Two-Bob-Andy would put on a

[7] Minutes of Special Meeting of BM, 2 November 1921.
[8] See *WAVP*, 1922–23, Vol. 2. Report of the Royal Commission on Hospitals.
[9] *Daily News*, 12 February 1923.

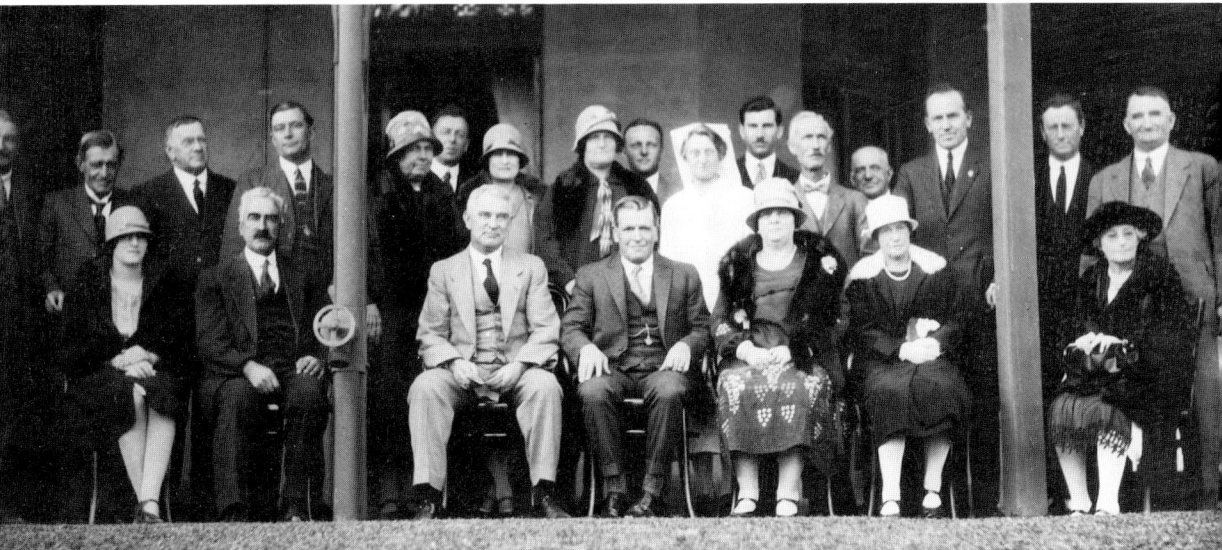

Photograph courtesy Fremantle Hospital

Plate 26.   The Ugly Men's presentation of £1,000 to Fremantle Hospital, 31 May 1927.

Standing: F. Rowe, M.L.A., W. A. Murphy (Secretary, Fremantle Ugly Men's Association), F. Instone, H. Hockley, Mrs Waddell, A. T. Hookway (Hospital Secretary), Mrs Jeffrey, Mrs Laidlaw, Dr Baker (R.M.O.), Matron Balding, Dr Macdonald (S.R.M.O.), F. Randell, J. Cobb, G. Potter, M.L.C., W. C. Sweet, H. Gray, M.L.C.
Sitting: Mrs Bremner, Cr J. M. Farrell (President, Fremantle Ugly Men's Association), A. McLeod (Chairman, Hospital Board), Hon. S. W. Munsie, M.L.A., Mrs Munsie, Mrs Gray, Mrs Bevan.

show for the required fee and Percy Buttons amazed with his acrobatics. Uglieland was good fun, but it was also a place where a man out of work could get shoes repaired, or a coat for his back until times got better. While clearing his block at Palmyra where he planned to build a dwelling out of bush saplings and flour bags painted with whitewash for his family's shelter, one man knelt on a scorpion. The resulting bite

> ... put him into Fremantle Hospital for about six weeks. At that time there were no such things as sickness benefits. While Father was sick there was no money coming in. There was a Society called The Ugly Men's Association. Those people found out about our problems and very kindly helped our family through those bad times ...[10]

[10] M. Lane recollections, Acc. No. 994.IF, FCL. For references to the Fremantle Ugly Men's Association, see notes by S. Jones, FCL, Ref. 791.068. Also *Fremantle Herald*, 31 January 1919; *West Australian*, 21 February 1927, 7 May 1979, 4 June 1979; *Fremantle Gazette*, 28 July 1982; *Sunday Times*, 26 March 1933. The Association continued until 1933, when the W.A. Lotteries Commission was established. See also H. R. Laudehr, interviewed by J. Brodsgaard and M. Scott, date unlisted, FCL. In the first fortnight of December 1922, the Ugly Men's Association helped in 63 cases of need: financial assistance was given to 38 people; beds, bedding and food were supplied in 21 cases; clothing and blankets were distributed to many others in need of them, *West Australian*, 16 December 1922.

recalled the man's daughter. The secretary of the Fremantle Ugly Men's Association, James Farrell, and the organiser's wife, Mrs W. A. Murphy, were both on the
hospital's board of management at different times.

Many more individuals donated time, means and funds to the hospital. At clubs
and pubs men dropped coppers into collecting boxes which could yield between
eleven shillings and £11 but usually up to £7. Church congregations made donations
in cash and in kind. The lumpers sent £50 each year and cases of fruit or tomatoes
when they were in season. Chen Hop, who had sold fruit to the hospital, donated
£10 in 1921 and the sum was supplemented by about 60 other Chinese, who sent between them over £35. Christmas was an annual reminder about benevolence and
caring. More than once in the 1920s, Mr Butson offered the takings from his choir's
singing of the Messiah, while Mr H. Bleatle gave a day's proceeds from the Blue Boy
pantomime matinee and evening sessions played at the Town Hall. At the beginning
of 1922, after granting another necessary £500 to keep the hospital going, the colonial secretary offered £1 for every £1 donated and the incentive inspired a promising
flash of philanthropy. Plays, community singing, football matches, balls, panto-
mimes, concerts and sweepstakes were held to raise funds for the hospital.

By September, however, the financial situation was once more so bad that the
minister promised another £400 to ease the situation. There were anxious months
with the accounts unpaid before it was received. Perhaps to encourage their efforts,
the colonial secretary agreed again in 1923 to match amounts collected by members
of the community. This time there was a greater response. Donations ranging from a
guinea each sent by the Melbourne Steamship Company and the Buffalo Club and
Bon Marché Stores, to £50 from the Honourable R. J. Lynn, M.L.C., were received.
Mrs Gill of the board recommended an appeal to the Chinese and offered her
father's help if this was agreed to. The board gave nurses permission to help in
Uglieland and the hospital's own fete raised over £117. A performance by a Miss
Tiffy Cook netted over £8 and the bazaar organised by Misses Florrie Nichols and
Iris Harper raised eight shillings. Special church collections on Anzac Day also
boosted the amount. In mid-April the hospital appeal fund totalled £203.10.0. By
the end of April it was over £464 and by mid-May the board was jubilant with no
outstanding accounts and a credit of £269. Donations from the community between
30 April and 27 June totalled in all over £1,134 which was supplemented by another
£1,000 from the colonial secretary's funds. Secretary Arliss Robinson happily
reported a credit of £1,007.9.0. with no outstanding accounts to be paid. It was a
propitious time for Benbow the engineer to request a raise in salary to £5 weekly.
Although the impetus of giving slowed, from August 1923 the lumpers picked up
their pay in one hand and with the other sorted out their bronze coins and dropped
them into hospital collecting boxes placed at pay offices for the purpose. Few complained at this union directive which, it was calculated, would raise £100 a year for
their hospital.[11]

The credit balance did not last long. 'Financial aspect not too bright,' noted the
secretary in September 1923.[12] By the end of the year the aspect was positively dim,

[11]   Minutes of BM, 15 August 1923.
[12]   *Ibid.*, 19 September 1923.

when over £3,000 had to be written off as 'bad and doubtful debts'. Some of the hospital accounts could not be paid. In early 1924 finances were boosted by a special grant of £1,000 from the colonial secretary's office, but the Jacktar Art Union consultation cards and buttons organized by the hospital to coincide with the visit of the naval fleet realised only a little over £7. By mid-1924 the hospital could not meet its accounts. This was the year when schools gave to the hospital—Presbyterian Ladies College and scholars from Princess May, the latter support continuing for decades. In August 1924 bad and doubtful debts totalling over £4,000 were written off and in October the government finally increased the subsidy from £5,000 to a more realistic £6,000. Despite this, finance was a deep concern for the new board in 1925 when Chairman H. J. Locke deplored the financial position of the hospital and declared it the board's chief trouble. 'Each month the institution is getting more and more in debt to the extent of about £200.'[13] A committee consisting of Messrs Farrell, Rowe, McMahon, Locke and the secretary was organised as a special appeal body.

Board chairmanship was not a good experience for Locke. Len Bolton had been a popular chairman since Mill's death in 1916 and had Bolton indicated that he wished to remain on the board, he would have been re-elected as chairman in 1925. At an adjourned meeting, when it was found that Bolton would not consider reappointment, Locke was elected with McLeod as his deputy and Dr East and Mrs Waddell once more on the house committee. On few matters could the four agree and finding the position intolerable, Locke submitted his resignation in March. In a secret ballot there was nothing between Woodhouse and Angus McLeod, until Acting Chairman Woodhouse gave his vote to McLeod, who served as chairman until 1928. No one was surprised when votes established Woodhouse as deputy chairman and the committee settled conscientiously to the task of administration.

In April 1925 the accounts were £800 behind. Chu Lung carted in three bags of his vegetables for the patients, the Fremantle prison gave four bags of onions and the immigration home sent a case of grapes. Gramophone records, flowers, milk, eggs, and even a vaccuum cleaner were donated to the hospital by different individuals and associations. Coogee Church brought fruit and vegetables and the Fremantle Uglies gave £500, which the colonial secretary doubled. In June, the Fremantle District Council of the Australian Labor Party presented the hospital with £530.[14] In its own effort to augment funds, the board introduced a scheme whereby visitors were charged sixpence to see a friend or relative during the visiting hours between two and three in the afternoons and six-thirty to seven-thirty at night. It seemed to the staff that visitors were a necessary bane. In a move strongly supported by doctors it was decided to restrict daily visiting in the children's ward, a practice which was introduced gradually to avoid upsetting the current patients and their families.

Although the need to improve and extend the hospital was great between 1920 and 1925, tightly pulled purse strings meant that only basic maintenance could be carried out. One visiting committee in 1924 despaired: 'We realize the futility of emphasising the defects and the unsuitability of most of the buildings, being cognizant that

[13]   *Ibid.*, 18 February 1925.
[14]   Members of the deputation included Curtin, who would become Prime Minister of Australia in 1941, Gray, Kitson, Hogarth and Sleeman. See Minutes of BM, 10 June 1925.

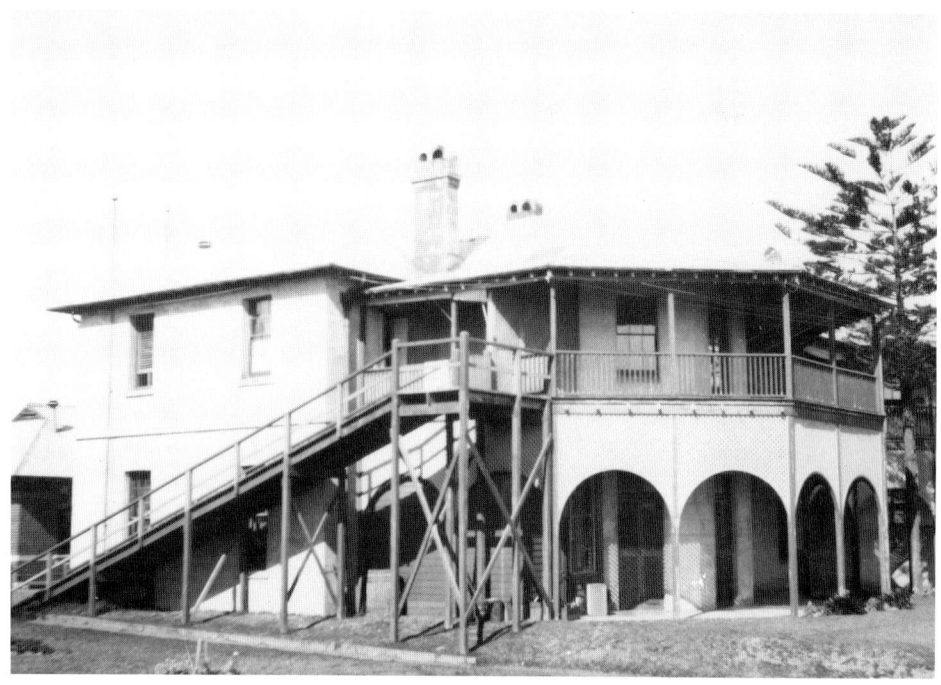

Plate 27.   The Knowle, *c.* 1920s.

... it wasn't the edifice that sort of caught one's imagination, it was the environment and the community really, which made it all worth while.

Mr M. Minchin.
Honorary Surgeon, 1950s

our greatest need is money and more money.'[15] Extensive renovations were needed, recognised Colonial Secretary Sampson in 1923, 'and at no distant date, the cost of rebuilding the male wards in brick will have to be faced'.[16] It was a period of repair and make do. Each month's elected board visiting committee of two inspected the premises and talked to the staff, and each of their monthly reports listed some new disrepair or discontent. Occasionally it might be as easy to remedy as cobwebs in the lodge waiting room or the need of a coat of kalsomine. More often there were problems with the hot water service or the dilapidated condition of buildings and fittings. In a typical month, Frank Rowe and R. Carter reported:

> We visited the various Wards and found several defects, complaints being heard on all sides about the scarcity of linen, pillow slips, towels etc. the position being deplorable as far as these various requirements are concerned. The Canvas blinds on the Verandahs are in a very bad state and require individual attention before the winter sets in.

[15]   Minutes of BM, 9 July 1924.
[16]   *Daily News*, 12 February 1923.

One blind in Medical Ward being missing altogether. Some of the sash frames have perished the result being the windows cannot be opened or closed with any certainty. Complaints were also made on account of a scarcity of lounges for the convalescent patients. The roof of verandah on Medical Ward leaks in several places. Patients have to be removed inside during wet weather. We inspected the Nurses Quarters and found them in very good order and condition ... We noticed several lockers in various wards, are in a very bad condition the doors of some being practically useless—there being no hinges. We would recommend that the outsides of Medical and Surgical Wards were painted as they are in a very shabby condition. We have much pleasure in stating that the children's Ward reflects the greatest credit on those responsible.

We also desire to draw the attention of the Board to the dirty condition of the Verandah caused through the stabling of a Motor car and we recommend its removal as soon as possible.

In conclusion we inspected the gates at Main Entrance and think the least said about them the better ...[17]

In mid-1920 'great inconvenience [was] caused to Kitchen, Theatre and Women's Ward owing to no hot water supply ...'[18] Not until 1921 was hot water from the main supply connected to the men's medical and surgical wards and the children's ward to replace the large gas rings that burned there continually to heat water, and only when the nursing staff wrote to the board about the dearth of hot water in their quarters was a bath heater granted—with the admonition that '... if burnt out through carelessness will have to be repaired by them'.[19] Only when no more than a trickle of water ran through the plumbing, was peak main water supplied from Alma Street. The sieve-like formation of the roof iron on the verandahs of the men's medical and surgical wards became more apparent each month and the surgical ward needed a new door to the verandah, new blinds and lattice work, a new corner post and attention paid to the verandah floor. In blustery weather there was nowhere for patients to sit except huddled inconveniently around a wood stove in the middle of the ward. 'We are of the opinion that this building is quite unsuitable for a hospital ward', advised the visiting committee in 1922.[20] A year later nothing had been done and a different visiting committee noted that there was a large hole in the surgical ward verandah, 'the outcome of which will be patients will be admitted suffering from a broken leg'.[21] In the children's ward, some full-length beds were provided for those who were above average height for their age, but one or two children's beds were urgently required for the comfort of infants too tall to lie straight in a cot. Experience had also shown the need for cots with upright bars closer together. New flywire was fixed over ventilators, and headrests were made for the 'morgue' after one visiting committee report. This was not as a result of a report made by the women on the board. When it was their turn to inspect the hospital Mrs Carpenter and Mrs H. E. Bolton avoided the area and always left the mortuary for the 'sterner sex' to inspect.

[17] Minutes of BM, 19 April 1922. The visiting committees were appointed monthly until February 1930, when the Advisory Board considered that they were unnecessary.
[18] *Ibid.*, 21 July 1920.
[19] *Ibid.*
[20] *Ibid.*, 20 September 1922.
[21] *Ibid.*, 19 December 1923.

A visiting committee recognised the effect of working conditions on employees when it described the old kitchen as 'very dirty' and 'most discouraging to persons working there'.[22] At another time the kitchen could be reported as spotlessly clean, but the kitchen staff worked continually to keep it that way. They frequently complained about the ashes which fell from the scullery fire, raising a dust which covered 'the crockery and everything in the place' and cook often had to order plates to be washed before being taken to the dining room. The situation was not eased by the build-up of ashes in the kitchen furnace, which was supposed to be emptied by the orderlies who 'were much dissatisfied because they had no place to rest when off duty'.[23] Usually the task was done at an inconveniently late hour in the morning, just before dinner, and the dust caused the kitchen maids great inconvenience. They looked forward to the arrival of orderly Myers each day for the diligence with which he alone carried out his duties.

Glass window panes remained unreplaced for ten years at the hospital and the sea gales that blasted off the ocean continually ripped verandah canvas blinds to shreds. But most government repairs took time—a great deal of time. No matter how minor the renovations required, the hospital had to advise the Medical Department, which wrote to the Public Works Department. That department then contacted its Fremantle representative, who inspected and assessed the work, estimated the cost of the replacement and reported back to headquarters in Perth, where it was decided if the work was necessary. Then the Medical Department was consulted. If it agreed to the repair, the Public Works Department would be directed so by letter and the work eventually carried out. To the board it was a frustratingly slow procedure and Chairman Bolton remonstrated with the Medical Department: 'the delay caused by sending to you, and then awaiting a finality through the usual red-tape methods, means that by such time as the request is granted another long string of items requires attention'.[24] The gates were a point in question. In November 1920, the W. D. Moore Company donated a handsome set of large wrought-iron gates to the hospital to replace the old dilapidated ones, but left their erection for the board to arrange with the Public Works Department. Six months later, no action had been taken by the government department, but in June the principal architect visited the hospital and submitted plans for a new main entrance. In August 1921 the secretary of the Medical Department reported that he had the matter in hand, nevertheless the gates remained propped up in the hospital grounds. In January 1922 there was a telephone call from the department advising that £100 would be forwarded for the erection of the gates. Tenders were called by the board and the successful contractors, Messrs Potter and Hancock, commenced their task. By April the gates were hung, but the lock was on the outside and so heavily did they drag on their hinges, that the gates had to be lightened. When by mid-1922, painting was finished and the lock altered, it seemed that the money had been well spent. However, the secretary was heard to mutter that '. . . the same laxity obtains whenever requests for works are desired'.[25] The gates were locked after 10 p.m. and a nurse from the medical ward,

22 *Ibid.*, 17 November 1920.
23 *Ibid.*, 21 June 1922, 16 August 1922.
24 *WAVP*, 1922–23, Vol. 2. Report of the Royal Commission on Hospitals.
25 Minutes of BM, 16 August 1922.

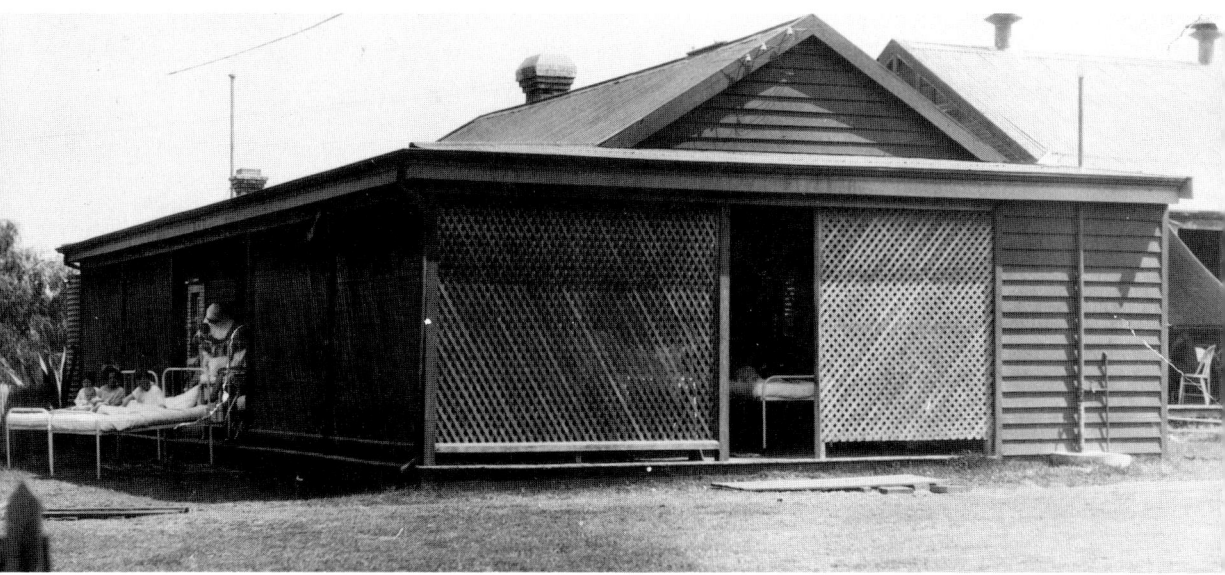

Photograph courtesy Fremantle Hospital

Plate 28.   The children's ward, 1926.

> The ward was so tiny. I think there were only about five or six patients inside and that was crowded with that number. There were no beds, they were all cots ... If an infectious case was brought in, the Isolation Ward was opened immediately and a nurse sent up to look after that patient and you did twelve hours a day.

Matron Olive Jones

summoned to open them by a bell outside, still had to wrestle with the heavy gates to get them open for the ambulance or for an emergency case or perhaps a nurse returning late.[26]

Work was always necessary and some of it was eventually done, although not always by the Medical Department. Staff at the Fremantle Foundry gratuitously fixed new pressure gauges to the theatre sterilizers when the work was urgently needed in 1923 and a patient painted the children's ward. From time to time prison workers were obtained from the gaol to paint buildings and fixtures, to clear the high dry grass which was a fire hazard around the nurses' home, and to blast the capstone around various buildings to level the ground. But if their labour was needed in the gaol, or warders were ill, the hospital work would be left abruptly. Painting of wards and lockers was put off by the Medical Department long after it was essential and in the interests of economy one coat only was often applied, which quickly peeled and required further attention. As years passed, flywire was replaced in different areas—particularly the scullery and the kitchen. Paths and roadways were laid down but irregularly maintained and the hot-water systems were replaced only when wards, the laundry or nurses' quarters had been without for some time.

[26] See *Ibid.*, 18 February 1925, 11 March 1925.

Equipment, too, was constantly needed. A few new surgical and medical instruments were bought—but there was little chance of keeping abreast of new discoveries and advances when funding was the issue. In the kitchen and laundry, in the wards and in the grounds, tools and equipment regularly needed repair or replacement. For years the board delayed an outlay from its meagre funds for new cane lounges for use by convalescents on the verandahs, hoping that ships' officers or local citizens might donate some. Only when the remaining few resembled 'string baskets' did the board give in and order some from the School for the Blind.[27] A water bed looking like a huge hot water bottle was obtained from Perdew Rubber Company in the early 1920s. In the same period a splendid table was donated for the nurses' dining room, but could not be used for want of chairs. Not until 1928 were 'proper telephones' installed throughout the hospital to replace the inter-hospital communication system of telephonettes.[28]

At various times kitchen and laundry renovations and improvements could be put off no longer. A new gas stove was installed with a hood and vent in 1920 and, although use of the wood stove continued and kitchen work was still hot and heavy, this was an improvement. For four years the kitchen slowly deteriorated despite plans to have it renovated, and by 1925 newly employed kitchen staff were quickly resigning to obtain better positions. A visiting committee urged, 'the sooner the kitchen is demolished and a new one erected, the better it will be for the Institution and for the Staff'.[29]

The constant use of the laundry also took a toll of the facilities there. The old laundry which was demolished in 1920 had boasted one great asset—a large-capacity rain-water tank and Benbow was forever concerned about the discoloured water used to wash the 134,630 articles, not counting the thousands disinfected, during 1921.[30] A new tank was eventually supplied but until 1923 it lacked an efficient filter. The laundry was engineer Benbow's domain. He willingly patched various parts of the machinery to keep it going and fretted on returning from annual holidays to find the boiler neglected and tubes leaking because an inexperienced man had been placed in charge. With his specialised mechanical skills, he was a valued staff member and as such could lay down certain conditions for his employment which were granted. In 1924, when new fire-fighting apparatus was installed, he assured the board that he had inspected it and would ensure that it was always ready for use: '. . . this you can always rely upon me doing, providing the work is left to me without interference'.[31] His concern for the hospital extended to fund raising and in 1925, with the help of his fellow members in the Ancient Order of Druids, he conducted an art union to raise funds for a new theatre trolley.

Conditions in the laundry were far from ideal. It was years before a vent was built at the rear of the ironing machine where the temperature was unbearable for women at the irons. They shut their eyes and tried not to breathe deeply while washing the foul linen, a most disagreeable task, as despite Benbow's request for one, the hos-

---

[27] See *Ibid.*, 20 September 1922, 12 November 1924.
[28] *Ibid.*, 17 August 1928.
[29] *Ibid.*, 12 November 1924.
[30] *Ibid.*, 15 July 1921.
[31] *Ibid.*, 13 August 1924.

pital had no mechanical foul-linen washer, the principal medical officer considering it 'not an imperative necessity'.[32] Like the housemaids and kitchen-maids, the laundry maids lived at the hospital. Only in the mid-1920s did matron report: 'Laundry Staff sleep away from hospital'.[33] Work increased steadily. In the new laundry's fifth year (1924), 143,719 articles were laundered, in its sixth year, a record 146,506. The workers took pride in their laundry, polishing the brass work until it was a credit to them. In 1926 Mrs Waddell and Mrs Laidlaw from the board suggested that the employment of domestics and laundresses should be taken from the matron's list of responsibilities and placed in the hands of the house committee. Most men on the board opposed the principle involved and the motion was lost.

In the mid-1920s Mrs Waddell took the interests of the domestic staff to heart. There were 12 on the staff, working in the main kitchen, ward kitchens, and the quarters, or polishing and cleaning floors in the wards. For those who worked in a ward kitchen it became 'my kitchen' and woe betide the nurse who did not clean up after herself. The maid cooked the broths and, under the ward sister's direction, prepared any special diets. Members of the domestic staff were required to sleep at the hospital and, like the nurses, had to request a late pass for an evening out. The lamp light, flashed on their faces during nightly bed checks, warned against fracturing the rules. At work, maids wore a long uniform, over which they tied a large white apron.[34] In 1926 Mrs Waddell organised a Domestics Comforts Fund for the maids, and arranged the renovation of their quarters and the preparation of a tennis court for their use. When asked, the staff decided that they would like a piano from the proceeds of their fund, but the board rejected the idea and the girls concluded that books and pictures for their quarters would suffice. However, Mrs Waddell did not forget the original request and some months later apologised for her absence at the house committee meeting of 15 November 1927, 'as she was buying a piano for the Domestics' Quarters'. It was a gesture so appreciated that the staff took up a collection and presented their benefactor with a beautiful silver teapot suitably engraved.[35]

For many years the X-ray department was a neglected area of the hospital. When W. S. Priestly returned from the war, he was appointed radiographer and dispenser on 8 July 1919, leaving Arliss Robinson as secretary. Little had changed in the X-ray department in his absence, and the X-ray plant which had been in use since 1907 was showing its age. Undeterred, Priestly set to work taking frames for diagnostic work and conducting deep therapy treatment for cancer sufferers. Whereas only 16 X-ray cases had passed through the department in the five months between 1 February and 30 June 1919, which preceded Priestly's appointment, 201 were recorded in the five months between 1 November 1919 and 31 March 1920. (No X-ray work was recorded during Priestly's first four months when the Spanish influenza was rife.) So satisfied with his progress was one of the deep therapy cases of the early 1920s that

---

[32] *Ibid.*, 12 November 1924.

[33] *Ibid.*, 18 February 1925.

[34] Recollections of Jean Kingswood (née White), wardsmaid in men's medical ward from 1917 to the early 1920s, as told to M. McPherson, her niece. Notes held at FH.

[35] Teapot held in Fremantle Hospital archives. Donated by Mrs Waddell's great-niece, Mrs Dean Lang (a former Fremantle Hospital nurse).

he gave Priestly the first of a planned annual donation. One Perth patient transferred his treatment to Fremantle and others expressed gratitude for their treatment.
In 1921 there were 19 such patients. The long treatments taxed the tubes of the
apparatus but the work was considered generally satisfactory. However, in other
cases the old plant was often unable to provide a helpful diagnosis, especially in
locating foreign bodies in an abdomen. A search for a bullet in the chest of a patient
brought in one Monday night in June 1922 was only one of three instances that
month when unsatisfactory results were obtained. Even with the apparatus turned to
full power the location of the obstruction could only be roughly estimated. Nor was
the plant reliable. Towards the end of 1920, when it gave more trouble than usual,
Priestly overhauled the equipment and found the electrolyte worn and useless. It was
a contingency he had foreseen but the new fitting ordered from the Medical Department and repeatedly requested had not arrived. Five days later a new valve was obtained from the Tramways Board, which was always willing to share equipment and
expertise. 'Efforts have been made to obtain prices for altering this apparatus,'
Priestly told the board, 'but [it] is not effective enough for modern requirements.'[36]
There was not even means to regulate the current. The radiographer urged the installation of an interrupter apparatus to save wear and tear on the tubes, but the board
was less concerned with the apparatus than with the ledger, which the radiographer
was not keeping up to date, and he was summoned to an interview over the unsatisfactory state of the X-ray department.[37]

The financial side of the department certainly needed revision. Not only would
patients often detour straight out of the hospital gate instead of seeing the secretary
about payment following treatment, but the continuous treatment cases receiving
five or six minutes' exposure paid five shillings compared to an ordinary patient who
paid two guineas for an X-ray lasting between five and 15 seconds. In an effort to
redress the department's financial wrongs, a year later the board concluded that if a
patient had to pay for the X-ray before it was taken, the problem would be solved.
The plan worked for those with means, but the ill or injured poor, who were still the
majority of patients, had to take their X-ray order form from the hospital doctor
and find a board member to obtain his confirmation of their poverty, before re-
tracing their steps to have the X-ray taken. The young house surgeon, Joe Stubbe,
strongly objected on their behalf to having 'the correct treatment of the patient subservient to the financial side of the department' and the practice was discontinued.[38]

Early in 1922 the induction coil burned out and for three months no X-ray work
could be done. Mr Bold from the Fremantle Tramways came across to the hospital
to give practical advice, and the coil was eventually rewound by the government
department. Never was there a more opportune time for a representative of Watson
& Son to call and try to sell the hospital a new plant. Priestly's envy at the work that
could be done with the modern machines knew no bounds and he continued to press
for new equipment. At the end of 1922 the colonial secretary granted the hospital
£400 for a new plant and the board ordered a 'Solace interrupterless Apparatus with
twice 10 inch spark transformers, 120,000 volts' costing £567, and added a Potter

[36] Minutes of BM, 25 August 1920. See also *Ibid.*, 15 September 1920, 17 August 1921.
[37] *Ibid.*, 20 October 1920.
[38] *Ibid.*, 19 April 1922.

Bucky Diaphragm from Gilberts Limited.[39] Before it arrived the last tube on the old apparatus gave out and work once more ground to a halt. Although not complete, the new plant was installed and working by mid-April 1923, with the house surgeon's assistance. The original makeshift table was unusable with the new equipment so Priestly and engineer Benbow roughly adapted it. It still wobbled so Priestly worked on the design of a new fixed table similar to an expensive proprietary model but able to be built locally, and the board outlaid £25 for its construction. Having an X-ray taken could be a frightening experience. The accompanying blue flash of electric flame was usually hidden from a patient's view, but there was always a loud din and acrid smell from the open mechanical rectifier that no wall or screen could hide.[40] Although figures varied from month to month, hospital cases invariably far outnumbered those referred by private doctors. The ratio of 229 to 40 in 1923, was not unusual.

On 30 June 1924, Priestly resigned as radiographer and dispenser and Dr Frederick Clark, who as the hospital's house surgeon had carried out X-ray work when Priestly took annual leave, was elected as the honorary radiologist. He swept into the position with reforms and improvements. Even with the new apparatus, conditions were far from ideal. When the black-painted X-ray room was closed and darkened, light still came in through ventilators, under doors and between window casings, and the pale coloured furniture reflected light into the operator's eyes when the tube was glowing. As part of renovations undertaken, the furniture was also painted black. Clark then directed his attention to finances, suggesting an increase in the five-shilling fee paid by the therapy patients. Next he called for one orderly to clean the X-ray room, who could be taught to handle the equipment carefully, and 'replace things in their right place instead of anywhere' rather than 'anyone at random as at present'.[41] He planned the purchase of a new fluorescent screen and a medium-focus tube before turning his attention to the efficiency of the department. Clark maintained that a nurse should be in attendance while people were treated, as 'many cases are bandaged up, many are women' and he suggested a greater control of X-ray patients, who came at any time and had no notion of what treatment was required.[42] A patient treatment request card issued at casualty or the office and taken to the X-ray department, was organised, and the films on glass plates with a patient's record of past attendances and reports, were filed for future reference. When his period of appointment expired in June 1926, Clark's influence continued although no honorary radiologist was appointed immediately in his place.

When Dr C. Roger Dunkley took on the position in October, the room still admitted light from many sources, tubes still needed replacing, and fluctuations in the current sometimes caused damage to the plant. The purchase of a mobile X-ray unit in late 1927 expanded the facilities and increased the effectiveness of the department but in late 1928 the honorary staff were calling for an urgent overhaul of the X-ray plant by its makers. Dunkley felt that he lacked the expertise to continue in his posi-

[39] *Ibid.*, 20 December 1922.
[40] See J. W. Bruce, 'West Coast Radiography', in *The Radiographer*, Vol. 21, No. 5, December 1974, p. 135. See also section on Fremantle Hospital, p. 137.
[41] Minutes of BM, 10 December 1924.
[42] *Ibid.*, 11 March 1925.

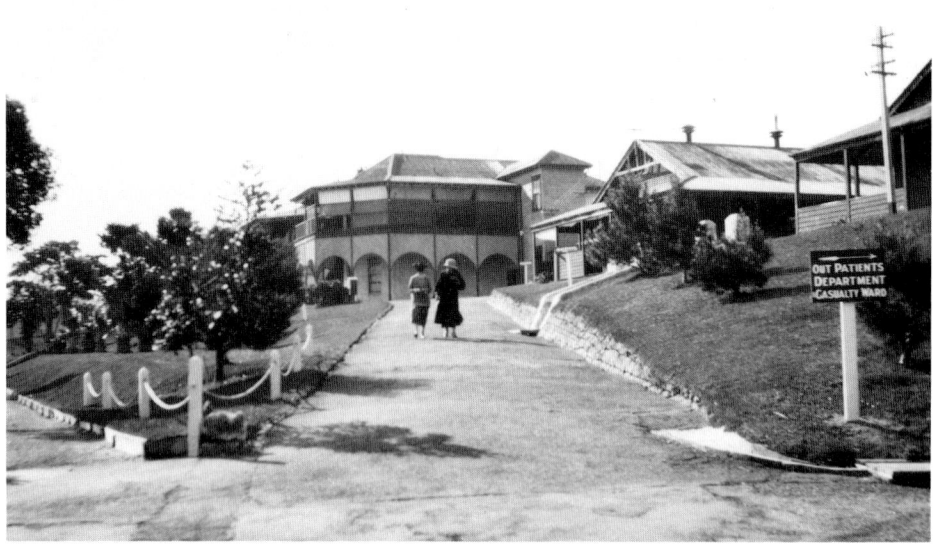

Photograph courtesy A. Orloff

Plate 29. Fremantle Hospital, c. 1920s.

Now Male Medical was one of two wards, both of galvanized iron. They were long iron wards, connected at the back. The connection at the back really was ... a 'breeze way' all right ... It was pretty primitive and the wards were very, very hot in the summer as you can imagine and the men that were in these wards they were not—well, some of them were pretty down and out and some of them weren't ... the people who went to Fremantle Hospital at that stage had to be the 'sick poor'.

Victoria Hobbs
Nursing Sister, 1935

tion and when Mr C. G. Wood, who had come to Perth from Adelaide to work for the Hospital Electric and Radium Company, became available, he was appointed radiographer with responsibility for the plant and its maintenance, as well as for patients' records and the smooth, speedy transition of cases through the department. Like many early radiographers, including his own brother in Adelaide, Wood suffered radiation burns to his right arm, which had to be amputated the following year in 1930.[43] Dr Arthur Gibson, who had studied radiology after the war and set up a practice in Perth, was appointed as honorary radiologist and planned to reconstruct the department in 1929. First he installed a new developing tank and an X-ray tube. Then he called on the Perth Hospital X-ray department for advice. An honorary radiologist from Perth Hospital, Dr Alan Syme-Johnson, came down and

---

[43] Minutes of HC, 13 October 1930, 14 November 1930. See Bruce, 'West Cost Radiography', p. 137. The orginal glass plates used by Priestly, Wood and the other early radiographers were found years later when the department was renovated.

for a time was enthusiastic about taking over the department at Fremantle, suggesting that Dunkley act as his assistant with the aid of a nurse trained in X-ray work at Perth. With the assurance that the nurse would still be under her direction, Maida Balding suggested young Olive Jones for training, but the nurse resigned the position in March 1930 after three months, and the vacancy was advertised at a charge nurse's salary of £150 a year. Sister Shirley quietly considered the idea, and offered to undertake the training, but nothing was done as Sister Robinson, a radiographer from the Children's Hospital, advised that she would be available in five months. Syme-Johnson looked at the facilities and threatened that unless an up-to-date tilt table was ordered, the hospital would not obtain his services. The ladies' auxiliary set to work to raise the funds and provided the table, but for almost two years until 1932 Dr Maurice Johnson, not Syme-Johnson, served as an Honorary Radiologist at the hospital. With the department desperately understaffed and in a state of disorganisation, Sister Shirley was approached to see if she still wanted the position of X-ray nurse. For some weeks from June 1930 she trained at Perth—sometimes at the hospital, sometimes in Dr Maurice Johnson's office—until she had learned the basic techniques and was appointed radiographer at Fremantle Hospital. For a few days, until it proved unworkable, Sister Shirley was also placed in charge of the outpatients and casualty departments, such was the board's zeal in effecting economy wherever possible.

On Priestly's resignation as X-ray technician and dispenser in 1924, the board decided to separate the responsibilities. A visiting committee in 1920 had found the dispensary unoccupied and was not impressed with either the cleanliness or the tidiness there, and were of the opinion that there was room for improvement. Priestly checked doctors' prescriptions, weighed and mixed powders such as opium and morphine, ground smooth pastes with a pestle and mortar, rolled and cut pills, and pounded compounds into liniments and ointments to make the hospital's medicines. He then distributed them to in-patients and out-patients in corked bottles or lidded jars with hand-written labels. Cod liver oil, arsenic, digitalis, salicylates, castor and paraffin oils, salvarsan, strychnine, quinine and paraldehyde were among ingredients commonly used.[44] Wine was still an important medication in the 1920s and an auditor's report urged the closer supervision of 'dressings, bandages and wines and spirits' to reduce costs.[45] In 1923 another visiting committee found the bottles in the dispensary and bulk drug room very dusty. Tucked away as he was, however, on the northern side of The Knowle near the casualty and out-patients departments, the dispenser was usually taken for granted as long as he filled the required prescriptions. Three men applied for Priestly's position when he resigned and Mr Sallur was engaged at a salary of £5 a week, rising to £5.10.0 after six months' satisfactory service. His coming was not without some conflict. Not long afterwards, Dr Clark submitted complaints to the house committee about the dispenser—he arrived late for work, took extra time for lunch and neglected his duty. The house committee recommended Sallur's immediate discharge with a month's salary in lieu of notice. The board concurred and the position was declared vacant. The new dispenser did

[44]   See Stubbe, *Medical Background*, Preface, p. xxv. For general background, see E. Jacobson, *Tinctures and Tact*, 1982, pp. 19–20.
[45]   Minutes of BM, 11 January 1922.

not take the action meekly and defended himself before the board at its next meeting. Dr Harpur, who had been at the hospital since December 1923, first as the junior, then the senior resident medical officer, could find little fault with the dispenser and Sallur was placed on three months' probation under the direction of the senior resident doctor, having to record his hours on and off duty in a time book. Between 9 a.m. and 5 p.m., except for a lunch hour, and on Saturday from 9 a.m. until 1 p.m., Sallur dispensed under the guidance of a list drawn up by Harpur, and also did some X-ray work when necessary. There were no more complaints and his position was confirmed. When Sallur resigned on 9 February 1927 the position was filled by J. K. Christie. Twice a week at night, as part of their duties, first Sallur and later Christie dispensed for the hospital's venereal diseases clinic.

There was probably no time when the colony had not had sufferers of gonorrhoea, syphilis or soft chancre among its inhabitants and through the years the afflicted were urged to send for various promising treatments delivered in anonymously wrapped parcels. In 1872, colonists were advised that they could purchase for ten shillings and sixpence the book *Constitutional Syphilis*, illustrated with 20 beautifully coloured plates and written by Dr James Beanie, the former surgeon to the Melbourne Hospital and Her Majesty's Troops in the Crimean War. The press lauded the publication and regretted that its information could not be conveyed to all young men on entering life.[46] The movement of infected men, at first to the goldfields, and between 1914 and 1918 from countries at war, plus the coming and going of infected sailors from ships, increased the incidence of venereal disease and a room at the Fremantle Hospital was set up as a 'V.D. Clinique' in 1917. It seemed that every one at the hospital knew it was there but most feigned ignorance of its existence. Two honorary medical officers were appointed on a government honorarium of £68.10.0. to attend the clinic. In 1920 Drs Kerr and Gibson were responsible, but when Hilda Kershaw joined Dr East as an assistant it was seemly to appoint them to treat the afflicted females and males respectively. Young Dr E. R. Dermer succeeded Kershaw. There were many in the community who shared the moralistic opinion of two board members, that the Venereal Diseases Clinique was 'an unsavoury place' and it was the last area considered to need upgrading, although the cubicles at times were dirty and required attention.[47] The anguish of some of the affected soldiers returning to their homes can be imagined, and one hospital patient with the disease newly diagnosed, tried to take his life rather than face his family.

Most of the regular patients who came by night to the venereal diseases clinics in the out-patients' department were Fremantle residents. They were joined by sailors when their ships were in port, as such diseases were classified as notifiable. The fact that he was a member of a ship's crew was no excuse for a sailor to miss treatment. Shipping companies were responsible for seeing that infected sailors attended clinics at each port for treatment, and police were asked to arrest those who tried to avoid the ordeal. A doctor diagnosing syphilis or gonorrhoea had to report the case to the Medical Department but statistical anonymity was retained as long as the patient submitted to medical treatment. If there was a lapse in attendance, the department

[46] *Inquirer*, 16 October 1872.
[47] Minutes of BM, 20 September 1922. See also 21 February 1923.

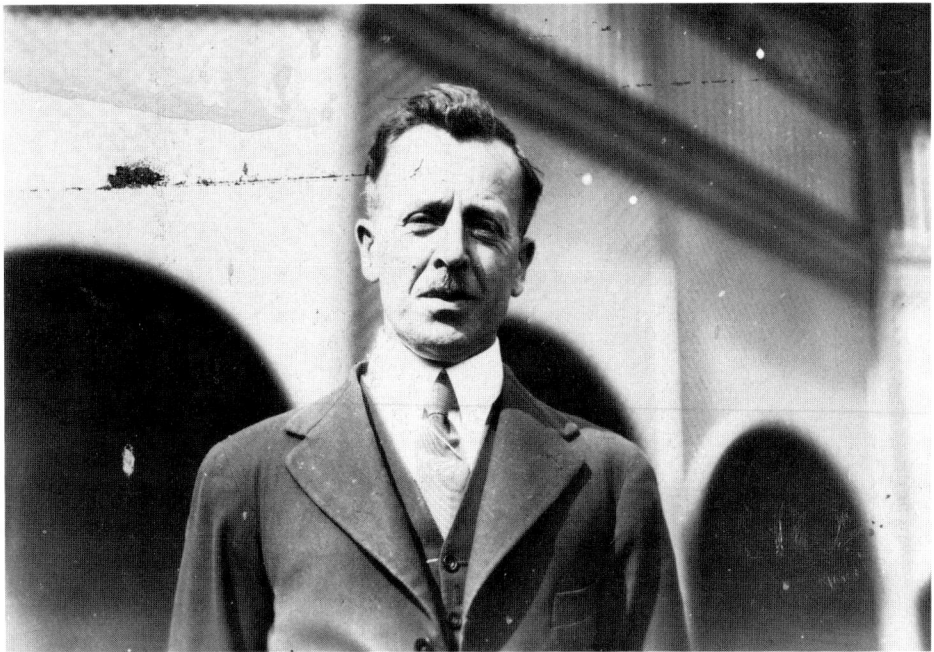

Photograph courtesy Fremantle Hospital

Plate 30.   Mr A. T. Hookway, Secretary of Fremantle Hospital for 22 years, who retired in 1948.

Mr Hookway was the secretary at the hospital and he had a very, very tough time there try-ing to square the ledger. He was not helped by the Medical Department who were under Mr Huelin who was very demanding. Mr Hookway survived and we managed, shall I say, to crawl through. It was a dreadful business.

Dr H. Uther Baker

had to be informed and if a patient continued to refuse treatment, hospitalisation for the very ill or gaoling by police for compulsory treatment, usually by a warder, ensued. The top-floor cubicles of the women's home in Finnerty Street, Fremantle, carpetted and made comfortable—while the lower floors where the old women waited out their time were bare—were used to confine such women under remand.[48] Treatment was lengthy, unpleasant and not always effective: 'Salvarsan and mer-cury ointment to run in' for male syphilis cases; washouts for gonorrhoea patients. Women endured washouts and swabbings and the painting and cauterizing of their cervix.[49] It was not surprising that some tried to avoid the treatment. Re-infection was not uncommon. From April 1925, Sallur stayed after work and dispensed for the night Venereal Diseases Clinique for a small fee. With a reorganisation of the department in 1926, dispensing for the 'VD clinic' was changed to regular hospital

[48]   Recollections of Barrington Knight (interview). The doctor visited the elderly, ill ladies in the women's home when he was a resident medical officer at Fremantle Hospital in the early 1930s.
[49]   *Ibid.*

hours. Thinking of its budget, the board decided not to pay Sallur the usual extra amount for prescriptions he dispensed for the venereal diseases patients. This decision angered the dispenser and he took the matter up with the board demanding either a return of the fee or an increase in wages. Neither, however, was granted.

In 1925, Arliss Robinson was confident in his position as secretary, yet may not have given the co-operation expected of an employee in charge of finances at the hospital. During a board meeting in August 1925 he was asked to retire and at the end of the meeting to resign. He did so from 18 August. From 54 applicants for the position, a tall, dark young man named Hookway was selected and commenced on 28 September 1925. Finances became a central concern for him, just as they had for each of the hospital's previous secretaries. Although he did not organise it, Hookway became involved in running the motor car art union for the hospital. The first instalment of £100 for the vehicle was donated by the Honorable Robert Lynn; books of 22 tickets sold for £1 a book. Hookway also worked hard for the 1925 combined hospitals' Saturday and Sunday collection fund. His services were appreciated and the house committee told the board that:

> Mr A.T. Hookway is carrying out his duties in an able and efficient manner. At the outset, he took the stand that in all matters connected with the staff, the Public, and the Patients, he represented the Board of Management. The house committee endorses this view and believe economy without impairing efficiency will be practiced to a greater extent in the institution.[50]

His position was one that Hookway took seriously and with the help of Mr Cousins and Mr J. Turner in the office, he administered hospital affairs in a commendable manner throughout the next difficult decades.

In 1925 there were also plans to form a ladies' auxiliary committee. With the enthusiastic support of Lady Campion, who had attended the nurses' ball and inspected the hospital, Matron Balding asked the house committee for the names of likely women who might respond to an invitation to join. On Friday, 28 August, Lady Campion chaired a successful meeting at which Mrs Gill was appointed as a temporary president, and many names were collected to form a committee. They were women of standing and status in the town. The first meeting of the ladies' auxiliary committee was held at the hospital on Friday, 4 September 1925. Mrs A. White was elected president, with Miss J. McKay as secretary. The women decided to hold a bridge afternoon at Mrs White's on 19 September, the proceeds of which would 'start the fund for commencing the work'.

The 'work' was urgently needed. The wards were filled to capacity in mid-1925 and even the full-sized beds occupied by children were eyed covetously for the women's ward. The daily average of patients in hospital in mid-May 1925 was 67. There were 71 at the end of June, 73 in mid-July and by the beginning of August there were 73.3 patients, an increase of almost ten on the previous year. The growth taxed all facilities and emphasised the deficiencies. There was no provision for keeping patients' meals hot between the kitchen and the wards, and no food-carrying trolley; the kitchen staff had to make several trips with meals to the different wards.

---

[50] Minutes of BM, 11 November 1925.

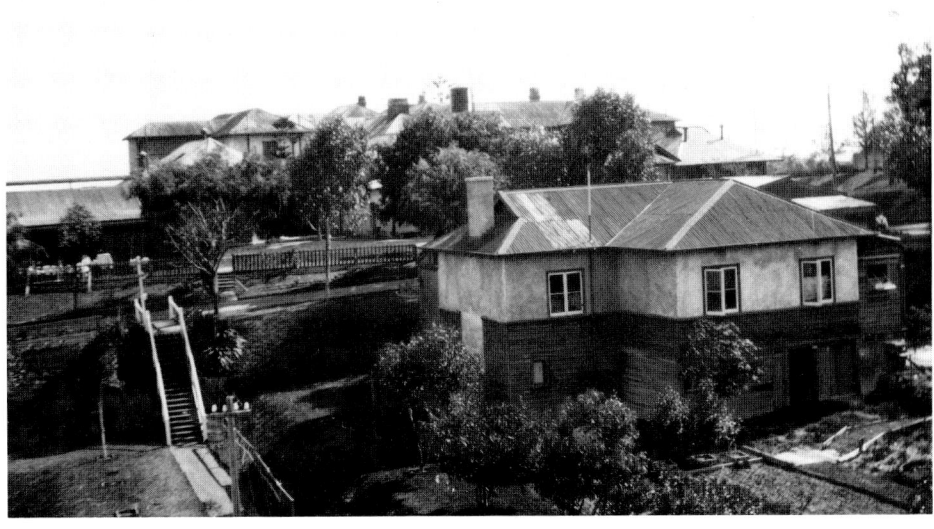

Photograph courtesy A. Orloff

Plate 31.   Nurses' quarters behind The Knowle, *c.* 1920s.

In the new quarters everyone had single rooms, upstairs and down. Very nice, and we had very nice lounge rooms and we had our first get together in a dance, which we went to Matron about, and said we'd like to invite our friends . . .

Marjorie Lund
Nursing staff

Ingredients for cooking could not be weighed in bulk for there were no large scales in the kitchen. There was no mattress airer, and mattresses taken out of the fumigator were not always dry before use. The 12 live-in maids even had to heat water on a gas ring for a bath in their quarters, and were only supplied with a chip heater because they used the gas 'extravagantly, very often'.[51]

Under the Collier Labor Government, between 1924 and 1929 hospital finances remained shaky, but there was an end to the long period during which no building work was carried out. An extension to the nurses' home was a priority. In January 1925, matron was trying to accommodate 31 nurses when she had only 30 beds, and in August two of the nurses' beds had to be placed in the women's ward. Plans for the new work costing £3,250 were finalised in December 1924. The following March a pile of bricks was delivered. By April work was underway and, in order to get some peace, the night nurses were moved to the vacant isolation ward. Matron wanted the plans amended to include a gas ring for the new quarters so that the nurses could make themselves a cup of tea when off duty, and somewhere where they could do their small laundry and personal washing, which they usually smuggled up to the wards to do when on duty.

[51]   *Ibid.*, 18 February 1925.

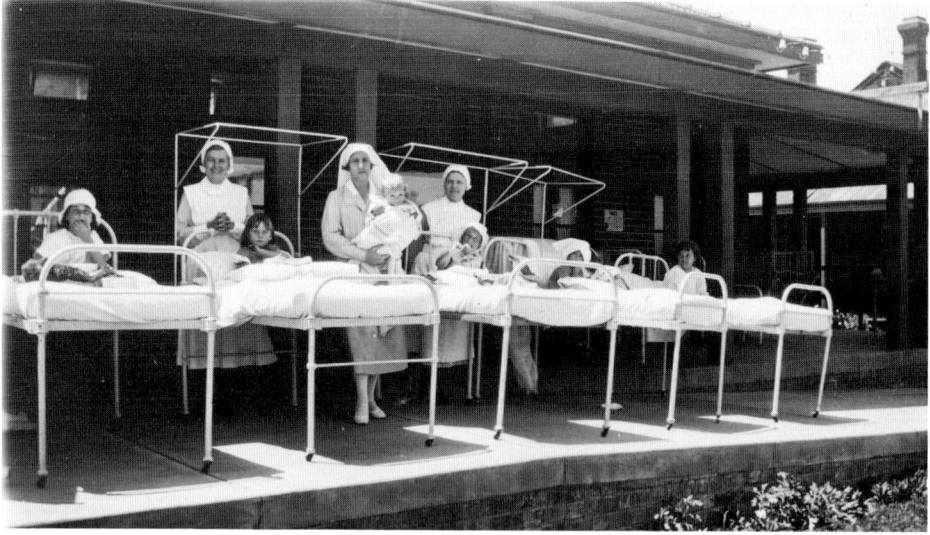

Photograph courtesy Mrs Edinger

Plate 32. *(Left to right)*: Nurse Draper, Sister Freeman and Nurse Murray on the verandah of the original Adelaide Samson Children's Ward which was opened in 1927. A patient of 1935 recalled time spent there:

> I had the bed near the fireplace. Of course I was in traction in those days—I had many operations . . . they used to drill and try to drain the wounds, and to keep you still they put in traction to make you stay that way . . . when I came out of traction—went out on to the verandah and we used to be able to look up and see the undertaker's vehicles.
>
> Bill Wilkinson
> Patient and Hospital Telephonist

With the nurses' quarters underway, when the Minister for Health visited the hospital in April 1925, the board decided to stress its need for a new surgical ward. Great was the satisfaction at a favourable response and a special committee comprising the chairman, vice-chairman, Dr East representing the honoraries, Dr Harpur as the resident medical officer, Matron Balding and the secretary were appointed to consider plans for the new ward. By early 1926 it was obvious that the children's ward, which had been the emergency dining room set up seven years earlier for the influenza epidemic, was the worse for wear. In planning the new surgical block it was decided to place the surgical cases on the lower of the two floors of the new building and the children upstairs, together with any overflow from the women's ward. It was clearly a temporary solution to the overcrowding and when the new board was announced in January 1926, and Angus McLeod and Harry Woodhouse had been re-elected as chairman and vice-chairman, the board decided to build a new children's ward with a bequest left to the hospital by Adelaide Samson.[52] In

---

52 Adelaide was the second daughter of Hon. Lionel Samson, who settled in Fremantle in 1829. She died on 19 September 1921, aged 72 years. See *Fremantle Gazette*, 19 August 1981; Stubbe, *Medical Background*, p. 54.

August 1926, the month that the board decided to sink its own well, it also approved plans for the two new ward blocks and a kitchen. By August 1927, the sewerage pipes, inadvertently broken when the well was sunk, had been repaired; materials from the old surgical ward had been sold for £50 which helped towards furnishing the nurses' quarters and the children's ward; and the board decided to name the new children's ward—which was rapidly taking its final shape—the Adelaide Samson Ward, on behalf of its benefactor. Work was finished in October, a month before the official opening and the small patients were carefully transferred into the spacious, well-ventilated, £3,000 building which could accommodate 24 beds and provide the wonderful sound of a wireless. When the ward was officially opened on a sunny Sunday afternoon on 6 November 1927, many of the new patients watched from the shady verandahs and clapped Mayor F. E. Gibson, Chairman McLeod and the Minister for Health S. W. Munsie. They cheered as Mrs L. Evans, a niece of the kind, late Adelaide Samson, officially unlocked the building's new front door and declared the ward open.[53]

The sound of hammering and sawing continued to echo into 1928 as the two-storeyed surgical ward and the new kitchen took shape. Another member of the community was equally busy. As a baker at Broken Hill earlier in the century he had supplied striking miners with bread; as a citizen of Fremantle he organized a unique drive to raise funds for the hospital. Mr E. H. (Harry) Gray, M.L.C., appealed for people to donate goods of all kinds which would then be sold for a shilling. It was an inspired plan: 'Everyone got a prize which was valued at at least one shilling. Even the children at the schools donated fancy work, books, etc. Donations of goods came from everywhere.'[54] An empty shop was loaned as headquarters, street collections were conducted by the appeal committee and many in the community became enthusiastically involved. On the night before the opening of the new ward, however, Harry Gray read in the press that it was anticipated that he would donate £2,000 to the hospital. He was £60 short. Undaunted, on the following morning he asked one, then another, and another for a contribution, until he had over £70. At the official opening of the ward on the afternoon of 23 September 1928, Harry Gray presented the chairman of the hospital board with just over £2,000. The wards, which cost £10,500, were Nightingale in shape, with male surgical cases on the lower level and female surgical patients on the upper floor. Without the surgical beds in it, even the women's medical ward on the first floor of The Knowle seemed spacious. The Minister for Health, Mr Munsie, with pleasure declared the new wards open and also took the opportunity to urge that school children should have their teeth examined regularly as a means of reducing the number of medical patients in hospital by at least ten per cent.[55] Among the large crowd were many Fremantle people, not just to witness the event but as proud contributors to the appeal organised by Gray. By

[53] *West Australian*, 7 November 1927.
[54] Notes supplied by Mrs E. H. Gray, March 1987. See also *West Australian*, 24 September 1928.
[55] *West Australian*, 24 September 1928. Although there had been talk of starting a dental clinic for Fremantle in the hospital's old isolation block in 1931, it was not until 1936 that a clinic was established through Mayor Frank Gibson and Mr J. Gustafson, at the Union Bank Chambers in High Street. In its first four years, 3,078 young patients of low-income families were treated. In 1949 a system of scaled fees was introduced so that children of between six and 14 could continue to be attended to, and by 1951 the centre was being called the 'Gustafson Children's Dental Clinic', PHD File 825/31.

the end of the following September, plans were being made to close in the verandahs of the new wards. Sunshine and fresh air were all very well, but enclosures meant an increase in accommodation and more usable ward space in inclement weather. It was inevitable that the board planned next to reorganise the central administrative portion of The Knowle, but almost as inevitable that funds from the Medical Department were unavailable. Renovation of the old male medical ward was started, however, and the Medical Department muttered about plans for an urgently needed out-patients' department, but so softly that nothing was done.

Patients in the hospital experienced not only different ailments, but were treated by different staff at different times in the decade between 1920 and 1930. Most appreciated the care shown to them. A visiting committee in 1922 reported patients' praise of nurses '... for kindness and attention given to them while laid aside. We mention this because people when ill, so often find something to grumble at—we felt that such expressions of gratitude must indeed be genuine.'[56] One patient at Perth Public Hospital put his thoughts to paper in a verse which was greatly valued and circulated amongst nurses at the metropolitan hospitals:

'THE NIGHT NURSE'

The ward is closed, the lights are low
Some of them draped in red
A case is on the danger list
The nurse must softly tread
The pulse beats slow on a strong man's wrist
A wreck in a snow white bed.

Silence reigns in the quilted cot
A light dread fills the scene
What is time to the sleeper
When destiny hangs between
The hours go by like a drifting mist
A case lies on the danger list
Of the verge of the great unseen.

The patient nurse alone in the night
With the lengthening shadow creeps
In the after glow of that soft red light
Out west where the dream waves sleep
Drifting slow are the threads of life
Can she pilot his weary soul tonight
Back from the Western Deep.[57]

Doctors, too, received accolades but it was the nurses who worked constantly and closely with the patient, often for weeks or months when a person was vulnerable and needing care. Strong ties of concern and respect were often made. In 1926 the number of patients in hospital for six weeks or more was on one occasion six, but

[56] Minutes of BM, 21 June 1922.
[57] Found pencilled carefully in the front of a Children's Hospital nurse's textbook in a second-hand bookshop. Dated 17 July 1928.

usually eight or ten, and at the end of the year was 14 or 15. In 1930 the number was still between eight and 15. In August 1933 it rose to 20, and Secretary Hookway was again pointing out the urgency of the need for a convalescent home 'to relieve the hospital wards'.[58] Four patients were in for further operations, two for diathermy and massage, six were serious medical cases and four were major surgical cases, while Dr Radcliffe-Taylor's orthopaedic patients, made cumbersome with splints or plaster, numbered four.[59] The house surgeon explained:

> One reason for the lengthy period of treatment required is that orthopaedic cases are usually in hospital for a very long time. The other patients are suffering from chronic ailments. As our wards are continually overcrowded this is becoming a serious problem and one extremely difficult of solution.[60]

By January 1934 there were 27 long-term patients. Several should have been sent to '. . . an institution for incurable diseases,' urged Dr Cass, the senior resident medical officer, but 'until such arrangements can be made they must remain here'.[61] Accommodation at the Home of Peace was limited and the chronically sick poor often had nowhere to go. Among the 26 patients in hospital for six weeks or more in June 1937 were cases of tuberculosis, diabetes, cancer, rickets, back injuries, fractures, osteomyelitis and a patient with a gangrenous knee.[62]

Not all patients wanted to stay. Olive Acton was eight years old when she had her tonsils and adenoids out under a general anaesthetic at three o'clock one afternoon in 1933. She was placed on a lounge on the Adelaide Samson Ward verandah with two other children under the charge of a nurse who left briefly to perform other duties after her patients fell asleep at six-thirty. Olive only drowsed and was thinking about going home. The longer she thought about it, the better the idea seemed. So quickly did she move that when the buildings and grounds were searched 15 minutes later there was no trace of her. The senior resident medical officer rang Olive's father to tell him the news, only to learn that the child was home and that the father wondering what he should do to avoid her taking a chill from exposure.[63] Olive was not the only one to abscond after a tonsillectomy. Nick Silich recalled

> . . . being taken to the Fremantle Hospital. We were lined up in a room, to take our turn. The eldest brother Vic went in first, then I could hear the gargling and after he had gone under the anaesthetic—'Okay, next please'—in went Nick in a lather of sweat. I was placed on this table and they put the hood over my nose and I could hear the angels singing and buzzing in my ears, and I eventually remembered no more. Next thing, I was in bed with a sore throat, in one of the wards, and the other brothers were also done. I understand Vic didn't like this, and living so close to the hospital, he just went walkie. Next thing, they dug him from home and brought him back to the hospital, to see his couple of days out [Nick was 7 or 8 at the time] . . . we were all rather

58 *West Australian*, 10 August 1933.
59 House Surgeon's reports are contained in Minutes of BM, various volumes; House Surgeon's Report Book, 2 June 1930, 15 July 1937, FH.
60 Dr Cass, SRMO, House Surgeon's Report Book, 15 to 28 September 1933.
61 *Ibid.*, 5 January 1934.
62 House Surgeon's Report Book, 15 July 1937.
63 House Surgeon's Report Book, 3 and 10 November 1933.

young and it was considered at that time, with such a sore throat and regularly recurring, that we should have our tonsils out.[64]

Another minor operation which was considered the 'in' thing, was circumcision for male babies. The infants would often be brought from Hillcrest Salvation Army home by car, operated on and the affected part bound round with ribbon gauze dipped in zinc cream, olive oil and thymol. Some surgeons preferred friar's balsam. An ill baby, or one who needed a Wassermann test for congenital syphilis, or perhaps a mother needing a caesarean section, were also admitted from Hillcrest.[65]

The death of a fellow patient was not a hidden ritual for patients in hospital. With few spare rooms where the dying could be taken, a wooden or an iron screen with white curtains, placed around the bed, was the usual privacy. Until 1927, when the council agreed to make Attfield Street a serviceable road and a back gate was built near the morgue, everyone from patients to the butcher, the ambulance and visitors, shared the same hospital road with the hearse on its way to the morgue to collect bodies. As there was no cooler in the shed-like structure with its two large lead tables in the middle and where, if there was a third body, it had to be laid on the floor, prompt burial of a body was advisable. When the town crier, Yorkie Creswick, died and through an administrative hitch lay from one hot Wednesday afternoon to Saturday, the press protested vigorously at the delay.[66] Occasionally, recalled a doctor, 'nobody else would bury [poor] people that used to die in the hospital and the Salvos would always bury them'.[67] The dead would be dressed in shrouds made by nurses from coarsely woven cotton, stiff with dressing:

> . . . Ooh, terrible stuff. White powder all over you. We just put . . . a band around the neck and picot edged the frill of the shroud . . .[68]

Most patients came from the Fremantle area and were not too upset at having to pay the farthing rate struck by the Fremantle Roads Board in aid of hospital funds in 1925.[69] In a not atypical month in August 1933 when there had been 317 inpatients, 271 came from Fremantle and sister districts, 18 from between Buckland Hill and Swanbourne, 11 lived at Perth and Claremont, two at Midland Junction, seven came in from the country, four off ships and another four were hospital staff.[70] Occasionally there was a patient from the gaol and in 1926, to everyone's consternation, a life-sentence prisoner escaped from a ward.

Visitors were usually welcomed by patients. Churches, lodges, service groups and organizations such as the Fremantle Labor Party, the Lumpers' Union or the Fremantle Labor Women's Organization were able to get a visitor's pass from the hospital board so that their members could be visited regularly, but most visitors from 1925 had to pay their sixpence.[71] Because of the lack of chairs in the hospital they

[64]   N. Silich, interviewed by L. Stevens, 17 and 24 September 1983, 14 January 1984.
[65]   Barrington Knight, interview.
[66]   Sunday Times, 22 December 1912.
[67]   Barrington Knight, interview.
[68]   H. Heath, interviewed by C. Jeffery, 15 May 1984, FH.
[69]   Minutes of BM, 8 July 1925.
[70]   House Surgeon's Report Book, August 1933.
[71]   Minutes of BM, 11 May 1926.

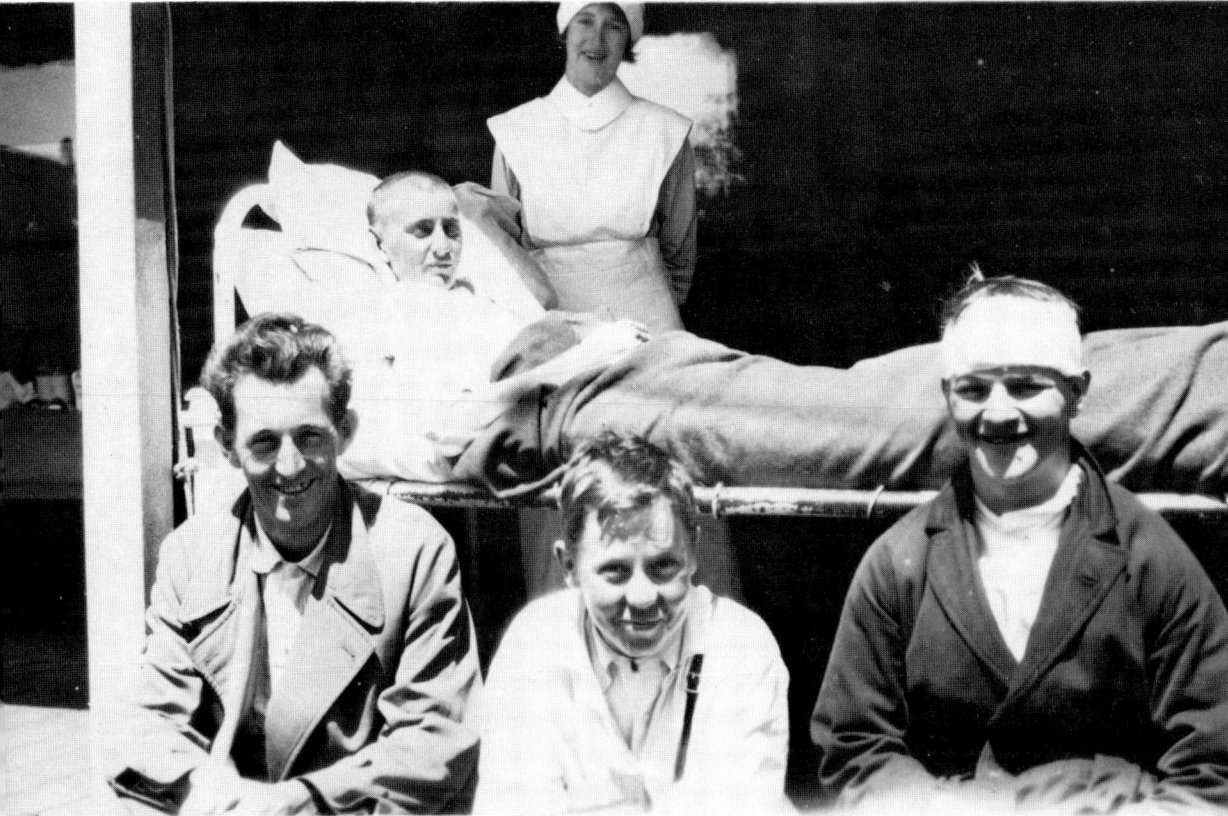

Plate 33.   Patients in Fremantle Hospital in the 1930s.

often had to stand. Visiting hours were strictly enforced unless there were exceptional circumstances, even for husbands and wives when transport or work may have made visiting within the prescribed hours difficult. Changes were suggested at different times by honoraries, the ladies' auxiliary, resident medical officers and the nursing staff. Dr Kerr wanted strict regulation of visitors by the rules in 1926, and in 1927 Dr East tried to reduce visiting hours but did not have board's support. In 1929 visiting hours were changed from two to two-thirty for an afternoon visit, and from six-thirty to seven in the evening to suit the charge nurses, as the hours were not convenient for the work of the wards.[72] A nurse's care was considered of more importance to a patient's recovery than the stimulation of a visitor and in 1933 matron pressed for a reduction in the hours and was supported by the senior resident medical officer: 'The length of visit allowed should be reduced from one hour to

[72]   *Ibid.*, 16 August 1929.

about forty-five minutes. This would give the nursing staff more time to attend their patients before going off duty at 9 p.m'.[73] The migrant visitors 'didn't understand and came in anyway'.[74]

Favourite visitors in the children's ward were the bun lady and the chocolate man who came weekly. 'She [the bun lady] was an old dear that used to make buns and bring them up to the kids' ward every Wednesday. She used to come up with a basket and make these little, very plain little cakes with hundred and thousands and things on them.'[75] The chocolate man was the Church of England minister, Canon Collick, who cycled to the hospital and brought comics or penny Nestle's chocolates in their distinctive red wrappers on Thursdays. Neither was he ever too busy or too tired to attend a sick patient. Patients and visitors alike in 1929 were treated to a series of concerts in the hospital grounds by Mr Ingram's Fremantle Citizens' Orchestra. So enthusiastic about the performances was Angus McLeod from the board that he suggested that the orchestra should be known as the Fremantle Hospital Orchestra but, when put to the board vote, the motion was lost. The orchestra crowded into the children's ward on Christmas Eve and returned to play for the adults on Christmas Day. In 1927 a different visit delighted patients and staff alike when the Duke and Duchess of York (later King George VI and Queen Elizabeth) were driven ceremoniously around Fremantle Oval to cheers from an enthusiastic crowd. A ramp was built over a dip in the hospital wall and everyone who could be moved was taken onto the bank opposite. Excited nurses placed children into cane pushers, and helped carry some patients—bed and all—onto the oval, where they were granted a special royal wave in their direction.[76]

Many people trekked through the out-patients' door under the sharp eye of Mr Hookway, who checked that only the eligible were amongst patients who paid the two-shilling fee to the lodge keeper. Some came for dental treatment by the honorary dentist—George Emmis in 1921, and Claude Terry from 1923, who was joined by P. J. McAuliffe in 1929. The resident medical officer would ring the dentist from the out-patients' clinic 'and he would come to the hospital and I would say, "There is a person here that has got some dental problems, would you come up and have a look at them?"' An ether anaesthetic removed much of the discomfort of major dental surgery but going home after a night in hospital with a throbbing, swollen mouth was not pleasant. The old retired miners from the Goldfields house near South Terrace often rejected the expertise of the honorary:

> Their main feature was they wouldn't have any new fangled ideas. They wanted their teeth pulled out. They wouldn't go to the dentist, they would come to the hospital and you had to pull the tooth out without needles. None of these new fangled ideas. 'No doctor. No. Just pull it out.' And you would pull it out.[77]

Many out-patients came to consult a doctor, but most came for treatment following hospitalisation. As there was some talk by the Medical Department in 1927

73 House Surgeon's Report Book, 28 September 1933.
74 M. Murray, interviewed by J. Lancaster, 15 November 1986, FH.
75 Barrington Knight, interview.
76 R. Buzza, interviewed by J. Lancaster, 1987, FH.
77 Barrington Knight, interview.

about a new out-patients block, little was done to improve the old quarters in The Knowle. It was the same in the casualty area, where glazing on the windows was so worn that there was no privacy for patients under examination, and the horse-hair mattress on the examination table prickled where the leather was worn through. A conciliatory coat of paint was applied to walls in 1927 but the doctors still had no examining cubicles:

> We just pulled a curtain around a place in casualty and there was a table in the middle where you did all the dressings and it was—it was really hard work, getting through the work in the conditions we had. You see we only had four places for people to sit down and have their dressings. We had one couch that people could lie on for examinations. A bit grim.[78]

The organisation of theatre and out-patients was the responsibility of a single charge sister, usually the senior in the hospital.

A long wait before seeing a doctor was usual, and out-patients had to remember to bring their own bottles and jars for medicines and mixtures from the dispensary. In July 1933, Christie, the dispenser, prepared and distributed 1,755 prescriptions for the 2,645 out-patients who attended that month, as well as 519 prescriptions for in-patients and 296 lotions.[79] In May 1932 he was commended by the board for his good work. Over 70 out-patients attended monthly in 1930 for treatment by the masseur: for massage, for manipulation, or for electric current therapy, to have muscles stimulated or relaxed, the blood supply to an area increased, or greater mobility restored to a stiffened limb.[80] Miss Jean Lewis resigned as hospital masseuse in 1921 to go to the goldfields and was replaced in 1924 by Mr Chivers, to whom out-patients paid one shilling for each treatment. Miss M. M. Beamish took his place as honorary masseuse to the hospital in 1925 and was relieved when necessary by Mrs Shepperd until the end of the decade. When there was no masseuse at the hospital, nurses sometimes carried out the task. The work of exercising or pummelling was physically demanding, but the purchase in 1926 of a faradic battery able to provide electronic stimulus, diversified the treatment that the masseuse could give. Sometimes special splinting was needed before a limb was ready for the masseuse and splints were made by the blacksmith down on the wharf front:

> ... He'd be there and I would go ... down there and the old blacksmith would say 'What do you want doctor?' Even a special iron frame Thomas splint with movable joints at the knee, were within the tradesman's ability. The bill sent to the hospital would be only a few shillings. Usually the blacksmith was 'glad to do something for the hospital'.[81]

Patients who needed crutches paid a deposit of 12 shillings and sixpence which was refunded when the crutches were returned.

The old, fear-filled days when a whole boatload of 430 passengers exposed to

---

[78] *Ibid.*
[79] House Surgeon's Report Book, 10 August 1933.
[80] See A. M. Ashdown, *A Complete System of Nursing*, London, J. M. Dent and Sons, 1924. Sections on Massage and Medical Electricity, pp. 627–49. This book was the FH nurses' text book from 1926.
[81] Barrington Knight, interview.

smallpox had been quarantined under canvas on Carnac Island for 14 days, when townspeople passed well to the lee side as Fremantle's Mr Carroll galloped a small-pox victim in his wagon—fitted with the special cover and with a yellow flag stream-ing—to the quarantine station, and when Mary Nicolay moved down to Woodman's Point to nurse the victims, was long past, thanks to vaccination.[82] However, illness was yet of great concern:

> People were very troubled at their advent [sicknesses] and such epidemics as polio, influenzas, diphtheria etc, left a very uncertain, subdued and even frightened feeling. Doctors had limited medicines at their disposal, [which] could not often be afforded, so parents battled with old remedies as long as they could. Doors and windows were often kept shut even on the finer days. To relieve chest infections, a paste of hot antiflo was smeared over the chest, covered with a piece of cloth, and left there for a day or two. Castor oil was a favourite standby, and to clear a flu-blocked nose we leaned over a bowl of hot water with camphor in it, covered our head with a blanket and sweated it out. It is difficult nowadays to convey the strange uncertain approach to sickness that existed then.[83]

There was still a need for a local infectious diseases hospital. The urgency was underlined each time there was an outbreak of diphtheria.

In 1928 the North Fremantle Council agitated for the reopening of the hospital's infectious diseases ward. The honorary medical officers agreed to the idea in prin-ciple but not in the old ward which was now considered entirely unsuitable, it having been discovered that the corrugated-iron walls were affixed the wrong way round making it impossible to clean properly. At discussions between the council and the hospital board, concern was expressed, but little was resolved. In 1930 the hospital's senior resident medical officer, Dr Ferguson, admitted a very ill three-year-old who needed an immediate tracheotomy to save its life. Although the child and Nurse Hannaford, who contracted the disease while looking after him, were later sent to the West Subiaco Infectious Diseases Hospital, Ferguson stressed the importance of having a local infectious diseases hospital, preferably outside the hospital grounds, where cases would be less of a menace to staff and children. His voice joined with those of other doctors and councillors[84] but funding was a problem. By 1933, with the health act requirement that local councils were to pay half the cost of infectious diseases hospitals, the voices had changed tune, calling for a new metropolitan infec-tious diseases hospital at Subiaco to replace the group of tin shanties there, where convalescents and the contagious were bedded side by side. Not until 1939 was this achieved.

The diphtheria problem was eventually confronted by the councils of the Fre-mantle district through a concerted immunisation programme.[85] Operating from the Fremantle Hospital, which agreed to accommodate and provide equipment, and extending to school clinics, 10,530 treatments were commenced. Only 3,109 were

[82] *West Australian*, 15 and 18 February 1897; Minutes of FLBH, 14 April 1893, 17 May 1893, 26 May 1893.
[83] J. Raffa, *The Happy Children*, 1984, p. 25.
[84] See *West Australian*, 23 August 1930; Minutes of BM, 17 August 1928, 7 November 1933.
[85] See *West Australian*, 6 August 1935, 11 March 1939, 5 May 1939, 12 May 1939, 7 June 1939.

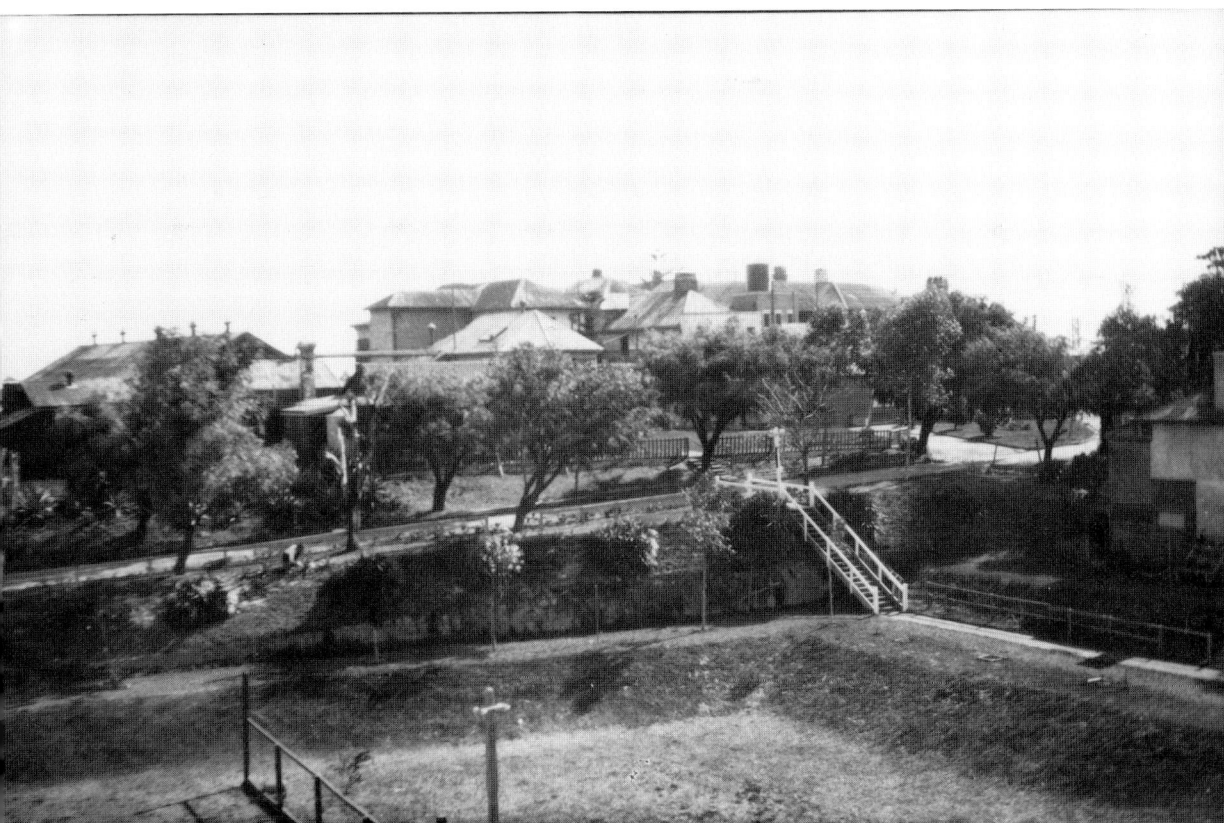

Photograph courtesy A. Orloff

Plate 34. Fremantle Hospital, c. 1920s, taken from the east.

The buildings are important but they are not the whole—the morale of the hospital was high and nursing had always been high, thanks to the first Matron, Miss Balding and then Matron Jones who was a mighty fine person backed up by good old Sister Fuller.

Dr John Rowe
Medical Superintendent 1953–62

completed, but none of the fully treated children contracted the disease. Four years later, in 1939, Dr E. S. Atkinson, the commissioner of public health, praised the Fremantle district's diphtheria immunization clinic committee. 'You stand out as an example to every local authority in the State.'[86] Before the immunisation campaign in 1935 and 1936, there had been 195 cases of diphtheria (23 per 1,000 of the child population); in the first year of the campaign the number dropped to 142, then to 128 and in 1939 there were only 100 cases (11.7 per 1,000 of the child population).[87]

[86] *Ibid.*, 17 August 1939.
[87] *Ibid.*

From mid-1939, the parents of any children admitted to the children's ward were given the opportunity of having them immunised while at the hospital, and clinics were established at 12 of the district's 20 main schools, with eight doctors and two nurses engaged in the work. Results were encouraging but there was still residual opposition to immunisation, mainly from the anti-vivisectionist leagues. Although in the 1930s immunisation was given with only the painful prick of a needle, there were still many in the community who could remember that early in the century death occasionally followed vaccination. Others recalled the compulsory smallpox vaccination given to a child under seven years of age, usually on the outer side of a leg, below the knee, where the skin would be scored in a cross to take the vaccine. Then there would follow severe illness and, for infants and babies, the fitting of a wire cage to stop them touching of the area of vaccination.[88]

In the early 1920s, the hospital's honorary doctors—White, Blackall, Anderson Kerr, East, Stubbe, Gibson, Tregonning, and William Dermer's son, E. R. Dermer—were general practitioners treating both medical and surgical cases. Specialisation was limited to the honorary dentist and the honorary masseur and to Dr Claude Morlet, who treated the eye patients. Appointment to the honorary staff was still an honour and dependent on the board vote following a reply to advertisements in the press, but the number of positions was expanded by the board as new and skilled doctors moved into the area. In 1924, when Stubbe and Clark applied for a vacant, advertised appointment, the number of honorary appointments was increased from six to seven, to accommodate both; Stubbe joined the staff of honorary medical officers, and Clark was appointed as honorary radiologist. The honoraries approached the board in 1928 about expanding the number of appointments once more, and creating junior and senior posts: 'We recognize that as considerable experience is necessary for major operations this experience can only be gained by an apprenticeship as junior,' the honoraries reasoned. 'We recommend that each junior should be attached to a senior to gain experience in operative work.'[89] The board was amenable. The older honorary doctors ranked their honorary assistants in order of seniority and experience, and Stubbe, Cook, Dunkley and Dorothea Parker respectively were allotted to the corresponding senior doctors. In 1929 there were ten honorary medical officers—Blackall, Kerr, East, Gibson, Dermer, Stubbe, Cook, Dunkley, Parker and Hallion. This was a period of increasing specialisation in medicine. The eye specialist was still Morlet, while Caldera concentrated on ear, nose and throat cases; Dunkley was the honorary radiologist, Dorothea Parker the honorary pathologist, and Kerr and Dermer were allotted the Venereal Diseases Clinique. There was still an honorary dentist, and an honorary masseuse. Moves to increase the number of specialists on the staff also came through the honoraries—an honorary dermatologist in 1931 in Jason M. O'Donald and, ironically, in the heavy carpentry section of surgery, tall red-headed Marion Radcliffe-Taylor was appointed as honorary orthopaedist, a position she retained for many years. There was still no honorary gynaecologist but only because there was no spare room in the outpatients' department. When senior honorary medical officers resigned, as East did in 1929, and Kerr in 1931 when Alan Bean took over his practice, they were invited

88   CSO File 672/93; Anderson, interview, BL.
89   Minutes of BM, 11 January 1928.

back as honorary consultants. The honorary appointments were made three yearly and the turnover of officers was limited, most remaining in practice for years in the Fremantle area and becoming familiar figures to those who lived in the town.

With the knowledge that the hospital's efficient functioning depended greatly on the honorary medical officers' goodwill and advice, the board usually treated the doctors with respect. Likewise, the honoraries acknowledged the board in its position of authority at the hospital and there existed a mutual regard. The board might wrangle internally over an honorary appointment but honorary requests were usually granted. Only occasionally did tension exist between the medical and the lay men. When, in 1925, the honorary medical officers requested increased representation on the hospital board to two instead of one, the board discussed the move and prudently decided it hadn't the power to accede to the request and passed the decision on to the Medical Department. As a result, Kerr joined East on the board within the month. However, when they requested it, the board did grant the honoraries direct representation on the powerful house committee of four which made decisions and passed them to the board for their confirmation, and in this way the doctors influenced the direction of hospital policy and planning. For their part, the board submitted the names of prospective resident medical officers to the honoraries for their recommendation, which was always followed. The honoraries requested necessary equipment for the hospital, and it was bought when funds allowed. They also urged the 'proper record system of recording in-patients'.[90] Their requests were not always altruistic. In 1930 the honorary staff wanted the board to refuse to admit shipping cases, an assured source of income for them as the shipping companies paid the fees.

From the honorary medical officers came the essential help to get through a crisis when there was a lack of resident medical officers at the hospital. The turnover of resident doctors was high. Young men freshly graduated from medical schools at Sydney, Melbourne and then Adelaide were sought by all hospitals to live in and work, thus consolidating their practical knowledge and gaining experience in the profession before moving on. Most preferred appointments in larger hospitals, where experience was expected to be more diverse, and Fremantle was often last on the list of a young man's hospital preferences. Nevertheless, the experience at Fremantle—the only hospital in the metropolitan area where both children and adults were nursed, where all manner of operations were done, and where greater responsibilities rested because of the smaller staff—came to be valued. For most of the decade of the 1920s, two resident medical officers were appointed at Fremantle, the senior earning £300 a year, the junior £125, and many juniors stayed on for a further term as the senior. For a brief period from 1928, three residents were appointed, but the Depression quickly curbed such enthusiasm. Each of the young resident medical officers of the 1920s, including Abernethy, Stubbe, Cuttle, Corr, Clark, Richard Green, Malcolm Harpur (who had to be directed to wear gloves in the X-ray department), Dunkley, Jacobs from Bendigo, MacDonald, Uther Baker, Tepper, Ferguson, Gray, Caulfield, Crowley, Hustler, Dunn and Bossence, influenced life at the hospital in some way and some stayed in the area, later to receive honorary appointments on the staff.

[90] *Ibid.*, 12 October 1927.

The availability of medical officers fluctuated and depended on numbers graduating from Melbourne and Adelaide. The period after examination results had been released was most propitious. Once, there were 12 applications for a junior position—usually there were two or three, but sometimes, as in 1930, no applicant could be found. Resident medical officers were recruited through medical journals, through university medical schools, through the agent Neilson Hancock in the Eastern States and, when Australian sources were dry, through the agent general in London. There were no set hours of work. There were, however, anatomy or bandaging lectures to give to nurses, and there were nights of interrupted sleep to be endured when casualties were brought in needing treatment. There were honorary doctors' patients to see. 'I did all this work,' recalled one doctor: '. . . looked after all their dressings and things like that, and used to see their patients.'[91] There were also operations to perform, and anaesthetics to give. Medical knowledge was as yet limited: 'We knew nothing of genes, hormones, platelets, fibrinogen, electrolytes, viruses, Rh factors and dozens of other data now elementary in the curriculum of the medical student,' mused another doctor who had been a young resident in 1920.[92]

Little changed for nurses between 1920 and the 1930s. A simple education test in English and arithmetic had to be passed at Perth Technical School before a probationer was accepted for training. There was still the initial interview with Matron Balding, stern and inflexible behind her desk, the wait to become a probationer, the medical examination by an honorary, the issue of yards of material to make the long uniforms and the dozen accompanying aprons, the trip to buy black shoes and stockings. Finally there was the journey to the hospital and work the next day. It was not unusual, as one nurse recalled of 1923, to go in on a Saturday night and commence on the Sunday morning:

> . . . I was frightened . . . I didn't know what to expect . . . . First thing take around the tooth mugs when you went on and then you had to start cleaning in the pan room. There was an awful lead sink to be cleaned, copper sterilizer. Then in between you had to help feed helpless patients . . . . We had to clean and wash down the lockers . . . with sand soap and water. Oh, there was an awful lot to cram into the morning. By half-past nine we had to be ready to sweep . . . the ward floor.[93]

Another nurse remembered spending her first year '. . . mostly in the pan lav. Cleaning the pan lav and attending to the requirements of the patients in that capacity . . .'[94] A junior learned quickly through observation and instruction from a senior nurse.

Second-year nurses started their morning by helping to sponge the bed-rest patients who had not been washed by the night staff. As a patient's stay was usually lengthy there was time to know each one. An appendix case would stay in bed for a fortnight and go home at the end of a month; major abdominal cases were probably in bed for nearly six weeks before being discharged or even allowed up. Sometimes it

91 Barrington Knight, interview.
92 Stubbe, *Medical Background*, Preface p. xxv.
93 O. Jones, interviewed by C. Jeffery, May to July 1984, FH.
94 M. Fuller, interviewed by C. Jeffery, 18 November and 13 December 1984.

was a battle to get sponges finished by lunch time. Then there were simple dressings to do and 'backs' to prevent pressure sores. Except for cleaning the hand basins and polishing the taps in the ward, the third-year nurse held more varied responsibilities. She received the report from the night sister and passed it on to the ward sister when she came on duty, did the daily dressings and prepared patients for operations. First, an ether swabbing of the surgical area was washed off with spirits of biniodide, then water. Next, the area was painted—'[gentian] violet ... was very fashionable in those days', and the appropriate part was covered with sterile lint and a binder before the patient was placed on a canvas ready to go to the theatre. Doses of atropine and morphia were given as premedication:

> The tablets were in ampoules and you had to sterilise a spoon over a spirit lamp and then boil the sterile water in the spoon, drop the tablet in, be careful not to boil it if it was atropine otherwise we were told you would cause the patient to vomit. Then it was drawn up into the syringe and taken to the bedside of the patient, the patient injected with that solution.[95]

Theatre nurses had special responsibilities. At 8 a.m. they went to the operating room. Sometimes the vapour of formalin and permanganate of potash used to fumigate the locked theatre overnight made their eyes stream and sting, especially when an orderly had been tardy in his task of opening the windows from the outside to air the theatre for an hour. While the charge nurse laid out the instruments for the day, the theatre nurse dusted, cleaned and polished the taps, then scrubbed the theatre walls with carbolic, one-in-twenty diluted with water, and sterilised the bowls. The removal of Dr Lotz' viewing gallery and a large gas bracket over the operating table meant that there was a little less to wipe over after 1917. Thread for suturing had to be sterilized:

> Well, the catgut we used to get in packets from the dispensary, also the silkwormgut. The silkwormgut we boiled in saline for an hour or more, then coloured it with methyl violet and stored it in ... one-in-twenty carbolic. The catgut was soaked in ether to defat it, then changed to biniodide and spirit ... for twenty four hours, and that was changed and ... then stored in spirit, ready for use. The suture needles were all stored in pure lysol. Also the scissors.[96]

Operations were scheduled three afternoons a week, usually two in number, sometimes three. As the decade passed the numbers increased. At the end of the day, if they were punctured, rubber gloves had to be patched with rubber patches and gum solution and then washed and boiled; dried gloves had to be tested for air holes and powdered for the surgeons' use. Soiled linen was soaked in carbolic and blunt instruments boiled. A theatre nurse was on call and it was not unknown in an emergency to work 24 hours straight. A final duty, especially if there had been a 'pusy' operation, was to fumigate the theatre:

> ... We turned on all the hot water taps in the theatre to fill it with steam and we placed an old dressing tray on the floor and on that we placed an enamel dressing bucket. We

[95] O. Jones, interview.
[96] *Ibid.* To preserve their keen edge, cutting intruments such as scissors '... were not to be boiled!'

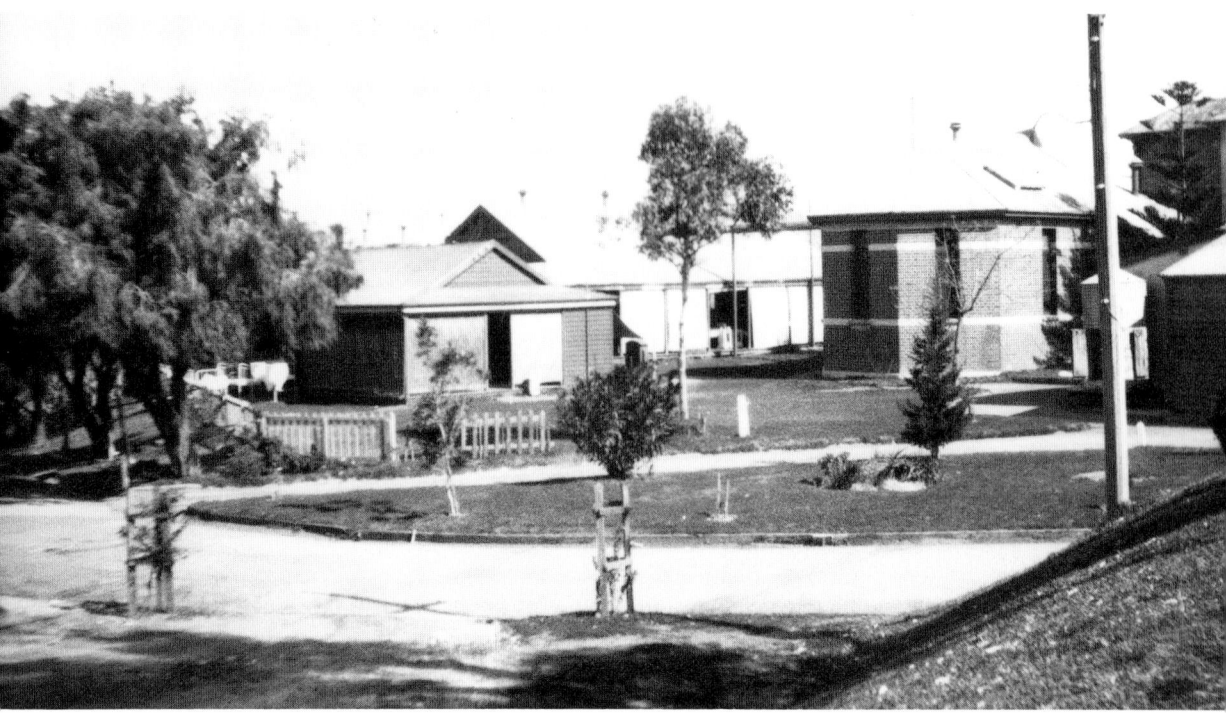

Photograph courtesy A. Orloff

Plate 35. *(Left to right)*: Children's ward, originally the temporary dining room set up during the 1919 Spanish influenza epidemic. The old operating theatre can be seen on the right.

> ... it was a conglomeration of buildings which appeared to be like an old tramp steamer struggling along and with no one from the outside giving it tender loving care.
>
> Dr John Rowe
> Medical Superintendent 1953-62

> put [in] ten ounces of permanganate of potash crystals and then poured over two pints of forty per cent formalin, then got for our life out of the theatre and closed the door.[97]

Nurses still wore uniforms of a fine, pink pinstripe with hemlines six to seven inches from the ground, and it was not unknown for matron to 'come along and put a ruler on you' to check the length.[98] Caps were still worn:

> Our caps had to be pleated to fit our head and if by chance you put a running thread in, intending to pleat it when off duty, Matron was sure to see it and ask you—if you wanted to put a running thread in your cap, why didn't you do your training in the government [hospitals]. Our third year caps were frilled and we took great pride in wearing them stiff and starched.[99]

[97] *Ibid.*
[98] Buzza, interview.
[99] Buzza, notes, 1986. FH.

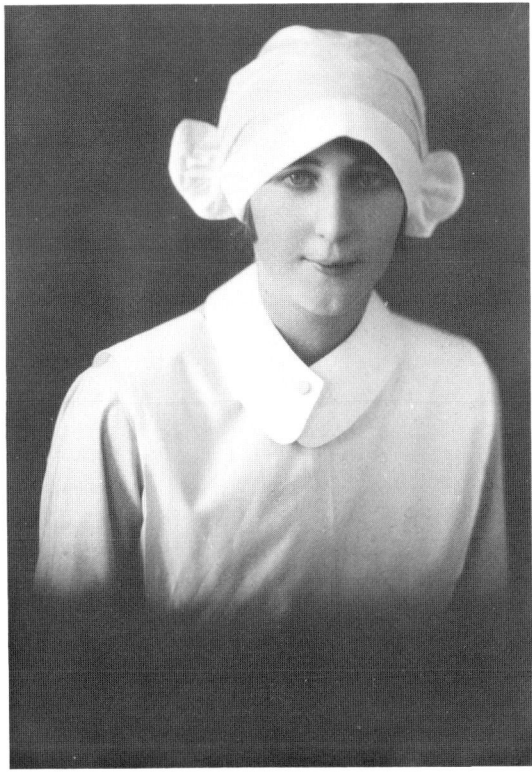

Plate 36.   Nurse Ray Buzza, 1930.

Photograph courtesy Fremantle Hospital

Hours were still long.

> We worked from 7 a.m. until 9 p.m. with a break during the day from 2 to 5.30. That's
> if you were on evening duty. But if you were on full day duty it was 7 a.m. to 6 p.m.
> with half an hour for lunch but that eventually, after a few years was lengthened to an
> hour for lunch.[100]

Probationers were rotated to a different ward after six or eight weeks or even after
three months, when it seemed that matron had forgotten a nurse's existence, and
there was an eight-week stretch on night duty from 9 p.m. until 7 a.m. Then there
would be a senior nurse in each ward but only one sister and a single junior for the
entire hospital. The latter was assigned the responsibility of getting supper for the
night staff: '. . . believe me it was a great hassle to try and make something out of
some scraggy chops, a potato and some sort of vegie'.[101] Ingredients were collected
in a large wicker basket from a safe outside the nurses' dining room in The Knowle
and carried to the wards. Sometimes a raid on the doctor's ice chest would supplement meagre rations. The junior night nurse also had the duty of washing up and

[100]   Buzza, interview.
[101]   *Ibid.*

putting away after the supper taken in shifts by the seniors, and helping with the heavier cases. 'Panning' had to be done before the day staff came on.[102] Sponging was started in the early morning after 4 a.m., but on a busy night, recalled one nurse,

> ... you would try to sneak some in before midnight and hope matron wouldn't come and do a round and catch you. Matron was very good really when she did those late night rounds. She carried her keys with her and she often jingled the keys so that you knew she was on her way.[103]

The early sponge was dreaded by patients. One man claimed that 'the fact of the nurses washing him in the very early hours had resulted in him contracting congestion of the lungs'.[104] Hurricane lamps dimmed with blue paper wrapping from rolls of cotton wool were used for light; squeaky floor boards were soon located and avoided so that a sleeping patient would not be disturbed. The night sister would do a ward round at 9 p.m. and take charge of the hospital. Then there would be a round with the senior resident medical officer at 10 o'clock and sedatives to give if ordered. In the morning, a report of patients' conditions, new admissions, and operations had to be given to Matron Balding, who had a phenomenal memory and knew all the patients' names and ages.

In 1927 Matron Balding taught that a nurse should 'be able to undertake individual and personal responsibilities and to accept things we are told to do and do not understand with confidence, that it is all for our good and try to understand the authority of the seniors'.[105] Obedience and deference were the foundations of a nurse's training and an unquestioning acceptance of a senior's authority was built into the nursing hierarchy. A junior nurse avoided the matron, the honorary medical staff and senior sisters when possible, but stood to attention with sleeves rolled down and hands behind her back as a mark of respect if she could not and was required to speak. One new probationer recognised a staff nurse previously known to her outside the hospital for many years:

> I passed her on the stairs and she snapped out 'Get down to the bottom of the stairs. Don't you know you never pass a senior nurse on the stairs?' I was going to ask her what was wrong with her but decided I'd better not.[106]

Another probationer nurse lost time due to rheumatic fever, then scarlet fever, and returned with the class below her:

> One of the nurses, a very domineering person, said to me 'I'm senior to you, you can go and do ... whatever it was. I took this for a while then decided to find out where I really did stand. So armed with a roll of toilet paper and the signing on book and a calendar I proceeded to calculate the number of days I was away and then convert them to months and weeks. When I had done that I got some good paper, set it all out and

---

102   P. Edinger (née Murray), notes, 1986. FH.
103   O. Jones, interview.
104   *Fremantle Advocate*, 12 August 1927.
105   Matron's lecture notes recorded by probationer Mavis Fuller, 8 June 1927, Lecture 1, FH.
106   Heath, notes, 1986, FH.

took it to Matron. Told her why I'd done it, so she checked it and found it correct. I said nothing about it until I came on day duty again and [was] again with this person, so when she said go and do so and so, I said, 'do it yourself, for now on I'm 2 months so many weeks senior to you and if you want to verify it, go to Matron.' I had no more trouble.[107]

Lectures were an important part of a nurse's training but practical instruction on the job was still the main method of learning. Charge Sisters Leo, Gill, Kiernan, Wright and Lane were fine ward teachers in the mid-1920s. Matron gave general nursing lectures, the resident medical officers the anatomy and physiology, while the honorary medical staff delivered the medical and surgical lectures. At times doctors didn't arrive, and nurses would sit 'nearly an hour and no doctor, no lecture and wasted all your time'.[108] In 1921 the resident medical officer, Dr Gibson, gave 14 anatomy and physiology lectures and matron delivered 14 lessons on general nursing to the junior nurses; to the seniors Dr East gave seven surgical and Kerr four medical lectures, while six lectures by Dermer and Kerr on hygiene and gynaecology respectively and four lectures on children's nursing by Tregonning completed the second-year probationers' course of study. In the following year there were still medical, gynaecological, anatomy and general nursing lectures, but Morlet gave ten lectures on ophthalmic nursing and Miss Buller organized ten invalid cookery lectures (theory and practice). Hospital examinations were set yearly and at the end of three years there was the Australian Trained Nurses Association examination to be taken at the University building in Irwin Street, Perth, and for many,

> That was a day and a half. All day Tuesday-medical in the morning, I think surgical in the afternoon. Wednesday morning was the general nursing and then we were supposed to return to the hospital on the Wednesday afternoon to go on duty.[109]

In 1920 there was talk of an interchange of nurses for part of their training, between the Wooroloo Sanatorium, where tuberculosis patients were cared for, and the main hospitals. But in a meeting between the matrons the idea was considered impractical.

At times, as in 1920 and 1924, there was a dearth of applicants for training and the whole nursing staff regretted the lack. Extra hours had to be worked, days off could not be taken and holidays could not be planned. One nurse of 1924 recalled coming off duty to find a note on her door, 'commence holidays tomorrow'.[110] Another remembered:

> ... after having a certain day off for week I thought it would be the same ... so I went home, not able to be contacted, but it wasn't so. Naturally I toed the carpet the next day at 9 a.m. sharp, and was given a stern reminder I was in the nursing world and nursing comes first.[111]

The lack of senior nurses in the hospital was a constant concern. In 1920, seven

---

[107] Buzza, notes, 1986, FH.
[108] O. Jones, interview.
[109] *Ibid.*
[110] *Ibid.*
[111] Buzza, notes, 1986, FH.

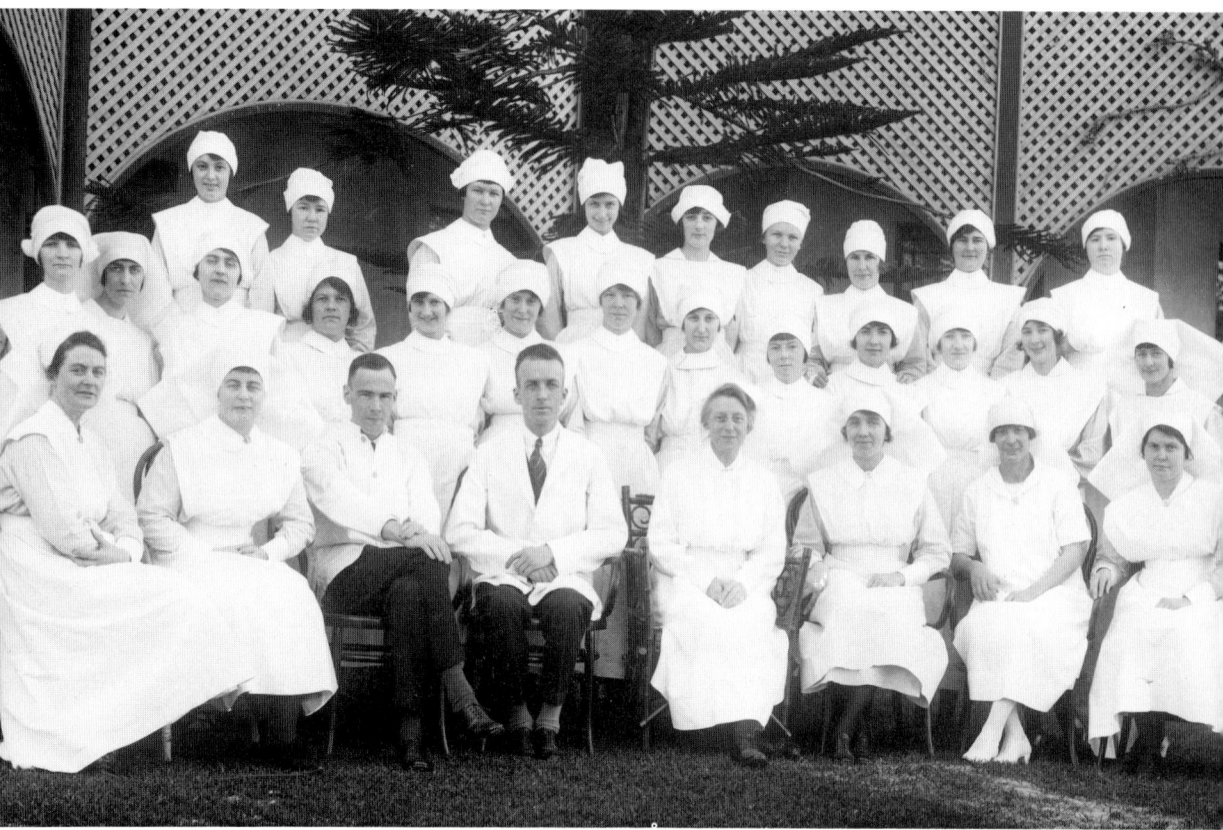

Photograph courtesy Fremantle Hospital

Plate 37.   Fremantle Hospital Staff, 1924.

Back row (left to right): Alice Erskine, Birmingham, Fathers, Amya Gray, Harrup, Irene Smith, Dot Perryman, Cullen.
Middle row: Carroll, S/N Young, Gjerde, Wray, Maisie Jones, Dorothy Johnson, Marjorie Hutchinson, Gladys Bishop, Ruth Butson, Olive Richards, Jean Lindsay, Dorothy Brooks, S/N Maudie Ryan.
Front row: Sister Irene Kiernan, Sister Rita Lane, Dr Malcolm Harken (J.R.M.O.), Dr Richard Green (S.R.M.O.), Matron Balding, Sister Leggatt, Sister Smith, Sister Vera Gill.

nurses completed their three years of training, five of whom remained to serve for a year as staff nurses. There were five charge nurses, one responsible for each of the wards, and when they were off duty, staff nurses took their places. Two years later, in mid-1922, the position was critical: there were five charge nurses, no staff nurses, and 21 juniors. By 1923, when Nurses Bishop and Woods passed the state registration examination in first and third places respectively, and two young probationers by the names of Olive Jones and Ruth Butson started work at the hospital, the number of senior nurses had increased only marginally to five charge nurses, and one staff nurse, with 25 probationers. In January 1924, with five charge nurses, two staff nurses and 23 pupils, of whom eight had started in the last six months, Matron Balding regretted the junior status of her staff: 'the pupils under three months are of very little nursing value,' she reported to the board.[112] Domestic work was indeed the main occupation of all first-year trainees and they were a cheap source of labour.

The matron calculated that without allowing time for holidays and emergencies, she needed a minimum staff of 32 at the hospital:

Charge Nurse and 2 pupils Cas & Theatre	3
Charge Nurse and 4 pupils Women's Ward	5
Charge Nurse and 3 pupils Surgical	4
Charge Nurse and 3 pupils Medical	4
Charge Nurse and 2 pupils Children's	3
Charge Nurse and 1 pupil Isolation	2
Daily Relieving 3 pupils	3
Charge Nurse and 7 pupils Night Staff	8
Total	32 [113]

In February 1924, when she had 23 on duty, four charge nurses were granted greatly overdue leave at different times, and when one of the new probationers left, and Nurse Craig was recommended three months' leave of absence owing to illness, Maida Balding protested: 'I cannot spare this nurse at present as my Staff is so short through sickness and annual leave of Nurses, unless extra help is procured ... and probationer nurses are not obtainable at present.'[114] To aggravate the crisis in that hot February, the admission figures rocketed from 79 and 82 in December and January respectively to 111, while the number of out-patients unexpectedly almost doubled to 1,739. Eight nurses were due for annual leave, there was little water getting through the nurses' quarters plumbing, and everyone was tired. The matter of staff shortages was referred to the house committee who condemned the matron for allowing senior sisters to take leave at the same time and threatened that if the position was repeated, that it would 'make a drastic recommendation to the board'.[115] To alleviate the position, matron took on the four willing probationers she could find and granted Nurse Craig leave before becoming ill herself. Two of the probationers, Misses Lindsay and Erskine, came without having passed the education test. They sat for it twice after entering the hospital and failed; the nurses' registration board would not recognise the commencement of their training. They sat once more in October, this time passing and officially commencing their training. Two months later, five senior nurses passed the nurses registration examination. At the beginning of 1925 there were 31 on the nursing staff, still less than the minimum needed to staff the wards and the same number as in 1923. Overcrowded nurses' accommodation contributed to the lack of nursing staff; not until the Medical Department completed new quarters in 1926 could staff numbers be increased appreciably.

Sickness was an occupational hazard for nurses of the 1920s. In April 1921, 12 of the nursing staff were off duty from between a few days and a month, and three

[112] Minutes of BM, 9 January 1924.
[113] *Ibid.*, 12 March 1924.
[114] *Ibid.*, 20 February 1924.
[115] *Ibid.*, 12 March 1924.

special nurses had to be employed to enable work at the hospital to continue. Nurse Streeter completed her three years' training in mid-1922, but had to complete the course of surgical lectures and pass an examination missed due to illness, while probationer Williams in 1923 passed both the hospital and state registration exams but had to make up 232 days' sick leave. Probationer Bishop's persistent cough in 1922 was reported by matron to Dr Gibson, who ordered the young nurse to take six months' rest from duty. In 1921 the house surgeon recommended compulsory typhoid inoculation for girls commencing training and suggested that the present staff also be inoculated. The board agreed to the first idea but left the second decision up to individual members. In 1923 all were inoculated against influenza but many during the decade of the 1920s were warded with diphtheria, especially in the bad year of 1927.

In 1921 a third-year probationer earned £36 a year, a second-year probationer £24 and a first-year nurse just £18. Increases were usually due to action by nurses or the matron. When Charge Nurse Phipps stated firmly that she was leaving due to an insufficient salary, matron told the board 'she is a very competent sister and I would recommend her to the board's consideration'.[116] The board immediately increased a staff nurse's salary by £6 to £66, and the salary of a charge nurse by £10 to £95, £100, £105 or £110 a year, depending on length of service. The matron received an increase of £12. By 1923, changes in nurses' hours and wages were being considered. As a result of a conference between all metropolitan hospitals, the board agreed to a 54-hour week for day nurses, and 60 hours for night nurses, with one day off a week for all. The wages of probationers and charge nurses remained unchanged but an increase for staff nurses was granted, bringing them to between £75 and £80 a year.[117] Following a meeting of hospital authorities in the metropolitan area to discuss an increase in nurses' salaries in 1926, first years received £26 with an increase to £34 in second year and £48 in their third. Staff nurses were granted £90 and charge nurses £110, increasing to £120, £130, £140 and then £150 with each year of experience.[118] Wages at other hospitals were a guide to the board at Fremantle and when salaries at Perth and the Children's Hospitals were raised, it was not long before matron informed the board and similar changes were made at Fremantle. Although appreciated, the new rates did not make much difference in a nurses' fortnightly purse. When trying to raise nurses' salaries in 1928, McMahon, on the board, faced opposition from Dr East and a bitter Chairman McLeod, who were thinking of their unbalanced hospital budget. The rest of the board agreed to increase the nurses' salaries by a welcome £13 a year for first-year probationers, £14 in their second year and £12 for third-year nurses. The board also voted to raise the secretary's salary—by £50 a year.[119] The entire staff of sisters was less fortunate in its request for an eight-hour day and an increase in salaries in 1929, when finances were tight. In 1930 the increase was granted but working hours were another matter.

With the move to their new quarters in 1926 other improvements for nurses were achieved. Matron gently persuaded the board to grant £25 to start a nurses' refer-

116   *Ibid.*, 18 May 1921.
117   Special Meeting of BM, 31 October 1923.
118   Minutes of BM, 14 April 1926.
119   *Ibid.*, 21 March 1928.

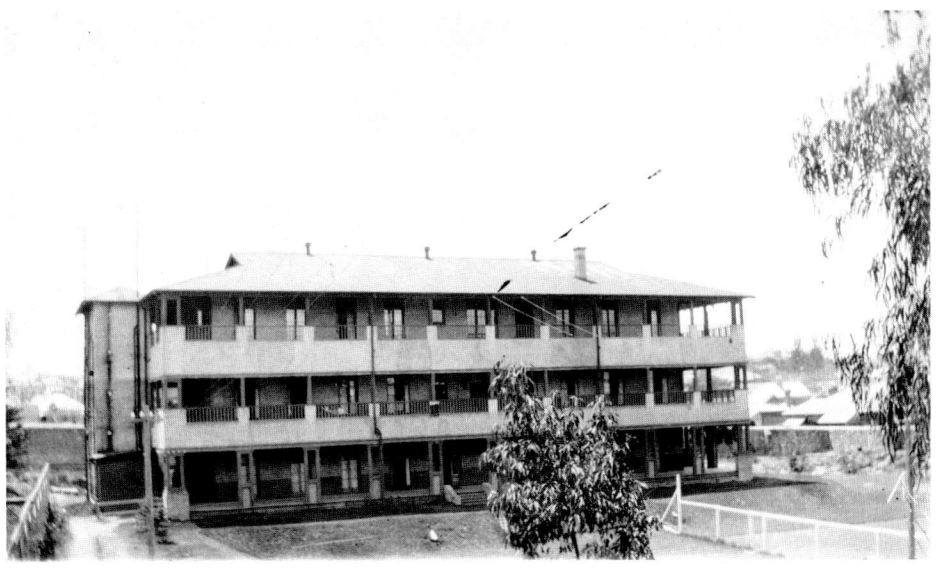

Photograph courtesy Ray Buzza

Plate 38.   Nurses' quarters 1929.

The quarters were a three storied building with the ablution block at one end of each floor. The rooms went off a central hall, with verandahs on three sides. The lounge room was the full width of the end of the lower floor. The rooms were comfortable as for those days a cyclone bed with horse-hair mattress, a combination wardrobe and dressing table, a marble topped wash stand come writing desk and a straight wooden chair. No bed lamp. The 1st year students occupied the lower floor-and we called it 'Pro's Alley' and the 3rd floor was the night staff quarters.

Ray Buzza
Nursing Staff

ence library under her control and responsibility. Dr Kerr suggested the appointment of a home sister for the new quarters, which was ignored, but the board did give enough for some extra records for the gramophone in the nurses' quarters. The house committee recommended the presentation of a gold medal, as was done at Perth Public Hospital, to the nurse doing best in her A.T.N.A. exams. Dr Kerr thought it should be for general proficiency but others advocated an award for the highest marks, which was easier to determine. Mr McMahon offered to donate the gold medal, which became a source of great pride to those who earned it in the following years. In 1926 it was Nurse Hutchinson, the following year Nurse Perryman received the highest marks in the examination. In 1927 the question of nurses taking the last two months of their training at the West Subiaco Infectious Diseases Hospital was again raised, and was recommended by Matron Balding at a joint conference between representatives of Perth, Fremantle and the Children's Hospitals. 'Our nurses'[120] were subsequently allowed to come back to Fremantle Hospital to

---

[120]   *Ibid.*, 14 September 1927.

sleep on nights off but the experience of nursing at Subiaco claimed its toll as more than one nurse became ill. Regulations governing nurses were also changed in 1928, when the board agreed that a charge nurse could be appointed at 23 years of age. This meant that a nurse could commence training at 19 years of age, instead of at 21. The age-limit ruling was not inflexible when probationers were needed, and young applicants were not always known to give a correct year of birth.

By the end of the 1920s Maida Balding had been matron for over 15 years. She was respected in her position by the nurses, including Sisters Leo, Freeman, Murray, Edis, Kiernan, Phipps, Olive Jones, McGaffin and others who became invaluable, dependable senior staff and who, she acknowledged, 'assisted me very ably in maintaining an efficient standard of nursing and discipline'.[121] Less impressed was the board, who checked her urgent requests for linen which were not found exaggerated and who, eventually, in 1925, after years of requesting, granted her a telephone extension so that she did not have to discuss hospital matters of a private nature at the public ''phone' in the hall. She might have been less highly regarded by probationers, had the nurses known that it was their matron who suggested that they should pay for panes of glass in the French doors of the nurses' home, broken through carelessness, and who introduced the scheme which would last long after her death of charging for broken thermometers. 'Her girls' were of great concern to Matron Balding and she agitated for increases in their meagre wages and for a night orderly so that the nurse from male medical ward would not have to open the heavy locked hospital gates at night when the outside bell was rung. She clashed with female board members in 1926 who tested her authority, moving that, instead of the matron employing domestics, she advertise such positions vacant and present details of applicants to the house committee for their selection. Again there was conflict when her duties had expanded so greatly that the matron appointed a nurse to assist her in 1927. The house committee demanded the return of the nurse to ward duties. In October 1928, Sister Fisher came as a charge nurse to the hospital and matron recommended her as a capable administrative assistant. Without consulting the matron, the board decided to appoint another as assistant matron to the hospital at the senior charge nurse salary of a £150 a year, and employed Sister Carpenter. The house committee was not entirely satisfied with the list of mundane duties that Matron drew up for Miss Carpenter, and Matron Balding was certainly less than satisfied at having to share her responsibilities with someone unknown and un-requested. Her anger at the house committee meeting in January 1929 was barely concealed and she stated categorically 'that there was no room for an assistant matron, the hospital only wanted the appointment of a house keeper—as put forward by her some considerable time ago'.[122] The schism between the women widened when Miss Carpenter found herself doing work that an unqualified nurse or maid might have done from a cramped, converted liftwell for an office, with bad lighting and ventilation. Eight months after starting at Fremantle Hospital, Sister Carpenter submitted her resignation. The house committee heard the complaints of both parties separately and together, and urged them 'to try to pull together for the

[121]   *Ibid.*, 19 October 1921.
[122]   Minutes of HC, 8 January 1929.

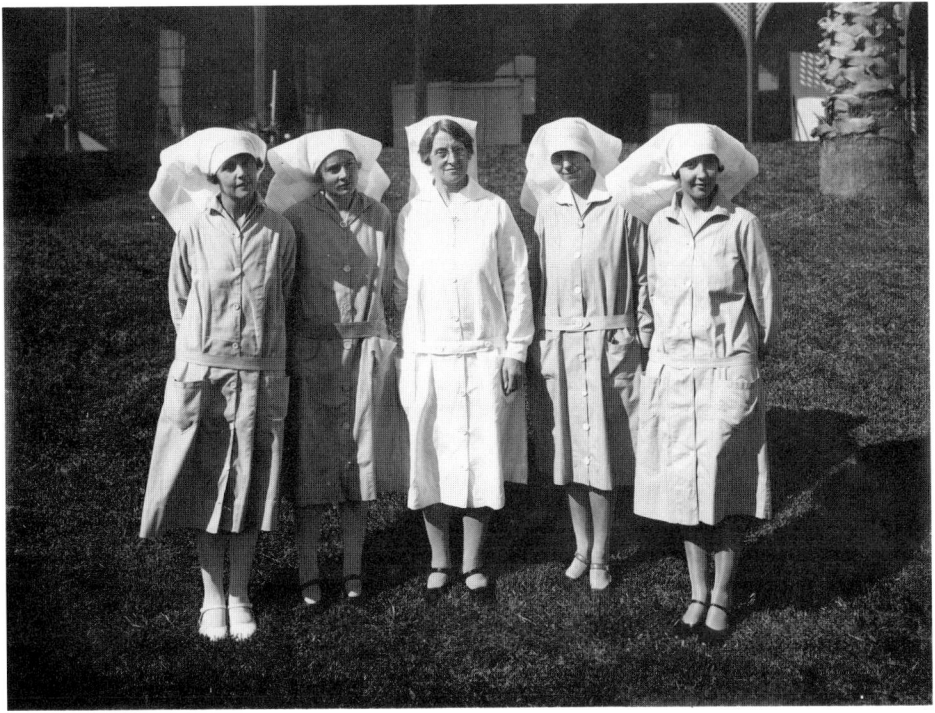

Plate 39. 'Keeping up with the fashions', 1928.

(Left to right): Sisters Rena Leo, Olive Jones, Matron Maida Balding, Sisters Edis, Irene Smith.

benefit of the institution',[123] but feelings ran too deeply. The board accepted the resignation but not without censuring the matron for her part in the matter. The following month matron suggested the appointment of a housekeeper but the request was ignored.

The cost involved in setting up and staffing the new surgical ward in 1928 was substantially added to by increased wages for nurses, the appointment of a part-time radiographer, and Miss Carpenter's employment as assistant matron. The community had responded magnificently to the hospital appeal, but it was too soon to ask again. The board learned that their request for an increase in subsidy could not be granted and once more the hospital's finances plummeted. Hookway predicted an increase of between £4,000 and £4,500 in hospital costs on the previous year and a deficit of £527 by the end of June 1929. 'Taking everything into consideration the financial position of the hospital is fairly satisfactory,'[124] reassured Chairman McMahon. Nevertheless, Christmas was celebrated conservatively with the finances in mind.

[123] *Ibid.*, 2 July 1929,
[124] Minutes of BM, 19 April 1929.

At the end of the 1920s the issue of private patients was a contentious one. As it had no intermediate ward, compensation cases or patients with means coming to Fremantle Hospital were usually advised to go to a private hospital, but those who were admitted in an emergency paid for accommodation and treatment, which was exactly that given to those who could not pay. The board set out-patient fees for treatments at ten shillings and sixpence for both anaesthetics and minor surgery ('such as amputations'); charged five shillings for suturing, splinting or minor throat surgery, and asked two shillings for the dressing of a wound.[125] There was much to be said for establishing a private ward. Local doctors could admit their own patients and the accommodation fees charged would boost hospital revenue. The old infectious diseases building was suggested and then rejected as a site for a community ward, and the idea of the new ward waxed then waned until another year had passed before the idea was raised and again dropped. There seemed little point in thinking of expansion when hospital finances were contracting.

Nurses strove together until the work was done, doctors usually worked for as long as their services were needed, but another group in the hospital organised to gain regulated wages and working conditions. As the Hospital Employees' Industrial Union of Workers, W.A. (Coastal Branch) the orderlies and domestics from the main metropolitan hospitals[126] united to forge an award in December 1922 and to revise it regularly.[127] It was a move born of discontent, when small wages compared to those outside the hospital were paid. In 1920 such employees had written to the board for wage increases. The shillings granted were only given in an attempt to curb the high staff turnover. The first industrial award fixed wages low—£1.7.6. for a waitress or housemaid, when those in the same occupations at coffee palaces and lodging houses earned £1.16.6. a week. It was set for only 12 months, for its proposers hoped that the financial position of hospitals would improve.[128] So scant were staff numbers that when in 1923 laundry workers were granted a 44-hour week and the other domestic staff a 48-hour week with one day off weekly, matron calculated the hours and advised the board that: 'I shall need two extra maids to enable me to grant this, as it cannot be done with my present staff.'[129]

The domestic staff was a small group and well known to the rest of the hospital's employees. Orderly Myers was universally liked for his co-operation with everyone and when orderly S. J. Moore died on 4 July 1923, the board sent a wreath in a case 'as he had been a faithful servant for many years'.[130] At times an orderly might be absent from duty and found 'more or less under the influence of drink'.[131] Such indulgence was discouraged, even when off duty. When one lived-in and could be called back on duty in an emergency, sobriety was esteemed. Sometimes the lodge

[125] *Ibid.*, 20 July 1928.
[126] Fremantle Public Hospital, Perth Public Hospital, Children's Hospital and King Edward Memorial Hospital.
[127] See *The Western Australian Industrial Gazette*, 1921–22, Vol. 1, 24 January 1923, pp. 165–7; *Westralian Worker*, 31 May 1929; *WAIG*, 1925, Vols. 3–5, 26 August 1925, pp. 127–9; *WAIG*, 1926–27, Vols. 6–7, 10 January 1927, p. 244; *WAIG*, 1929–30, Vol. 9, 21 March 1930, pp. 354–5.
[128] *West Australian*, 19 December 1922.
[129] Minutes of BM, 17 January 1923.
[130] *Ibid.*, 18 July 1923.
[131] *Ibid.*, 16 January 1924.

keeper was absent from his duty at the gate, but this was usually when he was called to help the house surgeon or to assist in an X-ray. In 1929 the board decided to allow married men on the orderly staff to live out if they desired.[132] In the same year, the board was requested to allow orderlies and domestics an extra day of annual holidays to celebrate the state's centenary, which was granted.

Many in 1929 glowed with quiet contentment upon the achievements celebrated at the centenary of foundation. Agricultural development was booming, Collier had been a good premier (since 1924) and the standard of living was not too bad. Some households boasted a vacuum cleaner and a motor vehicle, while trains across the Nullarbor, aeroplanes to Adelaide and ships from all over the world linked the state, albeit tenuously, with the rest of the world and with 'the East'.[133] There was wireless and new talking pictures and jazz, not to mention football, the races and many other sports. In his celebratory history of the state's one-hundredth year of British settlement, Hal Colebatch predicted exuberantly that:

> The end of another hundred years—no matter what vicissitudes of fortune may intervene—will find this state great and prosperous, the home of a happy and united people, stimulated by high tradition, qualified by inherited character, and determined, in love and patriotism, to hand on to their successors the choicest fruits of liberty.[134]

The cynical, looking back to their learning often born of ignorance and fumbling experience from the past, may have smiled at the historian's interpretation of their efforts as 'high tradition' and 'inherited character'. Most vigorously nodded their approval of the ideal.

[132] *Ibid.*, 15 February 1929; *Westralian Worker*, 1 March 1929.
[133] G. C. Bolton, *A Fine Country to Starve In*, 1972, pp. 1–66; Stannage, *The People of Perth*, pp. 335–7. 'The East' was the standard reference to the Eastern States of Australia; Crowley and de Garis, *A Short History*, pp. 69, 71–2.
[134] H. Colebatch, *A Story of A Hundred Years: Western Australia 1829–1929*, 1929, p. 476.

Chapter VI

We must look forward ... with restrained confidence,
using for our watchword 'Business as usual'.
A. T. Hookway.

Some predicted, but few really believed how close were the 'vicissitudes of fortune' which would affect most of the Western world. Then, in October 1929, news was flashed around the globe that Wall Street had crashed, toppling the communal complacency and the fragile stability of many individual lives. A glut of wheat and wool caused prices for these goods to plummet. Farmers, then businessmen and those in industries and the civil service were affected as work and wages lessened. The effects of Depression bit deeply. Hundreds applied for a single advertised job. At Fremantle in June 1930, 282 people were receiving sustenance relief and the press told of men sleeping in the open, of dole queues and soup kitchens. Charity turned from the poor in hospitals hidden behind walls to the visible thousands who thronged streets and towns and suburbs seeking work to keep themselves and their families fed and housed. In 1930 alone, Fremantle people gave £9,000 toward unemployment relief. Many of those who had been charitable in the past found that they could no longer afford the giving.[1]

Hospital needs all over the state increased with the Depression and the great number of newly indigent. It was an opportune time to reorganise state hospital finances and the Government's *Hospital Fund Act*, effective from 1 January 1931, was a move in the right direction.[2] Employers were directed to deduct a penny half-penny for each pound earned by their employees over £1 a week, but the income of £133,885 raised in the first year from those in work fell far short of the anticipated £200,000.[3] Tipping competitions and raffles which had involved so many in the community and which had contributed so much to hospital funds were also curbed by the new act. The financial situation at Perth and Fremantle Hospitals was parlous. In 1930 Perth Hospital estimated that in the following year it would have a deficit of over £6,000. So far behind were payments of the accounts at Fremantle Hospital that those of March and April could not be met until August. Towards the end of 1930, the board received a terse report from the minister for health: '... no [extra] funds are available for the management of the hospital'.[4] There were not

---

[1] See Ewers, *The Western Gateway*, p. 133 (sustenance figures); *West Australian*, 22 January 1931 (donations from Fremantle); Bolton, *A Fine Country To Starve In* (general conditions).

[2] *West Australian*, 22 December 1930.

[3] Bolton and Joske, *A History of Royal Perth Hospital*, p. 116.

[4] Minutes of BM, 19 September 1930.

even sufficient funds to carry out necessary alterations to the hot water boiler, but the house committee did order a modern water-softening machine costing £105 for the laundry. As it saved 40 per cent of the outlay for soap powder and some of the fuel costs, it paid for itself. When the tennis court needed top-dressing the staff met the expense by holding a tennis tournament to raise the funds. But nothing could prevent the contraction in trained nursing staff numbers which had to be made.

A special board meeting was called for 10 October 1930. All were present— McMahon, Mrs Kirby, Mrs Waddell, Locke, Frank Rowe, Turton, Dr Gibson, Knapp, Greenslade and Gray—and all listened to the secretary's grim forecast: '. . . we are going back financially at the rate of over £5,000 a year'; all knew that he was right in attributing the cause to '. . . stress of unemployment at present existing in Fremantle'.[5] Each deplored the proposed move to close the children's and male medical wards but there seemed no other option.

It wasn't as though the board stopped trying. So acute was the financial position, that a Melbourne Cup sweep netting £630 in November proved only a welcome drop in the ocean. The board tried to cut costs. Greenslade suggested buying fish and vegetables at the markets at market rates but it was too great an undertaking. It wasn't as though most patients weren't co-operating as best they could either, although there was a check on those who arrived in motor cars. Mrs McMonagle, the collector, was joined in her task by Mr Richards, Mrs Sweeny and Mrs Hopkins, but they collected between them only around £90 weekly before commissions were subtracted. Some patients paid two or perhaps five shillings a week, and the collectors' cards listed many accounts as 'unable to trace', 'gone to England or perhaps Italy', 'pensioner—widow', 'not in a position to pay', 'widow—two children', 'indigent circumstances', 'unemployed', or 'on sustenance and five weeks arrears in rent'.[6] The secretary was wary of false statements and even those patients claiming to be unemployed or on sustenance were checked on by the collectors to protect the hospital's interests. One patient offered carpentry and repair work to reduce his outstanding account. Those debts considered able to be paid were placed in the hands of the Crown Law Department. Some people promised payment when they could; many accounts had to be written off.

When the board failed to gain extra government help by January 1931, Hookway went to see both the principal medical officer, Dr Everitt Atkinson, and Huelin, the secretary of the Medical Department, to personally appeal for funds. He returned empty-handed. Just as unsuccessful was a visit by the finance committee. The Board of Management considered and concluded that there was no alterative other than to hand over direction of the hospital to the Medical Department. On 9 February 1931, it reluctantly surrendered its financial control and agreed to carry on in an advisory capacity to the department.[7] On the renewal of board appointments later that month

[5] *Ibid.*, 10 October 1930.
[6] Record book of Fremantle Hospital Collectors 1933–1944, FH. One account of £34.4.0. was paid over over a period of eight years in small, regular instalments between September 1936 and July 1944. It was not unusual for an account to last between six and seven years, with small amounts paid weekly or fortnightly.
[7] At Perth Hospital also, the Board of Management acted as an advisory committee between 1931 and 1936. Bolton and Joske, *The History of Royal Perth Hospital*, p. 116. See also *West Australian*, 17, 21

the advisory committee was little changed in membership and McMahon was returned as chairman. Turton was appointed treasurer of the committee and Mesdames Waddell and Kirby as a standing ladies' committee. The first task of the advisory committee was to push for the re-opening of the children's ward which, with the support of the honoraries, was granted. Its second task was the decision to delete the word 'public' from the hospital's title. The third move was to thank the Fremantle Road Board for assisting the institution to secure cheap firewood, and the fourth was to consider the large number of prescriptions sent to the hospital dispensary through outside medical practitioners. It subsequently advised the Medical Department that it wished to be known as the Fremantle Hospital Advisory Board. For its part the Medical Department directly involved itself in decisions about the nursing staff, increasing the age for probationers to 21 years; at a time when any employment was valued there was no lack of applicants. Next it appointed Miss S. Fisher as assistant matron at £160 a year. Some months later it limited evening visits to patients to Wednesdays and Sundays, and introduced free visiting daily for the half hour between 3 p.m. and 3.30 p.m. In May, much to the advisory board's relief, the Medical Department re-opened the surgical ward. In another move it opened the hospital's tiny old morgue, with its rear wall crumbling away, to the police, so that the police morgue could be done away with. The board's own banking account was given a good start by the sale of the donated block of land and a contribution of £72 from the Railway and Tramway Hospital Board. This was further increased by an anonymous £50 donation from someone calling himself 'Smiler'. The first confrontation between the department and the board was not long in coming. Matron Maida Balding, not the secretary, was informed of Miss Fisher's appointment and an indignant board 'considered it unwise for the department to have made such an important appointment without first obtaining the advice of the Board' and suggested that 'in the future the department should confer with the Board before making and finalizing such matters'.[8] The board was slightly mollified to receive the department's apology and explanation that the matter had been 'inadvertently overlooked'.[9]

It was inevitable that everyone in the hospital would be affected by the struggle to reduce costs. All were urged to reduce the amount of linen sent to the laundry. If washing was done only twice instead of thrice a week, savings could be made in soap and the cost of water. The pharmacist was requested to dispense only the drugs listed in the British *Pharmacopoeia* and the honorary medical officers temporarily co-operated with the board by not sending their private patients' prescriptions to the hospital dispensary to be made up. As one hospital resident doctor of the period recalled, 'We had to watch things carefully'.[10]

Many in the Fremantle community were affected by the Depression. Lumpers as well as market gardeners, shop-keepers and office workers suffered. Families often had no regular wage, many had to apply for sustenance and others were hungry or lost their homes. It seemed that some came to casualty

and 22 January 1931. Letter by J. R. N. Greenslade to Editor, *West Australian*, 21 January 1931; *Fremantle Advocate*, 12 February 1931.

[8]   Minutes of BM, 19 June 1931.
[9]   *Ibid.*
[10] Barrington Knight, interview.

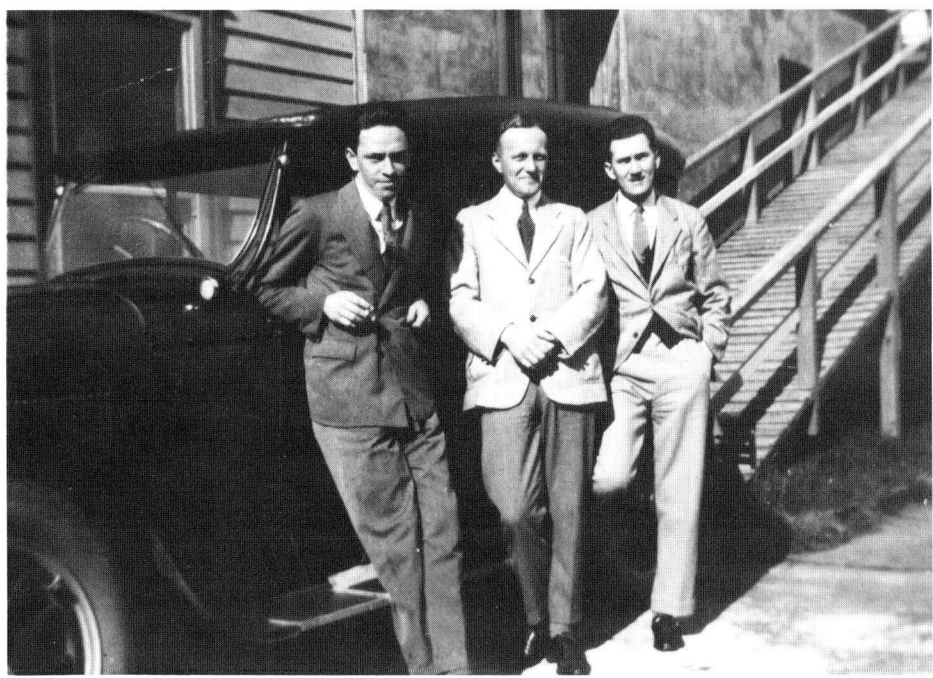

Photograph courtesy Dr Herbert Ferguson

Plate 40. 'Three bright young lads.'

(Left to right): Gus Christie (pharmacist), Harry Uther Baker and Herbert Ferguson (doctors).

Work was often hard and long as another young resident recounted:

> Many, many a time, when I was on duty for the weekend I've taken over on Friday morning. It was usual to have breakfast, [but] I never saw my bed on Friday night. On Saturday morning I just changed my clothes and went on, and the first time I would see my bed again would be Monday night.

> Dr Stanley Barrington Knight

> ... with all sorts of excuses. They really wanted a bed, but they had all sorts of complaints and Doctor Cass was then ... senior medical officer, and he was very sympathetic towards them. If he couldn't give them a bed he would give them money to get a feed.[11]

The numbers coming for treatment rocketed and hospital resources were stretched to the limit. In 1926 12,000 out-patients were treated; in 1928, 17,000; there were 20,000 in 1930 and in 1932, 24,811. 'We cannot treat the large number of out-patients expeditiously. Sometimes they cannot move in there', reported the secretary.[12] On one day alone, a doctor saw 67 patients. 'The existing out-patients' accommodation is so inadequate that the attendance of the public overflows into the

[11] Fuller, interviewed by C. Jeffery, 18 November 1984 and 13 December 1984.
[12] *West Australian*, 17 June 1933.

main corridor near the office of the secretary and staff', the *West Australian* found.[13] Nor did the public stay in the corridor:

> We are daily faced with the difficulty of people wandering all over the grounds and wards and it will be almost impossible to prevent this so long as the out-patients' department and the office remain in the present position—we have had notices placed in various parts of the hospital, but these are ignored, and the Sisters and the Staff cannot be expected to be continually driving people away from the wards.[14]

While the number seeking treatment increased, so did that of the nursing staff, but not appreciably. There was a staff of 50 in July of both 1930 and 1931 (12 trained nurses and 38 pupils); 56 in 1933 and 54 in 1934.[15] The increase was not proportionate to the number of in-patients. In July 1926 they totalled 141; there were 149 admitted in July 1930, but by July 1933 there were 264.[16] Finances curbed all but talk about major extensions—even for a desperately needed out-patients' department. The hard-working ladies' auxiliary, however, shared with the Medical Department half the cost of a new tilt table for X-ray, paying £25 as a deposit and £2 each month. They donated a new shadowless lamp for the theatre and were well pleased with their new tuck shop which had been completed at the rear of the old kitchen on 24 November 1929, and named after a benefactor named Grosser. Increasingly in the early 1930s, as one nurse recalled,

> ... there was a ... restriction on generosity in the hospital, both with equipment and food. There was not one thing ever wasted. We had to—if there was anything over from a meal, it had to be put away and heated up for the tea.[17]

Another shuddered: 'tapioca pudding, a roast of beef etc ... if [it] wasn't eaten, reappeared a few times ...'[18]

When the Medical Department requested a list of a dozen people suitable for appointment to the advisory board in mid-1930, the current members felt unsure of their restricted powers, and warily thought it 'inadvisable to nominate any names'.[19] During these years of Depression, little changed outwardly. The honoraries continued to urge the board not to admit shipping cases. Medals for nursing were presented to Nurse Dillon for success in exams and to Nurse Mavis Fuller for general efficiency in 1930, while Nurse Bowden and Nurse Robinson received medals in 1931 before the lack of funds caused a temporary suspension of the award. On a different occasion, some of the staff gathered in the boardroom to see Sister Smith receive an enlarged photograph of herself in appreciation for her work in the *Daily News* Charity Appeal. Nurses agreed to share the instalments for a wireless for their quarters, to which the board initially contributed £10, but two years later in July 1933, when salaries were reduced, the board also paid the outstanding balance total-

[13] *West Australian*, 26 August 1933.
[14] PHD File 260/1932.
[15] Matron's Report Book, 3 June 1930-17 December 1934.
[16] House Surgeon's Report Book.
[17] Fuller, interview.
[18] Heath, notes, FH.
[19] Minutes of BM, 20 June 1930.

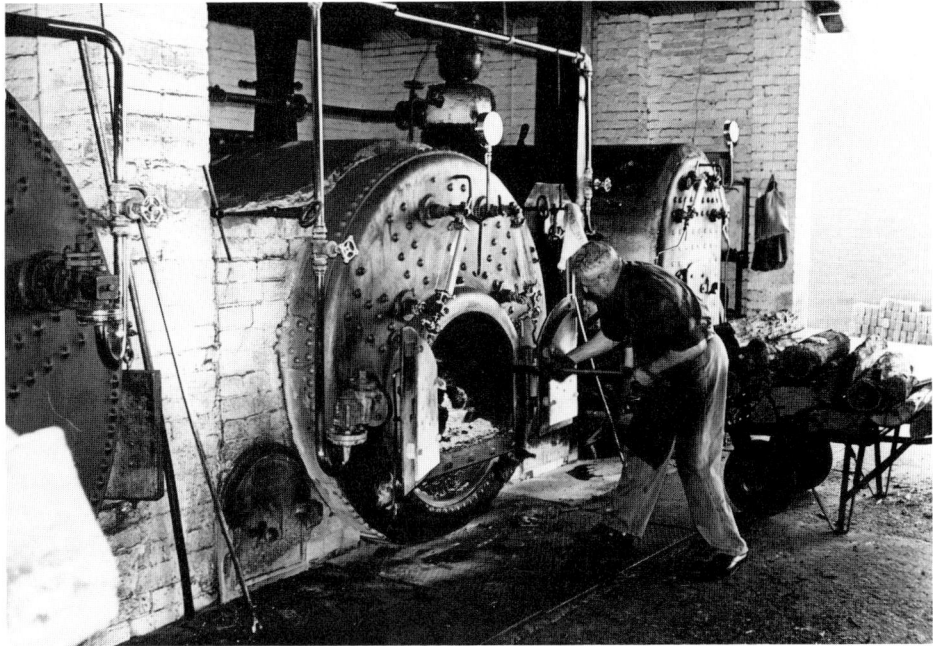

Plate 41.   Wood-fired boilers, used at the hospital until the late 1960s. Sometimes, one could find the boilerman on a winter's night

> fast asleep in the wheelbarrow ... he used to get his wheelbarrow and put the handles down on the ground, and he used to sit on the back tip of the wheelbarrow, put some old bags in there and he had the most comfortable armchair that you could ever find. They used to have to hawk these pieces of timber into the boilers.—Well the first thing they knew about them was when the boiler started to lose pressure and sounded the alarm!
>
> Bill Wilkinson
> Patient and Hospital Telephonist

ling the same amount. When nurses worked overtime, as they usually did, Chairman McMahon said 'something should be done', but nothing was.[20]

In 1933 the small regular payments allocated from the *Mirror* crosswords competition paid for the installation of the first refrigerator at the hospital which was 'of great value in the matter of keeping foods fresh'.[21] This modern advance was so valued that when the children's ward gained a refrigerator, the ward sister was allocated the work of its cleaning.[22] Another advance was brought about through great poverty in the area. In a gesture to what would later become the responsibility of an almoner, the board granted £50 towards a special fund controlled by the chairman to provide reading glasses or any special apparatus needed by the very poor.

[20]   *Ibid.*, 4 March 1932.
[21]   Matron's Report Book, 5 April 1933.
[22]   Hobbs, interviewed by C. Jeffery, 21 January and 5 February 1985.

With reduced employment in the town, working women with a husband in a well-paid job were regarded askance, and the Benbows were often mentioned in the conversations of objectors. Such was her competence in the laundry that Mrs Benbow's hours there had changed from occasional help in an emergency in 1924, to full-time as head laundress. Husband and wife had the hospital's interests at heart. They had once donated a lamp to be raffled to raise funds, and Benbow often used their motor car for hospital needs. When cockroaches overran the kitchen, Benbow was called from his work in the laundry to clear them away. He laid water pipes in the grounds, at which the plumber's union protested so vigorously that they paid a qualified plumber to do the work rather than have an unregistered man involved. The engineer coaxed the boilers into producing the hospital's necessary hot water and nursed the machinery in the laundry into effective old age. The first official complaint about the Benbows was lodged by the new board member, Mr Curly Molyneux, in October 1929. He thought that it was 'inadvisable that a married couple should be both employed by the hospital'.[23] The board discussed the matter at length and decided to call a new head laundress after secretary Hookway had recovered from a scheduled operation. Two months later, with nothing further having been done in the matter, the Fremantle Australian Labor Council challenged the hospital on the subject. The resulting focus of attention on the laundry only revealed that some of the laundresses had understated their ages to gain employment. Such was the need for her ability, however, that Mrs Benbow could not even take her holidays as no competent senior laundress could be found to replace her. In August 1930, as poverty among the unemployed increased, another deputation from the Fremantle Australian Labor Party protested to the board about the employment of both a married woman and her husband on the hospital staff. Not wishing to lose Mrs Benbow's excellent service, the board once more delayed finding a replacement until Maida Balding returned from England, and then the matter paled in comparison with the handing over of control to the Medical Department. Not until 18 July 1931 did Mrs Benbow leave the hospital with her record of 'excellent service during the period of nearly eight years'.[24]

In 1932, in a hard-contested game watched by supporters, South Fremantle League Football Club's captain and coach, Ronald Oldham Doig, received a blow to the head which caused a haemorrhage and resulted in his death. Such was the distress at the death of the popular sportsman, that members of the football club planned to raise funds for a memorial to their esteemed companion. The deplorable condition of the out-patients' and casualty departments of the hospital adjacent to their home ground was well known to the injured players and those who took them there for treatment, and a new department in memory of Ron Doig seemed most appropriate to the footballers. As the deputation from the football club left the hospital on 27 September 1932, Secretary Hookway, thinking of the £1,000 already set aside by the Medical Department for alterations and additions to the out-patients' department, rejoiced, '. . . They are prepared to launch the appeal immediately'.[25] Before plans were drawn up, the honorary medical staff submitted a long list of

23   Minutes of BM, 18 October 1929.
24   Matron's Report Book, 21 August 1931.
25   PHD File 260/1932. See also *West Australian*, 29 September 1932.

recommendations for the new department, based in part on their personal hospital experience and information from institutions in the eastern states. They met with the under-secretary and the principal architect, Mr Clare. Site, size, layout of rooms and theatre were considered in the two-level building. The honoraries also advocated the construction of a large reception hall at the entrance from which patients could move to consulting rooms, then straight forward to the dispensary at the exit. Conferences and considerations of costs shaped a final building totalling £8,350, an amount which had to be reduced. The electric lift was rubbed off the plan, and then the retaining wall, the steam heating, a collapsible entrance gate, and two small, light-giving windows at the entrance. The chocolate-coloured tiles were exchanged for red, saving £30.[26] Despite the necessary changes, the new building was a great improvement on the old quarters.

With the 1933 board appointments there was little change. The only new face belonged to Mr Greig. McMahon remained as chairman but with the hospital work expanding at a greater rate than the facilities, it was a taxing time. Hookway continued to pare expenses and actually reduced the cost per patient per day. Early in 1934, as the secretary termed it, there was an 'extraordinary increase in the number of patients admitted'.[27] Indeed, in the month of January there had been 320 in-patients altogether, with a daily average of 142. Two extra beds were added to each ward in a band-aid move to increase accommodation; with this increase in patients, more visitors came, and there was even talk of eliminating this privilege altogether.[28] It was obvious that a new ward was needed, and a new male medical ward to replace the old corrugated-iron one was an obvious choice. Out-patients recommended for admission had to wait hours before being allocated a bed. But children didn't mind the wait for a tonsillectomy on a lengthy small-operations list submitted by their school medical officer. So long was the list that throat, tonsil and adenoid operations were done by the medical staff on Sundays in 1931.

If the numbers admitted to the wards caused headaches, each day in out-patients was a nightmare. A man who had a seizure in the street was taken to the hospital at 9.30 one morning in June 1933 but was not treated until 1 p.m. A deputation to the board on his behalf admitted that during the three-and-a-half-hour wait, 'the staff was working at top pressure and they were doing a tremendous amount of work'.[29] A child suffering appendicitis was not even examined before being immediately referred to a private hospital because her father was employed and therefore considered able to afford the fees.[30] Another injured person, a member of the Western Australian Motor Cycling Association, was admitted to a ward but was overlooked for three days, such was the pressure on the only resident medical officer on duty.[31] Fremantle had always been a Labor stronghold, so it was not surprising that the Australian Labor Party protested about conditions at the hospital. It was told of the increase of out-patients from 12,000 in 1926 to over 29,000 in 1933 and were assured

[26] *Ibid.*; File 260/1932.
[27] *West Australian*, 16 February 1934.
[28] *Ibid.*
[29] *Ibid.*, 17 June 1933.
[30] *Ibid.*, 27 April 1933.
[31] *Ibid.*, 29 April 1933; Minutes of BM, 20 April 1933.

that if a third doctor could be found and the Ron Doig Block completed, things would be better. 'We cannot do justice and have not done justice to the suffering people of the district,' added Chairman McMahon. 'We hope before long that power which we had until recently, will be restored. When we had that power we did the job well.'[32]

The fact that they were under medical board control rankled with the advisory board members. In April 1933, Frank Rowe urged a return to administration under the old conditions, but did not receive whole-hearted support from his peers until June. At a special meeting called in July with the Minister of Health, S. W. Munsie, it was agreed that the board's managerial powers should be restored subject to two limitations: no new expenditure could be passed by the board without the authority of the department, and increases previously granted to nurses would not be agreed to unless other hospitals were placed on a similar scale.[33] The conditions were accepted and the board committed itself to 'a policy of efficiency and economy'.[34] In effect, however, the Medical Department maintained control to the degree that it granted approval for the employment of additional probationers and domestics. This proved unsatisfactory to the advisory board, who perceived the urgent need for additional staff, but who could do nothing to obtain it. In January 1934, Matron Balding travelled to Perth and met with the under-secretary of the Medical Department to explain the hospital's need for an additional maid. The department triumphed in the power tussle that developed with the board over the issue, and no maid was appointed. The board retired from the conflict resentful at the department's attitude, which it believed was quite unjustified.

In the ensuing reorganisation it was decided that the house and finance committees should amalgamate and be known as the executive committee, which would total four in number and control all the financial business of the hospital and hold the executive power of the board. The new committee comprised Turton, Wauhop, Greenslade and Dr Gibson. Theirs was a gently moral and paternalistic outlook. In a revision of rules, the resident medical officers were precluded from entertaining any visitor at the hospital after midnight; nor could visitors to wards set apart for persons of the opposite sex visit before seeking approval from the sister or nurse in charge. All in all, the board felt gratified to attend the laying of the foundation stone of the Ron Doig Block on 8 October 1933, with a modicum of restored status and power.

On that Sunday afternoon, 2,000 people, including Doig's mates from the football and cricket fields and those who had donated in his memory, gathered on the sloping front lawn of the hospital facing the sea to listen to the Fremantle Naval Band, to hear the speeches, to see the mayor and government officals and watch the Minister for Works, Alexander McCallum, lay the foundation stone of the new block, which was 'not too good for the man in whose honour it was to be erected'.[35] Already the Ron Doig Memorial Committee had raised £1,600 to supplement amounts of £4,000 from the Medical Department and £2,000 from the Lotteries Commission.

32   *Ibid.*, 17 June 1933.
33   Minutes of BM, 14 July 1933. See also PHD File 245/1931.
34   *Ibid.*, 21 July 1933.
35   *West Australian*, 10 October 1933.

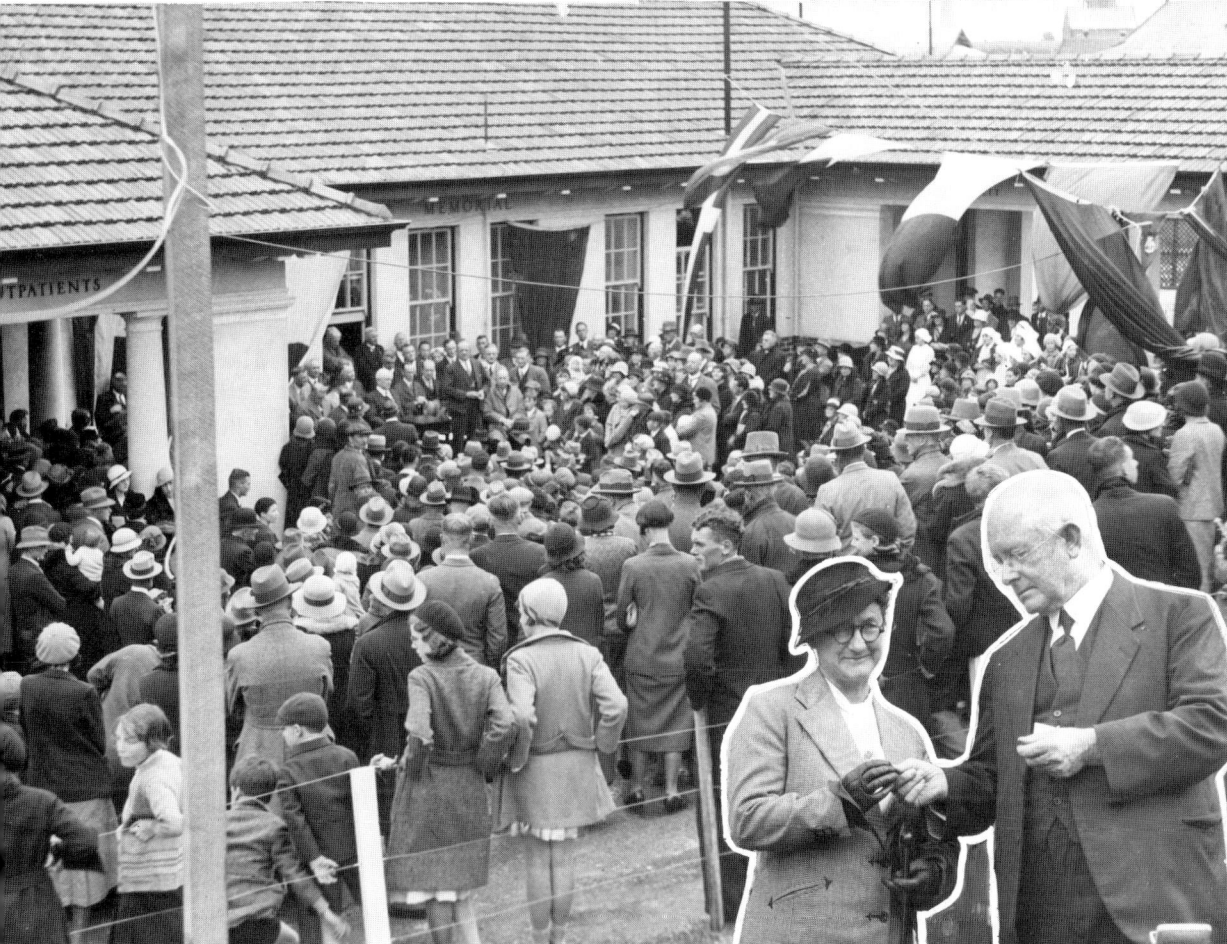

Plate 42.   Mrs Doig with Mr McMahon, Chairman of the Hospital Board, at the opening of the Ron Doig Memorial Block on 26 August 1934.

As work progressed, there was concern about the proposed access ramp between the new out-patients' building and the main hospital. The casualty officer, Dr Barrington Knight, went to a board meeting and took the members down to the building site.

I remember putting some bricks up and putting a plank on the bricks so I got a gradient of one in seven and I said to the Board, 'Now' I said, 'Walk up that. Doesn't that pull on the back of your legs? Well,' I said, 'it will pull a darn sight more if you tried to push a trolley up with a heavy fifteen or sixteen stone person on it.' So righto, we got Mr Clare down [from the Public Works Department] and he said, 'Oh, that will be all right'. I said 'Right Mr Clare,' I said, 'I have arranged for a trial' and I gave him the plank and I put him on the whatsthename and I said, 'Now walk up that'. I said, 'You can't do it Mr Clare. We will have to have a ladder—it will have to have a lift'.[36]

The cheapest means of providing a lift was chosen by the Public Works Department: a 730-lb. hand lift run by rope, pulley and hand power which was to be paid for by the board. But the board strenuously objected to such an obsolete lift in an up-to-date building and foresaw difficulties with its use. Not so Mr Clare and the medical mechanical engineer, who thought that to spend £800 on a lift which would be used only three or four times a day for a height of ten feet, was absolutely ridiculous. Although the board triumphed and an electric lift was installed and paid for by the hospital, the speed of the conveyance was disappointing: 'it would never disturb a patient. I mean if they were asleep at the bottom they would still be asleep when they got to the top. It went . . . as slow, as slow, as slow.'[37]

On 26 August 1934, a large crowd gathered outside the new Ron Doig Block to witness its opening, which was not before time. In January alone, 2,500 patients had been treated in the old casualty and out-patients' departments, often restlessly waiting three hours or more to see a doctor.[38] During the official ceremony showers dampened the people but not their enthusiasm, as Mr McCallum glowingly spoke of the work 'which had been backed up by the community as a whole' and which was the first public monument erected in Australia to the memory of a footballer.[39] Even Mr Munsie, who had haggled over costs, thought that 'every penny of it was well spent'.[40] The staff had their doubts at first when they tried the wonderful hot-water system to the basins, operated by foot pressure, which 'got hotter and hotter and hotter then finally it blew steam at you and no way—no way—could you get it cool'. After weeks of futile adjustments, the resident medical officer noticed that one of the big taps was turned off downstairs 'so we turned that tap on and we had no further trouble. The cold water tap was turned off.'[41] After the old quarters the new ward seemed palatial. On its first day a record number of 175 patients came for treatment and to approve the new extension to their hospital.[42]

Greenslade's appointment to the Charities Commission in 1934, two years after its inception, augured well for hospital finances. Except for emergency cases, patients were still interviewed by the lodge keeper and closely questioned about their financial situation and only those able to convince the interrogator of their meagre circumstances were admitted as patients, although they were expected to contribute what they could to the cost. With the introduction of the hospital tax, individual donations and subscriptions dropped—after all, people rationalised, weren't they now donating to hospitals every week through the scheme? In 1932 the medical department gained £55,142 less for hospital work than it had had the year before, and the number of beds for which it was responsible increased by over 70 between

36 Barrington Knight, interview.
37 *Ibid.*, PHD File 260/1932.
38 *West Australian*, 16 February 1934.
39 *West Australian*, 27 August 1934.
40 *Ibid.*, 27 August 1934.
41 Barrington Knight, interview.
42 *West Australian*, 28 August 1934.

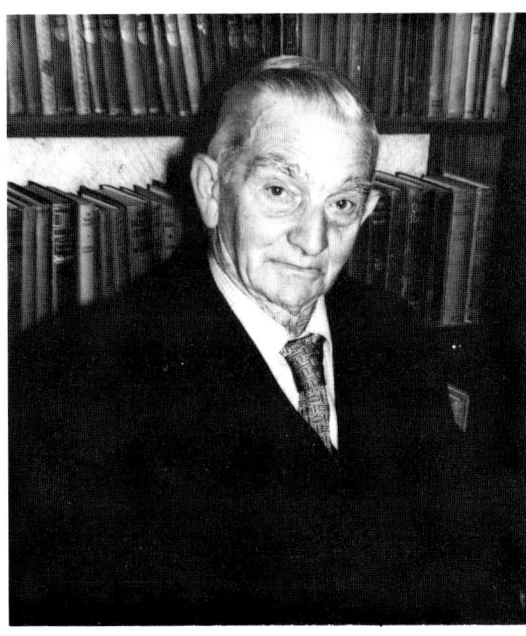

Plate 43. Mr J. R. N. Greenslade, J.P., was well known for his enormous amount of public service in local government, the Fremantle Children's Dental Clinic and the Lotteries Commission. He was a member of the Fremantle Hospital Board from 1932 to 1971. The Greenslade Wing was named in his honour.

Photograph courtesy Fremantle Hospital

1930 and 1933.[43] Under its control were four public hospitals in the metropolitan area, which admitted the poor or relatively poor; 25 departmentally-managed hospitals in the country; 61 board-managed hospitals in the country; five mental hospitals and Wooroloo Sanitorium for tuberculosis patients.

It was not surprising that Frederick Huelin, the under-secretary of the Medical Department, agreed that the Lotteries Commission was something of a fairy godmother to the department.[44] The Lotteries Commission wooed those with Cinderella hopes of overnight riches and dispersed the surplus between administrative cost and allocations to worthy institutions. Fremantle people were tempted by the possibility that a kind fairy might change their ticket '... into a cheque for £2,000 and transform a household drudge into a princess', or that even though there were no Aladdin's lamps, or Alf's bottles used by magicians to imprison imps, one could still win £1,000 with a two-and-sixpenny ticket.[45] Whereas donations to the hospital had helped to provide necessary building and equipment in the past, the task now often fell to the Lotteries Commission. At both Perth and Fremantle Hospitals, amounts were granted for social services departments. An advertisement for a triple certificated sister to establish this service at Fremantle in mid-1934 resulted in the appointment of Ruth Butson, an ex-Fremantle trainee then living at Mount Barker. For two months she trained in the social services department at Perth Hospital before taking up work in a basement room of the Ron Doig Block. Eggs, spectacles, splints and even a special voice box were sympathetically provided to some of the many who

[43] *West Australian*, 10 October 1933.
[44] PHD File 395/36.
[45] *Fremantle District Sentinel*, 4 July 1935, 19 July 1934.

came to the first social service sister. When Miss Butson left, Sister I. Smith carried on the work for the first six months of 1937, before Sister I. M. Gjerde's appointment in June.

The problem of patients who were able to pay for treatment had long been a source of concern to the secretary and the lodge keeper, who had to turn these people away when they came to the hospital. Likewise, the honorary doctors were concerned at not being able to continue the treatment of their patients once they were admitted into public hospitals. Early in 1935 the British Medical Association was publicly predicting that the old system of honorary medical treatment in public hospitals 'belonged to a passing social order and must pass before long into humble oblivion'[46] and the communal ideology, which maintained that the sick poor should be treated in a public hospital subsidised extensively by public charity, was gradually changing with the new system of hospital funding. A community hospital where indigent and paying patients could be treated in separate wards was seen by many as the ultimate solution. In 1934, Fremantle's honorary medical officers once more suggested the introduction of a community bed scheme. In mid-1935 they again supported the idea. This time, the board, the Medical Department and the B.M.A. discussed and agreed to the plan. It seemed to the board, that with the growing public acceptance of hospitals as centres to treat the sick and injured, that Fremantle's hospital 'should be open to all sections of the community irrespective of their financial position or circumstances'.[47] To all, the scheme seemed a workable one and a decision was made to adopt the system on 1 January 1936.

Townspeople reading their *West Australian* on 26 December 1935 learned that their hospital was to be 'recreated' and that everyone, irrespective of financial position, would be admitted when necessary. Some would pay all hospital charges and doctors' fees, some would pay 75 per cent of them, others 50 per cent, while the poor would pay hospital maintenance only. All patients were to be treated alike, but only those able to afford the fees could have their own doctor, who would bill them directly. The number of beds for paying patients in each ward was limited to ten, so that the impoverished would not be deprived. Now the employed could go to their private doctor and, if hospitalisation was indicated, he would ring the medical superintendent to see if accommodation was available. The initial estimated length of a hospital stay would be made by the medical superintendent and an approximate fee for a patient's treatment calculated, but the new community patients often found that in these respects the honorary doctors were not always co-operative. So large was the number of private patients, and so great the need for their beds, recalled a medical superintendent of the time, that a doctor

> ... would rush in ... all agitated, not a minute to go—wants so and so to come in ... and the following day, before anything could be done ... they were only just kind of settling into bed, Doctor would come in. 'Oh, must get so and so ... we'll discharge that one' ... so I said, '... I go to all the trouble working out what I estimate it's going to be and you just discharge them.[48]

46 *West Australian*, 10 January 1935.
47 Minutes of BM, 15 November 1935.
48 Barrington Knight, interview.

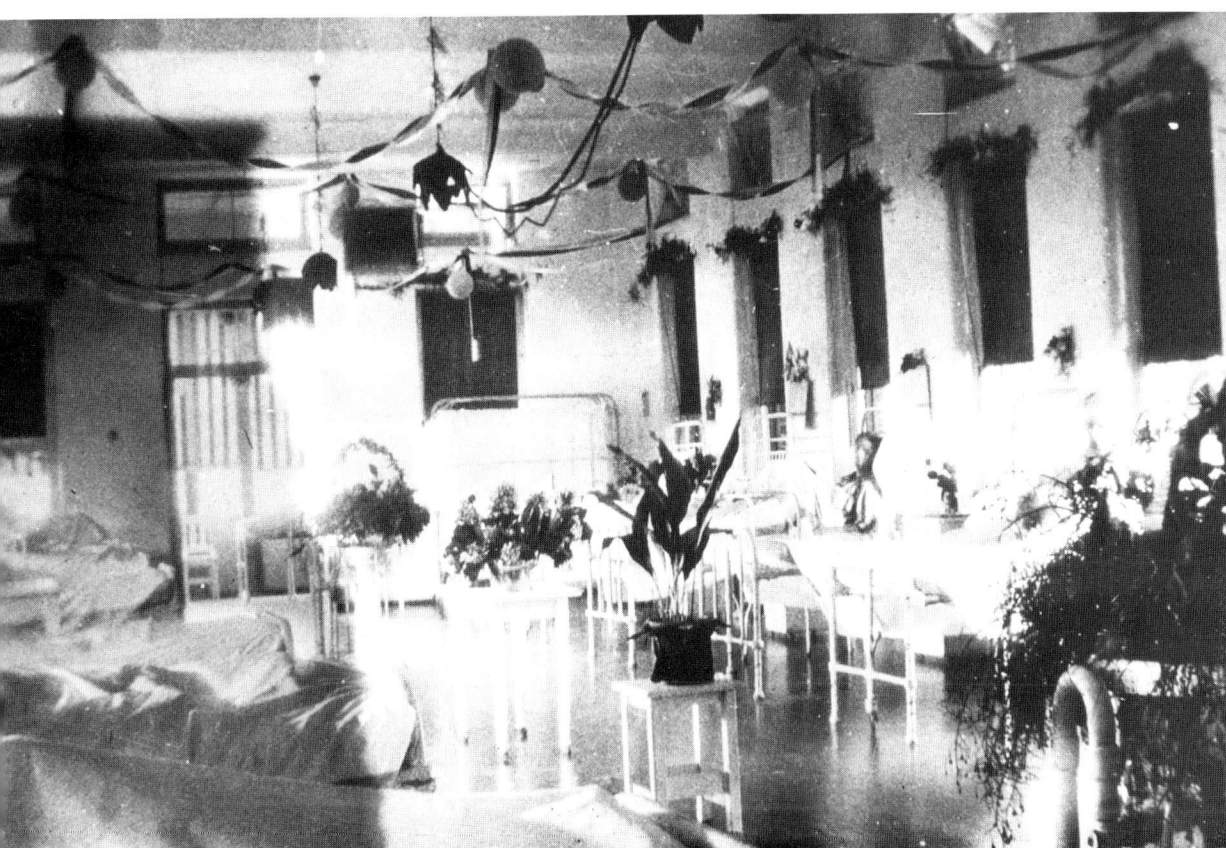

Photograph courtesy Fremantle Hospital

Plate 44.   Male surgical ward, Christmas, 1936.

In each of the five wards, community and indigent patients were nursed in beds side by side, without even a screen to segregate them. Female medical ward was still on the top floor of The Knowle, and in the surgical block to the south of The Knowle towards Alma Street, women were nursed in the upper ward and men on the lower level. Next to these wards, closer to Alma Street, was the old male medical ward with its rusting corrugated-iron roof, and the children's ward was on a bank roughly east of the main building. Decisions were made about the new class of patients—the masseuse could treat paying cases but not with hospital apparatus, and private, shipping and workers' compensation patients had to be billed for medicines supplied to them, for X-rays taken at the hospital, and for pathological examinations. Eight months later, 40 private patients had been admitted and the scheme was working well. As the *West Australian* observed:

> ... the best medical attention and hospital service with its many special departments

... besides being available to only the sick poor of the community is made available also to a great number of people who by their thrift have been classified in the category of those able to pay for private treatment.[49]

While accident or sickness could spell destitution for a low-income breadwinner with a dependent family through medical bills and loss of his wages, medical insurance had been available for members of Friendly Societies through various lodges since the mid-1850s.[50] Under the *Friendly Societies Act* of 1894 in Western Australia, the small weekly sum paid voluntarily by all members of such organisations was invested and, when the need arose, an amount of up to 20 shillings a week was made to the financial member or his family for medicines and medical attendance.[51] By 1934 the Medical Department was meeting with the three major hospitals—Perth, Fremantle and Children's—to discuss a hospital insurance scheme similar to that in New South Wales. For sixpence a week, a contributor could receive six shillings a day towards public or private hospital fees.[52] It was an arrangement, however, similar to one which had been advocated by Hookway for years, who called it his 'baby',[53] and was akin to a system successfully run by Perth Hospital since 1929. Although the board repeatedly tried to amalgamate with the Perth Hospital scheme in the 1930s, there was little encouragement from the city hospital and the time was thought economically inopportune to deliver Hookway's 'baby'. Not until the widespread acceptance of the Metropolitan Hospitals Benefit Fund of the early 1940s was hospital insurance freely available to people outside the Perth district.

Despite the fact that it was an area of the hospital which was in constant use, in 1932 the orthopaedic department contained only one examination couch, five ordinary chairs, a folding chair and other limited furniture and equipment. In December 1933 the orthopaedic surgeon, Marion Radcliffe-Taylor, argued for over an hour at a meeting with the board for the appointment of a full-time masseuse with higher qualifications than those held by the hospital's part-time employee. Her concern was for her patients, for there was a great need to improve and expand the orthopaedic department, and to bring it to a higher state of efficiency. Many on the orthopaedic list were motor car or motor cycle victims. Children who frequently played on roads and drivers who dodged around trams and each other often seemed not to have developed the road sense that the next generation would have, and 'the motor bike craze had just begun ... and many young, broken bodies were brought into Casualty'.[54] The board compromised by hiring, in conjunction with the Lady Lawley Cottage by the Sea, a masseuse from Adelaide named Miss Gwen Richards. It was not a favourable move for the young woman. Forced on her arrival to share her accommodation with rats in a lodging-house in Marine Terrace, Gwen fell ill and was admitted to a Fremantle Hospital bed. On her recovery, many hospital cases benefited by her treatment, but Gwen's enthusiasm did not stop at her patient's wel-

[49] *West Australian*, 15 August 1936.
[50] P. D. Reid, 'A Brief History of the Influence of Friendly Societies', Work as part of study at Graylands Teachers College, 1956, BL.
[51] *The Friendly Societies Acts and Regulations*, Perth, Richard Pether, Government Printer, 1896, BL.
[52] *West Australian*, 21 November 1934.
[53] PHD File 638/1931. See also *West Australian*, 5 August 1935; *Fremantle Advertiser*, 30 July 1931.
[54] Brown (née Fry), notes, 1986, FH.

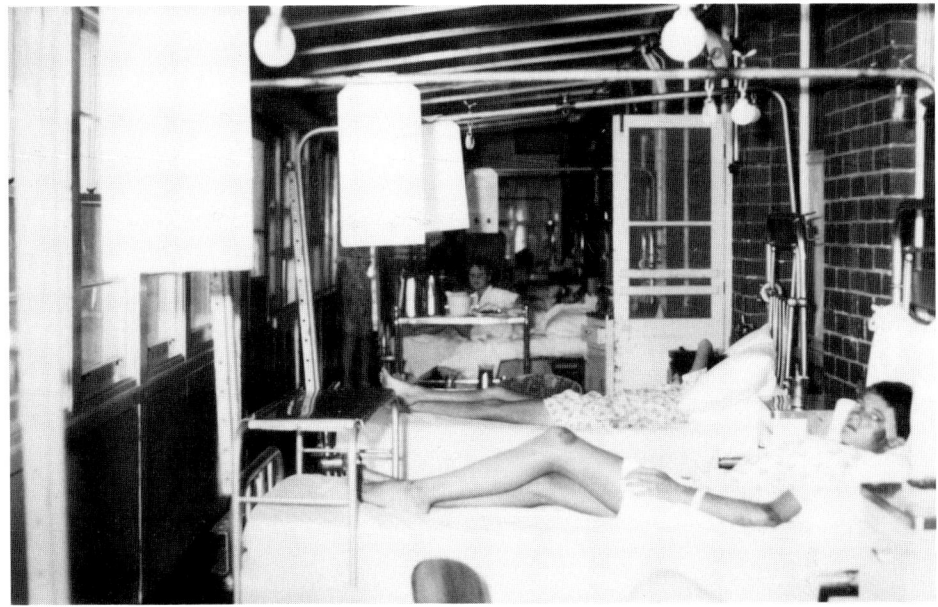

Plate 45.   The Adelaide Samson Children's Ward.

Additional bed space had always been obtained by closing in verandahs—at the Knowle, the children's wards, the old medical and surgical wards and the McCallum ward. The William Wauhop wing was different. Paddy Clare [government architect] used to get hostile if you built a verandah on any building ... 'All they do is to put bloody beds on it, so you don't build verandahs'. So we didn't have any verandahs on the Willy Wauhop wing.

Dr John Rowe
Medical Superintendent

fare; her gymnastic evenings for the staff, held in the Nurses' Home, were greatly appreciated by those who attended.[55]

Although the early 1930s at the hospital reflected depressed conditions in the community, there were changes. In this period the mortuary was shored-up and enlarged. The honorary staff was increased from 10 to 12 in number, and Dr Ferguson was appointed as an honorary anaesthetist. From March 1934 the title of senior resident medical officer was changed to 'medical superintendent', but Dr Sargent found that his duties altered little. Dr Day-Lewis joined the staff as a resident in September 1934 and was followed by Dr T. Harvey Johnston. To help with the increasing work in pharmacy, T. A. O'Donnell was appointed as an assistant dispenser. Despite the initial repercussions, when orderly Myers inadvertently stoked the laundry steam boiler while it contained too little water and seriously damaged it, he did the hospital a good turn, for a large efficient boiler had to be installed. Increasingly the Hospital

[55]   S. Gill, notes, 23 February 1987, FH.

Employees' Union intervened on behalf of a member—meeting with the board to protest at a dismissal, or supporting in a claim for compensation through injury. At the request of the medical staff, visiting hours were changed to two hours of free visiting on Sundays and Wednesdays, and to half an hour on alternate afternoons and nights during the rest of the week, when adult visitors still paid their sixpence, and children a silver 'thrupenny' piece.

With the increase in the number of in-patients, ward space was desperately needed and the ends of the male and female surgical wards were closed in by the hospital carpenter in 1934 for the very sick or those who needed to be isolated. The wide verandahs of The Knowle outside female medical ward were also closed in with blinds. Sometimes the disruptive patients were wheeled to these enclosures. A doctor explained: 'We would put them out there. We would even put them out in the passage or somewhere if they were rowdy and noisy so that they wouldn't disturb the rest of the patients.'[56] Such cases were often the result of addiction to alcohol which was not confined to patients. At different times, two of the resident medical officers were dismissed for their indulgence. Beds were acquired second-hand from Wooroloo in 1932 and nine more were obtained in 1933, bringing the in-patient accommodation to 154 beds:[57] the male medical and surgical wards and the female medical and surgical wards each accommodated 30 patients; there was room for 33 in the children's ward and for one in the nurses' sick room. Nevertheless on several occasions there were no spare beds and patients requiring treatment had to be turned away.

It was difficult to know who needed accommodation the most—the patients or their nurses. Eighty nurses shared 41 small rooms and some shared a wardrobe as well. In 1933, six wardrobes were ordered from a well-known cabinet maker of Fremantle who charged only £20.17.0. for his work. There was serious talk of taking over part of the old immigration building for nurses' accommodation, but as a temporary measure, in May 1935, the nursing home verandahs facing Attfield and Alma Streets were closed in. Plans were made to extend the nurses' home and in the interim, there was some relief when the old isolation ward was reconditioned as extra quarters.

Although there were some changes for nurses in the 1930s they still went straight to the wards. 'We didn't know a thing. It's a wonder patients ever got better—but they did,'[58] reflected a nurse of the time. They still performed the domestic tasks that were part of a nurse's training and which provided reliable cheap labour in the hospital's organisation. Parents still signed indenture forms at a daughter's commencement of training, but from 1935 the hospital secretary was authorised to sign the forms on behalf of the Medical Department. In September 1934 the Western Australian Nurses' Association Industrial Union of Workers was registered.[59] Until then improvements in wages and conditions at Fremantle Hospital had been negotiated between nurses and the board or the Medical Department, keeping in mind the salaries paid at the Children's and Perth Hospitals. Through the union a 48-hour

56 Barrington Knight, interview.
57 PHD File 260/1932.
58 Buzza, notes, FH.
59 Minutes of Executive Committee, 4 September 1934; Hobbs, *But Westward Look*, pp. 90–2; 237–8.

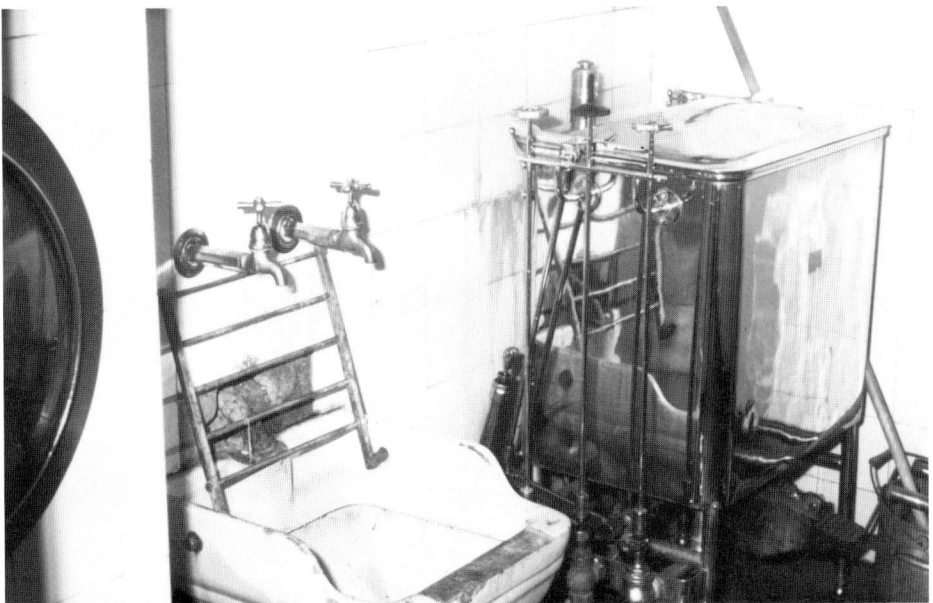

Photograph courtesy Fremantle Hospital

Plate 46. The first experience of a trainee nurse: the pan room with a 'slophopper' and sterilizer.

> As a first year nurse, you'd do a pan and bottle round depending on which ward you were in ... You would clean the Pan Room. You'd have to soak all your pans in a disinfectant in the big trough. Then after they'd soaked adequately, you had to wash and polish them all and stack them away.

Sister Bette Needle

week was demanded and also a re-scheduling of salaries which was granted in October 1935. The long-overdue changes posed financial and administrative challenges. Matron made out new timetables but could not avoid the spread of hours that required a nurse to alternate her scheduled periods on and off duty over 14 hours in the day, which the executive committee thought 'not quite fair to the nursing staff'. Twelve new nurses were needed.[60] The union pressed for increased nursing accommodation at Fremantle, for the provision of fresh fruit on the nurses' dining table once a day, and intervened when a nurse felt herself wronged. Nurse Draper's claim for two months' sick leave was supported by the union who persisted in the claim as strongly as the board resisted it before the amount was granted. In 1938 an award granting a straight eight-hour shift cost the hospital £285 in salaries a year for ten extra nurses. The senior probationers of 1935 did not go to Perth for the final oral and practical examination, for it was held at Fremantle Hospital, and from 1937 trainees no longer had to make their uniforms, which were supplied under the

---

[60] Minutes of Executive Committee, 10 January 1936, FH. For a comparison, see Bolton and Joske, *History of Royal Perth Hospital*, pp. 119–20.

nurses' award; nor did they have to go to the infectious diseases hospital when the board decided that the experience at Fremantle Hospital in this area was sufficient.

The Western Australian Nurses' Association in 1937 showed concern, both at the 'exorbitant amount of domestic work done by trainees to the exclusion of their gaining experience in and knowledge of actual nursing duties',[61] and at the use of nurses as cheap labour—cleaning windows, cleaning brasses, scraping plates, scrubbing and cleaning lockers and equipment. But it was felt by many that a nurse had to have a practical knowledge of domestic cleanliness. Sweeping the long wards three times a day often produced painful blisters that burst and hurt even more. The Fremantle board was loathe to intervene and a probationer nurse of 1939 recalled that she scrubbed wooden lockers, cleaned tooth mugs, folded linen, emptied sputum mugs and cleaned windows:

> I would like a penny for every window I have cleaned in male surgical too. The maids used to clean the bottom but they weren't allowed to climb, so on Sunday afternoons or something, I have, many times—you swing from the window sill and clean the top windows, inside.[62]

Another nurse similarly engaged on top of a ladder was reprimanded for the undignified action of having her shoes off. She replied with asperity that, 'as it wasn't dignified to have her shoes off, it certainly wasn't dignified to be perched on top of a ladder cleaning windows'.[63] Sometimes matron or a senior nurse would run a clean white handkerchief over a ledge to check for dust, or test the top of a door to see if it had been properly cleaned.

While the strong domestic leaning in a nurse's training was never forgotten, there were other memorable moments. From the wide verandah of The Knowle in the mid-1930s the wreck of the *Lygnern* could be seen out to sea, breaking up a little more each day as the sea pronounced an undisputed victory over the once-proud ship which had run aground.[64] There were many magic dawns and brilliant sunsets to remember. One nurse recalled the unforgettable beauty of daybreak seen from The Knowle. Despite her tiredness after night duty, she 'stood and looked out just at dawn as the fishing fleet was leaving the harbour and sailing towards the moon'.[65] At all hours gulls would soar in screeching circles but on some quiet summer evenings, the songs of Italian fishermen could be heard at the hospital as they sat on the sea wall together, mending their nets or enjoying the companionship.[66] Sometimes over the distinctive hospital smells—the whiff of the hurricane night lamps, the food cooking, the ether—there would come the sharp smell of the sea.

The sea brought new patients as well as memories. Ships that called often left either a passenger or crewman for medical treatment: an appendicectomy, broken bones from a fall or fight, perhaps an illness. Many of these patients spoke no English, and one long-term Norwegian called his hospitalisation, 'The Great Austra-

---

61 PHD File 841/36.
62 L. Allen, interviewed by C. Jeffery, 28 August 1985, FH.
63 Heath, notes, FH.
64 Hobbs, interview.
65 L. Moorhouse (née Baker), notes, FH.
66 H. J. Curran (née Strange), notes, FH.

lian Loneliness'.[67] Walking patients were expected to teach these other patients the 'meaning and usage of common words—"drink", "pan", "bottle" etc., with sometimes embarrassing results!'[68] A Chinese crewman knowing no English was put ashore and admitted in 1940. After two operations the man seemed concerned about something which no sign language could clarify. Eventually, when a doctor who could speak six Chinese dialects was located through the Flying Angel Mission to Seaman, it was discovered that 28-year-old Chong Tong was desperately concerned about his savings which had been brought from the ship. He was relieved to learn that they had been placed in safe-keeping at the hospital. For many weeks, the young Chinese Buddhist happily shared his room with an Indian Muhammadan.[69] Nursing such patients was not always easy. One nurse recalled the distress of a Lascar suffering with pneumonia: '. . . [he] just lay down and died. Nothing, I think, with all the care we gave him would have saved him.'[70] Another remembered that during the Sino-Japanese war she nursed a Chinese seaman bedded opposite a Japanese seaman, '. . . and as it was on night duty, I didn't much like walking between them'.[71]

While nurses often spent their off-duty times together—sometimes swimming at Leighton or South Beach, walking to the war memorial on a crisp winter morning after night duty, going to the pictures either in a parlour car to Perth or sitting 'in the gods' at Fremantle—it was good to be invited out. Male friends were not permitted in the hospital grounds and it was common to see a knot of young men waiting outside the Alma Street gate. The distrust of their young male friends was distressing to some and even after 40 years one nurse questioned the practice:

> He [fiancé] was so sweet and clean living and yet was never allowed to venture near the living quarters. We did have a concert party one night and our class did an act in old fashioned bathing costumes to the tune of 'Beside the Seaside'—our boyfriends and family were invited.[72]

Other parties in the quarters in the 1930s to which no one except perhaps the resident doctors or matron were invited, were the nurses' initiation ceremonies held when there was a large enough group of new probationers. There was:

> lots of fun such as dancing, singing and reciting in each corner of the room ... You were blind-folded, put your hands on a book and swore that you would never pinch anything out of matron's pantry ... and then you put your hands on your face and found when you took the bandage off, that you were covered in soot. Another time, one of the doctors was held down and given a spoonful of grated onion ... He was most indignant.[73]

One new nurse found her mattress on the rain water tank on the second floor, and

[67] *Ibid.*
[68] M. Hatch (née Borwick), notes, FH.
[69] *West Australian*, 15 February 1940.
[70] Heath, notes.
[71] Hatch, notes.
[72] Moorhouse, notes.
[73] Heath, notes and interview.

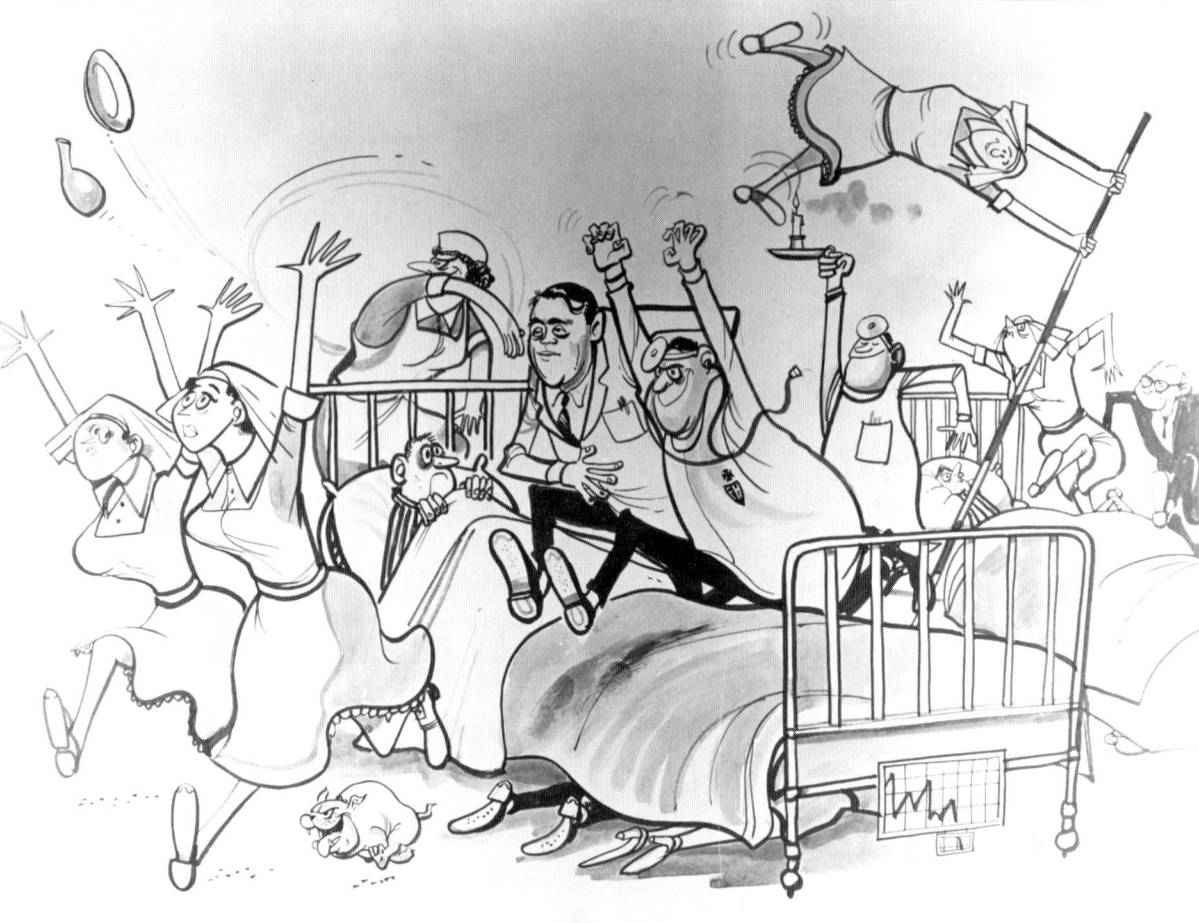

Fig. 15.   Fremantle Hospital Games, by cartoonist Rigby.

battled to retrieve it as no one would help her. In the nurses' lounge room the new initiates might have had to kneel balanced on a tussock with hands behind the back, and lean forward to kiss a rose on the carpet, but they invariably overbalanced. On the occasions that matron was invited, little sandwiches were sent for supper.[74]

By 1935 the matron was getting old. One evening, in her nightie and with her hair in pigtails down her back, she ventured from her room on the top floor of The Knowle along the corridor to the women's ward to get some aspirin for her rheumatics, and was mistaken for one of the patients. A nurse offered: 'Come on gran, back to bed dear'.[75] The response was prompt and outraged. In this year Maida

[74]   R. Buzza (née Bowden), notes, FH.
[75]   Hobbs, interview.

Balding completed 21 years as matron of Fremantle Hospital and was presented with an electric reading lamp by the board in recognition of her services. She had seen changes and made changes, faced challenges and overcome them, she worried about 'her girls' but rarely allowed them to know it and always acknowledged the help of senior nurses. In 1932 she wrote:

> The work of the charge nurses has been difficult. Credit is due to them for the good nursing results we have had and they have loyally supported me in endeavouring to maintain a high standard of nursing.[76]

Her ways were traditional and sometimes did not keep pace with changing hospital needs. Often nurses were redeployed daily, leaving some wards drastically under-staffed. Of the early 1930s a doctor remembered:

> She had a habit of changing the staff in any particular section, or ward or casualty, and then changing all the staff—every single jack one of them, staff nurses and everything else. Leave the main sister there but all the rest goes ... Of course this used to wipe everything out and you had an emergency and nobody knew where anything was and it was just a state of chaos until it had sort of settled down, especially in casualty.[77]

At times, the resident medical officer suggested to the matron that a partial change of staff would enable newcomers to be orientated, and would prevent the usual dislocation, but the matron persevered in her ways. The young resident was woken after one such change by a nurse wanting to know where the keys to the cupboard in casualty were kept:

> I got dressed and met matron coming down the stairs and just asked about this ... 'No one has ever questioned my administration of the staff or anything else'. Oh, she was most upset about it. Said I was bullying her and everything else ... and I did my best to convince her that she was the last person I would ever try to bully. ... She went into her office, shut the door in high dudgeon. I tried to go in, but no, she wouldn't see me. Then when I eventually got down to casualty, believe it or not, I had all the spare nurses in the hospital down in casualty. The place was running ... every person that was off duty she sent down. 'Mr Knight wants you down in casualty'. I had ceased to be Doctor. I was Mister and I got more staff than we knew what to do with. So I said, 'Well, you report back to matron.' 'Matron does not want to have anything to do with us at all. We were sent down for you to deal with.' 'So, righto', I said, 'We don't want you. You'd best take a day off'.[78]

For a long time relations were strained until one late night, the two were summoned in dressing gowns and slippers to hunt for a reported intruder at the nurses' quarters. The doctor recalled that after the hullabaloo, both returned in stony silence to The Knowle stairs. Matron looked at the young man and said:

> We are foolish, aren't we?' And I said, 'We are.' And she smiled. She had a lovely

[76] Matron's Report Book, 16 December 1932.
[77] Barrington Knight, interview.
[78] *Ibid.*

smile ... and I said, 'I was only trying to help matron'. And she said, 'I know you were'.[79]

There was even some foot shuffling and muted talk at board level about the matron's early retirement in 1935.

In 1935 Perth Hospital opened a preliminary training school for nurses. In May 1936 the under-secretary submitted proposals and held conferences to organise preliminary training for Fremantle nurses. Matron Balding went to see the lecture room and equipment at the Perth's new school and was impressed. The time seemed right for such a venture. In October 1935, nine probationers had been accepted for training, five commenced in September 1936, four in March and eleven in August of 1937. The board approved the purchase of equipment, and matron ordered anatomical models from London costing £76. Several times she nudged the secretary about a lecture area in which to set up the equipment, but there was no spare room. She did get a case made for the models in late 1937, and in early 1938, when Wooroloo Sanitarium started its preliminary training school, the only delay to the appointment of a tutor sister at Fremantle was the Medical Department's approval. Perhaps, hedged the under-secretary, Fremantle and the Children's Hospitals could start a combined school? Representatives of both hospitals met, argued, and agreed that an assistant matron could be appointed tutor sister if a housekeeper was hired for her former duties, but due to growing concern about the world crisis, the decision was shelved. When the subject was broached again in November 1941, the Fremantle Hospital Executive Committee felt that the time was 'not opportune to recommend expenditure in this direction'.[80] The board was not greatly concerned. Fremantle nurses' results from the A.T.N.A. in early 1943 had been good and Nurse Yates topped the state.

Early in 1936, the Lotteries Commission offered £5,000 toward the construction of a new medical ward. Not until plans were drawn up in 1937 did the Treasury promise £2,500 towards the cost. Construction was started by H. A. Doust, who had built the Ron Doig Block. The news spread and South Fremantle Football Club again approached the board with the idea of the block as a memorial—this time to Alexander McCallum, the late member for South Fremantle and former Minister for Works, who had taken such an interest in the hospital and who was respected as the mover of the compensation legislation. His death in July 1937 was regretted by many. The new building was not before time. Between mid-1936 and 1937, the total number of days spent by patients in hospital increased by 4,677. Staff numbers had to be increased to 135, and matron requested more probationers because of the shortage of staff nurses. Clerical staff, too, felt 'unnecessarily overtaxed' and they requested the help of another junior typist.[81] A second-hand duplicating machine was a welcome and well-used addition to their office.

Before the new, two-storeyed brick medical block began to take its shape alongside the surgical wards, the existing men's medical ward was loudly demolished. In keeping with new trends in hospital planning, long, narrow Nightingale wards with a

[79] *Ibid.*
[80] Minutes of the Executive Committee, 19 November 1941, FH.
[81] *Ibid.*, 19 May 1937.

row of beds down each side, had not been planned. The ground floor, designed to accommodate intermediate and private patients, boasted five single-bed wards, another room with two beds, one with three, and two wards containing six beds; the upper floor, for public patients, had only three single-bed wards, plus two rooms with six beds and an eight-bed ward. On the plans, balconies were glassed in. There were stainless-steel benches and sinks, Frigidaires, an electric food lift, a laundry chute, a call-bell system and wireless with earphones attached for the patients. The building promised the ultimate in efficiency and comfort. The foundation stone was laid on 31 July 1938 with an appeal for contributions to swell the McCallum Memorial Fund to £3,000. The community ward, it was said, 'made the appeal peculiarly applicable to the people'.[82] The people had supported their hospital before and once more they responded to an appeal. Large companies such as Woolworth's, W.A. Rope and Twine Company, and Kodak donated. Good Year Rubber Tyre Company assisted, and the Fremantle Trotting Club and Gloucester Park Association charity meetings raised nearly £1,500 between them. Small businesses and many individuals responded willingly. One person gave an electric reading lamp to be raffled, another a supper cloth. The Harbour Trust delivered sections of the old dismantled wharves and decking from ships as firewood to conserve hospital funds. Sweeps and dances were organised. Miss G. Best called on her way to England with a gift of £25 'in view of very excellent treatment received by her uncle about twelve years ago',[83] and during the year, through many small, regular donations, pupils from Princess May School raised £50.

A new ward meant that more nursing staff would be needed, and already secretary Hookway had been to the arbitration court to hear a complaint lodged by the nurses' union about crowding at the nurses' quarters. Plans to extend their building were drawn up; finance came not from the Medical Department but from the Lotteries Commission, who granted £5,000 toward the construction. Her work was the focus of Matron Balding's interests, and when plans for the new nurses' quarters with a special apartment for the matron were proposed she emphasised

> ... the importance of the matron being quartered in the Administration Building if constant supervision of the Wards and Nursing Staff, both day and night is desired—the Nurses' Home is a distance away from the main building, and is not connected with the Wards—I think Matron should be close to the active work if she is to be responsible for general conduct.[84]

The board agreed, partly because the idea meant that there would be more room for nurses' bedrooms. By June 1938 they were finished.

From November 1936 matron had three months' sick leave. A year later, while searching with an orderly for a prowler one dark night, she fell over a tap sunk in the lawn and broke her right arm. The board magnanimously overlooked the occasional tensions it shared with the matron. Applicants for training was an instance. Hers was the task of interviewing a young woman and making a recommendation to the

[82] *West Australian*, 23 November 1937.
[83] Minutes of Executive Committee, 13 April 1938.
[84] Minutes of BM, 9 November 1934. For nurses' quarters, see *West Australian*, 1 August 1938, 30 July 1938.

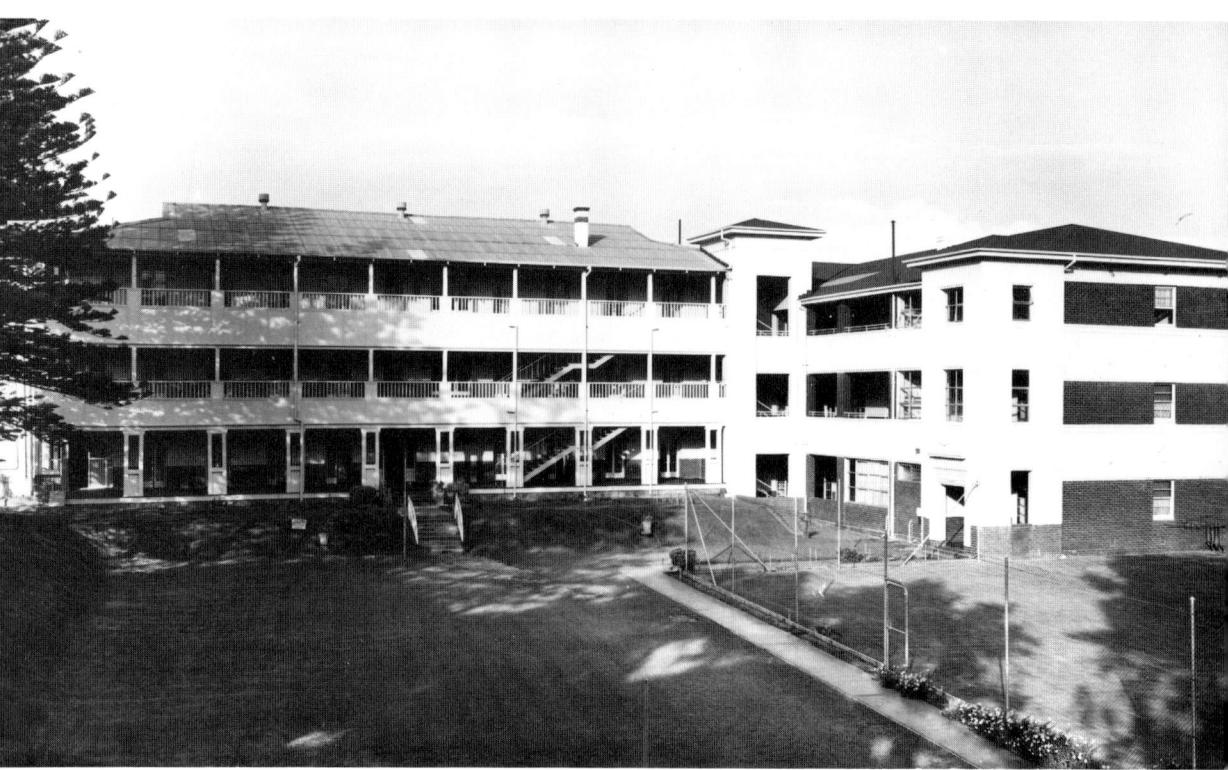

Photograph courtesy Fremantle Hospital

Plate 47.   The Balding Nurses' Home ...

where probationers were housed in the old part because the new part was exclusive to Sister Fuller, the sisters and the third year nurses. Very much exclusive. So, we were on the ground floor, which was the very base of the Balding Home, because then as you graduated up to first year you went to first floor and second to second floor. We were given our rooms and there were two to a room, but there were no beds in the room. There was a dressing table cum wardrobe each and a shoe box each and a straight backed wooden chair each. A mat on the floor in the middle, and then you went through a french door out onto a verandah that was an open verandah, with a canvas blind and the beds were all in a row along there.

Olga Hedemann
Director of Nursing

executive committee. It reported to the board who confirmed the appointment. Sometimes matron's decision about the suitability of an applicant was questioned, and at times she did not appoint those approved by the board in what they considered to be the correct order. Nevertheless, in 1937 the board overlooked their differences. Instead of paying her at half-rate under the terms of the *Workers' Compensation Act* for her broken arm the board granted their matron full rates. Although she suffered some permanent disability, Matron Balding returned to duty but again slipped and broke her hand on 1 July 1938.

Later that month, after the laying of the foundation stone of the McCallum Block on Sunday, 31 July 1938, the new nurses' home extension was opened, and an official celebration was held in the quarters which had cost £12,000. With impressive dignity, Mrs M. F. Hennelly, R.V.C.N., unveiled a commemorative brick let into the wall just inside the entrance. It was one of the many which had been carefully salvaged from Florence Nightingale's home and made available by the British College of Nurses to nurses' training schools all over the world.[85] While Mr Hookway read aloud the inscription on the silver plaque, Harry Gray, who had been elected chairman of the board in early 1936, looked across to the new McCallum Block under construction, and knew that there was a great deal more fund raising to be done for this new building. With her hand in a sling and her twenty-fifth year as matron looming, Maida Balding watched the celebrations and thought of the changes she had seen. With a sigh of satisfaction she determined to apply for reappointment as matron. In official minutes of the hospital the request, when it was received, was marked 'no action taken'.[86]

On 26 December 1938 Maida Balding would turn 65 and the Medical Department urged her early retirement so that all accrued leave could be taken before that date. But it was important to Miss Balding that she should stay until 6 February 1939 to complete her 25 years at Fremantle Hospital. The Medical Department strongly disagreed but was persuaded by a board deputation on the matron's behalf. She retired on 14 March 1939 with a pension of £245 a year. A fitting tribute was paid when the new Fremantle Hospital Ex-trainees Association, which had been formed early in 1937, suggested naming the new nurses' quarters after their matron.

In 1935 there was another who had been serving continuously at the hospital for nearly 25 years, and when Frank Rowe was not included on the list of those appointed to the board of management, there was 'severe comment' in the town, as it was well known that he wanted to complete a quarter of a century of service to the hospital. As the initiator of the ambulance service in the town, as secretary of the Lumpers' Union, as a staunch Labor man representing North-East Fremantle in the Assembly between 1927 and 1930, and as one of the most conscientious members of the hospital board, he was well known in Fremantle. Many protests by various organisations resulted in his reappointment to the board a few months later in July 1935.[87] Rowe resigned in 1937, just two years before his death.

The men and women appointed annually to the board often shared political and social interests as well as concern for the hospital. As the old stalwarts such as Lilly, Instone, Bolton, Mills, Wray and Mrs Carpenter retired or died in harness, other Fremantle citizens, often with local or state government responsibilities and usually with strong Labor connections, took their places at the board table. Two were usually women. In 1939 the local governments of Fremantle, East Fremantle, North Fremantle, Hamilton Hill and the Melville Road Board were represented by Davies, Wauhop, Turton, Willis and Cann respectively. Stubbe voiced the interests of the honorary Staff, Knapp the Fremantle United Friendly Society and Copelin the Hospital Employees' Union, while Gray was a member of the Legislative Assembly.

[85] *West Australian*, 1 August 1938.
[86] Minutes of Executive Committee, 25 January 1939.
[87] *The Fremantle Districts Sentinel*, 28 February 1935; PHD File 245/31.

Mrs Kirby and Mr Greenslade had less-obvious affiliations. Like Mesdames Waddell, Laidlaw, Beadle and Kirby, Mrs Edith Mannion was recommended for appointment by the Fremantle Labor Women's Organisation: 'Fremantle is a Labour stronghold and its Working Class Women should we think be represented,'[88] the organization had urged. In 1937 the board-elected executive committee of Gray, Greenslade, Wauhop and Stubbe were a strong and powerful group and after only a few skirmishes, notably in the board's move to have James Scrymgeour appointed as assistant to the secretary rather than someone of the executive committee's choice, the board left most of the decision-making to the competent committee.

The Alexander McCallum Memorial Block was formally opened on 12 March 1939 with customary dignity and complimentary speeches, and the turning of a key in its lock by Mrs McCallum. The £26,000 building brought the bed capacity of the hospital to 200, just under half that at Perth Hospital. Ironically, the ward was spoken of as 'an everlasting monument to Mr McCallum' and as sufficient to meet the requirements of the district for many years to come.[89] Almost as important was the simultaneous opening of the new pathological laboratory financed by the Lotteries Commission. The honorary medical staff had wanted such a department with a permanent officer since 1936 and had visited the Children's and Perth Hospitals to see the work done there. When Dr H. G. Breidahl was appointed honorary biochemist and pathologist in 1938, it seemed that all the available nooks and alcoves had already been converted into rooms. However, the tuck shop, sited conveniently near the Ron Doig Block, seemed a possible place for a pathological laboratory if the ladies' auxiliary was provided with new quarters facing the out-patient department in the Ron Doig Block. The enthusiastic ladies under Mrs Bell in 1938 who bought ten sun umbrellas for the children's ward, who presented a modern inductotherm costing £145 to the board, and for whom visiting hours were changed to suit their needs, were enthusiastic about the move. Subsequently the relocation was opposed by the board, but it did transfer the orthopaedic department to the Ron Doig Block, leaving vacant the original, small out-patients building which was behind The Knowle and adjacent to the children's ward.[90] Breidahl organised and ordered equipment and encouraged the executive committee to appoint Miss L. Boot of Sydney as biochemist, and young Richard Poole of nearby Hamilton Hill as a laboratory assistant. Twice a day the lad collected blood samples from the wards for testing, and took the samples from the out-patients' department to the laboratory, prepared them, and when they were done wrote up Miss Boot's careful findings. Ward staff brought down urine and faeces for examination. In July 1939 Breidahl resigned as honorary pathologist and in his place Dr Samuel Michaels was appointed. During the following year, Richard Poole reported that he had a sore

[88] PHD File 245/31.
[89] West Australian, 13 March 1939, 23 November 1937. See also West Australian, 30 July 1938, 1 August 1938, 22 February 1929, 11 March 1939. All too quickly the need for beds outstripped their availability, and the 'everlasting monument' was demolished over forty years later when new wards were built.
[90] For a comprehensive history of the Pathology Department, see N. J. Lane, 'A History of the Laboratory Services 1839–1985', FH, 1986.

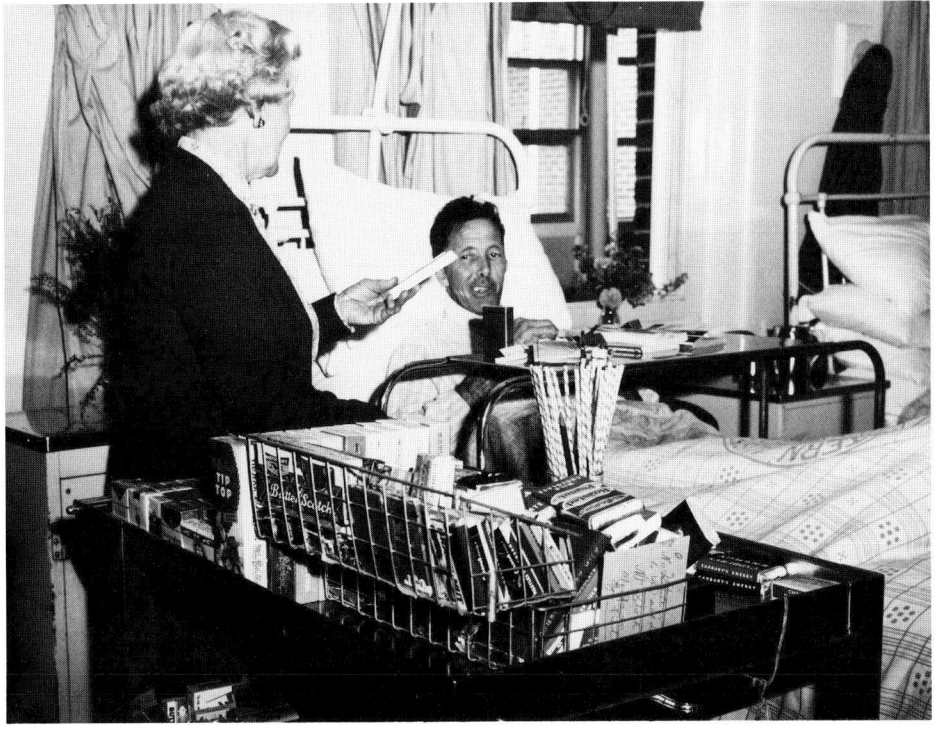

Photograph courtesy Fremantle Hospital

Plate 48. Ladies' Auxiliary voluntary worker.

The Ladies' Auxiliary continue their good work by providing amenities for the patients in hospital, all profits from this activity being used in improving the conditions for hospital patients.

Fremantle Hospital Annual Report
Year ending 30 June 1949

throat and was warded for three months with nephritis, a condition which caused his untimely death. Ken Cole then filled the position until 1942. Despite the fact that she was almost crippled with osteomyelitis contracted as a young girl, Miss Leo Boot worked hard to build a fine laboratory and proved herself a wonderful teacher. There was always work to do. All the glassware used in the department was washed for use again and again; needles were sharpened and resharpened, and

> ... there were no whiz machines to do the work—all titrations, calorimeter readings, blood counts, section cutting, etc., were manual, as was all staining. It may have been primitive by modern standards but we got the work done and while we may not have had the accuracy or the range of tests available today, in our own way we worked some minor miracles.[91]

[91] K. Cole, notes, 'History of the Path. Lab. FPH.', held at FH.

In the late 1930s the hospital was battling to keep abreast of advances in medical and even domestic equipment. A child had to be sent to the Children's Hospital because necessary instruments for an operation were not available, and Dr Cuthbert quoted £160 as a minimum for 'absolutely essential instruments',[92] including a bronchoscope and oesophagoscope, sphygmomanometers, suction apparatus, a colorimeter and haemometer, and for Smith-Petersen pins and an introducer. Outside the wards, a newly-bought petrol lawn-mower made the upkeep of the grounds easier. The kitchen staff valued a new toaster, a griller, the bread cutter, a wonderful peeler which could skin 24 lb. of potatoes at a time, and an electric mixer with a vegetable and fruit slicer and meat-mincer attachment. As the increased number of patients was always reflected in kitchen work and kitchen staff would not stay if work was irksome, the investment was well worth the cost.

When Maida Balding left the hospital, the key position of matron was not filled without a great deal of deliberation. Some on the board preferred Sister K. Fisher, some Olive Austin Smith, who had been assistant matron since mid-1936. In the end, following her successful application, red-haired Sister Sarah Jones, the matron of Taree Hospital, was invited to travel from New South Wales to take up the position.

On 1 September 1939, Germany invaded Poland, and the world exploded in a Second World War which changed the maps and lives and thinking of most of the so-called civilized world. Two days later, as the wireless crackled with static and 'Red Sails in the Sunset', the broadcast was interrupted by Prime Minister Robert Menzies pledging Australia's allegiance to the Allied cause.[93] At the nurses' quarters, one of the probationers burst into tears and ran from the room; others were stunned, wondering at the implication of the news. Once more the nation's great distance from the seat of war did not prevent her involvement. The impact was not immediate, but by 1940 Australian troops were marching across docks onto ships that took them to Europe and Britain and to exotic sounding places such as North Africa, Greece, Crete and Syria. Fremantle Hospital was not unaffected.

Little changed at the hospital at first, as life continued in its familiar pattern of challenges. Marmion's Cottage was demolished in 1939 and the board envisaged in the newly-created space, another much-needed entrance to the hospital grounds. On behalf of the domestics, the Hospital Employees' Union requested the installation of two washing troughs on the back verandah of the maids' quarters. Once more the board discussed the establishment of a home for incurables to help reduce the number of such patients in the wards; once more the idea lapsed due to the lack of finance. But the war was not far from the minds of most, and when The Knowle's roof had to be painted and repaired, a suggestion to mark it with a large, distinguishing red cross was earnestly discussed, before it was rejected. The hospital was asked to provide practical experience in nursing to sick berth ratings, and to arrange for first aid refresher courses. On one occasion, staff members were sent '. . . two school teachers from a convoy tied out of Fremantle on the way to the Middle East, to train as orderlies in three days. Fortunately they stayed seven days so Dr Dunkley

92 Minutes of Executive Committee, 11 August 1937.
93 E. Davies, notes, FH.

kindly took them into theatre for four days.'[94] A new type of patient began to arrive—young men eager to join the military but rejected on medical grounds. Some came for hernia, and some for appendix operations, others to be circumcised. 'We had a lot of those,' remembered one who nursed them.[95]

Although the idea of blood transfusion was not new in the late 1930s, its practice increased and more thought was given to its use in this period. A man with a seriously ill wife might still rush into the Life Saving Association's annual ball and presentation of trophies, to appeal for volunteers to donate blood for his wife's life-saving operation,[96] but there was a greater awareness of the need to have a pool of suitable and available donors. In 1936 Greenslade urged an arrangement with the Red Cross Society for such a scheme, and two years later the Red Cross was approached by the hospital wishing to obtain the names of willing donors in the Fremantle district. The Naval Department was singled out as a likely source of men willing to help. Under the impetus of war the hospital appealed directly to the community for volunteers—preferably young men of Fremantle—to come to the hospital between seven and nine on any evening to donate blood.[97] At the same time a blood bank was organised by the Red Cross in Perth, and in both centres a refrigerator was installed to store blood.

By 1940 the drain on staff was underway as orderlies, nurses, domestics, doctors and others volunteered or were called to the war effort. John Millar, the radiographer, was called up, as were Mr J. Crimmins from the dispensary, and Drs Cuthbert, Hillman and Percy White, the latter for the second time in a world-wide conflict. Hamersley, the assistant dispenser, and S. Caple, the hospital barber, went. Mr Richard Noble, the admitting officer, Claude Terry and L. Dodd, the honorary dentists, were not exempt. Ken Cole from pathology joined up. Doctors Stubbe, Moss, and Harry Hill, then Frank Whitton, the gardener, and Miss P. P. Graham and reliable H. Mutton, both from the office, left, as did orderlies F. Igglesden, G. Fletcher, Charles Fletcher (the head orderly) and Mr Wynfield, the collector. Many from the nursing staff joined the forces, including Louvima Bates, Marjorie Thompson, Ella Onge, Ada Jones, and Sisters Riley and Jean Wheatley.[98] Staff nurse Lindsay, the X-ray technician, and Hazel Bell, the masseuse, were taken. Dr Norman Rose, the resident medical officer, was called up, but five days later was returned still wearing his uniform after the board protested at his withdrawal, so great was their need for a doctor at the hospital at that time. Later, Rose left with the military. Short-sighted Dr Otto Mater, another resident medical officer, also joined up.[99] The demand for doctors to treat both those in the services and civilians at home, seemed insatiable. By 1942 it was reported that one-third of all Australian doctors had joined the forces but that 'no more doctors than necessary were being

---

[94] E. Roper (née Bell), notes. FH.

[95] Allen, interview.

[96] *West Australian*, 30 June 1939.

[97] *Ibid.*, 18 May 1939.

[98] For a list of nursing graduates from Fremantle Hospital known to have served in World War II, see Appendix 3a and b.

[99] Prior to the war, Mater, who could not swim, was once rescued by nurses after he accidentally walked off the end of a wharf after taking a wrong turn at the Oyster Beds Restaurant at Fremantle one black and rainy night. M. Hatch (née Borwick), notes, 1986, FH.

called into the army'.[100] As the months dragged by, the Hospital Employees' Union was assured that the positions of members called to war would be open for them when hostilities ceased. At out-patients, facilities were closed on Wednesdays and Saturdays except for emergencies, and patients were told that they were to be at the hospital no later than 10 a.m. if they wanted treatment. Honoraries once more helped out where they could.

There was still escape in the make-believe world of celluloid fantasy with films such as 'The Great Waltz' and Laurel and Hardy in 'Swiss Miss' providing a more bearable insanity to the one in Europe. It was said that if everybody in the world could see 'All Quiet on the Western Front' that there would be no more war.[101] The screen could remind of the real world too and ten men selected by the Perth post-master watched 'If Gas Came to Perth' in the course of their training in the newly formed anti-gas defence. The statement of the retiring consul-general for Japan in a farewell speech to the Australian people was quite convincing:

> . . . Japan has never been and never will be moved by any territorial ambition towards foreign countries other than that which is bound up with her own national security and the protection of her legitimate and political and economic interests. We have never dreamed of any such aggressive adventures on the continent of Australia.[102]

On a still, clear January day in 1940, eleven large troop ships called at Fremantle with 12,000 troops on their way to the front.[103] Many times, convoys of huge steamers such as the *Queen Mary* and the *Empress of Britain* with other naval vessels, lined up in Gage Roads ready to leave for the Middle East. The sight, particularly just as dawn broke, was an unforgettable one.[104]

At the end of 1941, Pearl Harbour was bombed, and with the entry of Japan into the war, a new dimension of fear was introduced to West Australians who had seemed so serenely secure in their isolation from the centre of conflict. By 17 February 1942, the press was reporting the fall of Singapore—'the darkest moment of the war for the United Nations'.[105] Three days later West Australians read with incredulity that 72 bombers with an escort of zero-type fighters had bombed Darwin in two separate raids; 15 had been killed and the hospital bombed and machine-gunned.[106]

In the event of invasion, counselled Mr Lazzarini, the country's Minister for Home Security, 'give all the help you can to our troops. Do not tell the enemy anything; do not give him anything, do not help him . . . Stand firm, carry on.'[107] Broome and Wyndham came under attack. At the western gateway of Fremantle, many feared an invasion. Throughout the metropolitan area preparations were made: public slit trenches were dug in streets, daylight and night mock air raids prac-

[100] *West Australian*, Statement of the Minister for the Army, Mr Forde, 10 January 1942.
[101] *Ibid.*, 26 and 27 May 1939.
[102] *Ibid.*, 23 May 1939.
[103] *Ibid.*, 13 February 1940.
[104] Davies, notes.
[105] *West Australian*, 17 February 1942.
[106] *Ibid.*, 20 February 1942.
[107] *Ibid.*, 5 March 1942.

ticed, search lights swept over Fremantle Harbour waters nightly and troops and guns were stationed on Rottnest Island. Passengers from liners told of ships being darkened for two nights before their arrival in Fremantle, and of wireless messages rigidly curtailed.[108] In all buildings at night, windows were darkened with black-out paper cut to size, or with wooden shutters, or black-out paper blinds which could be rolled up in the day-time. 'We always seemed to be living in the dark at that time you know,' observed one woman.[109] Butter muslin or cellophane was pasted with gelatin glue over windows to prevent glass flying. Householders were advised to keep sand in buckets to smother a possible fire, and many home shelters were dug and provisioned in back yards. The war was coming closer to Australia. In June 1942, Sydney was shelled from the sea. By August battles were being fought in the Solomons and at Kokoda, and Darwin suffered its twelfth night raid. In Fremantle on 10 August, 500 women provided the local participants of the biggest air raid exercise so far undertaken, with sandwiches, cakes, scones, rolls, tea and coffee. Two thousand 'casualties' were treated in a mock raid on the harbour, Perth and Midland Junction. Fremantle Hospital was allocated 25 stretcher cases and 37 minor cases, which in retrospect caused much concern—so enthusiastic were the voluntary stretcher bearers that had the injuries been real, 'much damage would have been done', to the patients.[110]

When Prime Minister Curtin, who was suffering gastritis, spoke from his hospital bed urging that 'all Australia must voluntarily answer the government's call for a complete giving of everything to the nation',[111] Fremantle people were behind him. Some collected urgently needed wattle bark to fuel the fires for the tanning of hides for military footwear, some collected aluminium scrap for the military to speed up aircraft production,[112] others made camouflage nets in their spare time until their fingers were raw. In official and unofficial capacities, women combined to serve in the community through the Red Cross and similar organisations. They visited hospitals, cheering, writing letters, doing shopping. They worked in canteens or work rooms, knitting and sewing articles for the troops: pyjamas, bedside pockets, calico pillowcases, and doctors' gowns and masks. Some volunteered for hospital work. There were shortages, notably of paper and tyres; clothing, tea, sugar, butter and petrol were rationed. Nurses' uniforms costing £1.5.6 could be bought for 12 clothing coupons, an apron took three, two coupons could purchase a pair of nurses' glazed cuffs, while a cape from Bairds required nine; many nurses extended the life of a worn pair of nursing shoes by cutting a sole from cardboard and binding top to bottom with lengths of zinc oxide sticking plaster stained black with Nugget shoe polish, and as new black hose was unprocurable, much time was spent darning and re-darning stocking feet and some nurses even painted a leg with ink at appro-

[108] *Ibid.*, 30 August 1939.
[109] A. Prior, interviewed by D. Brooks, 16 April 1985, FCL.
[110] Correspondence Dr Christie, medical superintendent FH, to Dr H. R. Nash, Perth, 13 May 1942, copy held at FH; Christie to the Director, WA Emergency Medical Services, 15 May 1942, FH.
[111] *West Australian*, 20 February 1942.
[112] *Ibid.*, 28 January 1942. It was said that if a ton of aluminium could be obtained from each municipality in Australia that 1,000 new aircraft could be made from it. Some people collected the metal by the sugar-bagful.

priate places to conceal a new hole.[113] Matron was kept busy working out the ration of butter, which was delivered in bulk to the hospital kitchen. At the hospital and in suburban homes, it was noted that bread deliveries were later due to the employment of older men who could not move as fast as the younger men now at war.

The decision to evacuate the hospital in 1942 was not made lightly, but was strongly indicated when anti-aircraft gun encampments were strategically erected on Scotsman's Hill, only feet away from the children's ward.

> We firmly believe that the time to move to a more suitable situation is *now* and to have our preparations complete and ready, and not to wait until our Hospital may be wrecked and then attempt to move, in a state of more or less chaos to a place that will not be, to say the least of it, in anyway prepared to function as a hospital . . .[114]

urged the board. Not only would the guns make the hospital a likely target to bombers, but their firing in practice shook and shocked ill hospital patients. There was also much to be said for dispersing staff, patients and equipment in two locations rather than concentrating them in one, in the event of an attack. The board resisted a proposal to evacuate the hospital to Santa Maria College, north of Fremantle in Attadale, preferring to have all of their charges and equipment at Heathcote Mental Hospital at Applecross, but the minister for health was adamant that 60 beds would be allocated at Heathcote and 50 at the Lucknow No. 2 Hospital at Claremont, available because of the building of the Repatriation General Hospital at Hollywood in 1941.[115] On 10 April, lorries and drivers from Daly Brothers—who would accept no payment for their service—and other master carriers of Fremantle, pulled up at the hospital to transfer equipment, while St John Ambulances arrived to shuttle medical patients and the children to Lucknow. A week later the procedure was repeated with surgical patients leaving for Heathcote. The very ill and community patients remained at Fremantle under Matron Sarah Jones. A mobile X-ray unit was provided at each of the new centres and the Lotteries Commission installed a Frigidaire in each. The pathology department had to be transferred to the Medical Department in Perth as neither Heathcote nor Lucknow had the space for it. The severe conditions at Heathcote under Mavis Fuller and Maude Grimes proved not as comfortable as at Lucknow, where Olive Jones was in charge. Nevertheless, the large old home was badly in need of repair and an obstacle course of buckets and basins had to be set out when it rained and the roof leaked.[116] At first there were no sterilizing facilities and the wood copper was resorted to. Both fuel and hot water were scarce. Here nurses were accommodated at Riverview House, the boarding section at Christ Church Grammar School and the domestic staff had the smaller Craigie House nearby, seven minutes' walk from the beautiful old hospital with its view across the river (now Bethesda Private Hospital). At night, blackouts between the buildings made the journey hazardous and 'you just could not see'. Olive Jones recalled how 'one night, walking over, I couldn't find my way and I walked into the

---

[113] *Ibid.*, 17 November 1942; D. Semmens (née Clark), notes, FH.
[114] Memo prepared by Hookway on evacuation, p. 4, FH.
[115] The bed numbers are those stated in Minutes of Executive Committee, 18 March 1942.
[116] O. Jones, interview; D. Semmens, notes.

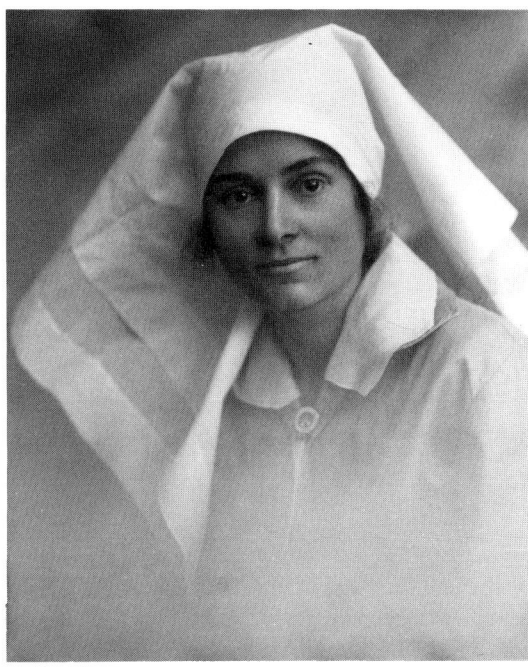

Plate 49.   Matron Olive Jones

I think that she was a very astute woman. She was very intelligent and she didn't run the hospital with an iron hand, she ran it with a warm hand. She was always courteous and polite to us as junior residents. If there was a particular problem, we would be confronted. The first troops that would go out would be the ward sister. If that one wasn't solvable, the next troop would be 'Gillie' [Sister Gill] and the next one would be Sister Fuller and of course, the last one to come out, you know, on the white horse would be Matron Jones herself and we were so terrified that we solved the problem long before it was her turn to come out.

Dr Peter Smith
Medical Superintendent

Photograph courtesy Fremantle Hospital

middle of a garden'. Matron Sarah Jones travelled by taxi to conduct her inspections at the two auxiliary branches, and at least once spent time in a slit trench beside the road during an air-raid warning.

Air-raid exercises proved challenging at Heathcote when surgical patients were in traction. Years later, a nurse laughed at the recollection:

> And the arrangement was when you had a bomb alert, that you took the patient out of bed, put them under the bed, and put the mattress at the end of the bed—so fragments wouldn't touch them. But at one stage I had three old ladies who all had broken legs, and of course they were all strung up ... so I put a mattress at the foot of the bed where they were all on extensions, and I used to sit between them and knit while the alert was on.[117]

One day after a newly installed electric sterilizer interfered with transmission from Whitford's radio station, a nurse received a call—'Can't you turn that bloody sterilizer off?—It's stopping the presentation of music from here'.[118] From that time, the bowls for surgical dressings were boiled at night. As the dispensary and the laundry remained at Fremantle, drugs and linen had to be transferred to both hospitals daily. For their lectures, nurses returned to Fremantle Hospital by ambulance. 'It was,' as Olive Jones recalled, 'a real upheaval.'[119]

---

[117]   Fuller, interview.
[118]   *Ibid.*
[119]   O. Jones, interview.

So thought the honorary staff, the medical department and the board, and on 15 July 1942 patients and staff were brought back from Heathcote to Fremantle Hospital, and from Lucknow by early October. An attack on Fremantle was not ruled out, however, and the medical superintendent, Dr Christie, was warned that '... whatever part of Fremantle Hospital may remain after a raid is over, may be called upon to work to capacity'.[120]

Because the big anti-aircraft guns remained on Scotsman's Hill beside the hospital, it seemed likely that the hospital would be a target if there was an invasion. Even when fired in practice the guns made 'a terrific noise'.[121] At its first blast, all the windows in pathology and the children's ward shattered, and the big demijohns in pharmacy fell off the shelves and broke. Troops were quartered in the vacated children's ward and one night caused a diversion when some came home 'a bit blithered' and tried to do a round in the nurses' quarters. There was an uproar with soldiers knocking on doors and nurses in curlers and nightgowns running and shrieking.

> They just opened the doors and had a look in and of course, Pat Giles woke up and saw—you know, 'What in the wide world are you doing here?' Sister Ure came out and sent them packing ... It was really funny but the joke was a couple of days after when the Army encased all the children's ward verandah with chicken wire ... the poor boys were standing up behind their chook wire, looking at us.[122]

The settlement later paid by the Army to the hospital included £45 to repair damage from the gun blast, £140 as rent for the children's ward and £40 for damage by soldiers to the premises.

Air-raid shelters were built in 10 strategic positions around the hospital grounds. Two were dug to the left and one to the right of the cement steps leading down to the Nurses' Home, another two were sited down the bank from the board room and X-ray department, facing the ocean; there was one at the wall beside the wattle bush at the back of the maids' quarters, and one under the fig tree south of the maids' quarters. Others were dug under the peppermint tree beside the school wall, to the left of the path leading to the orthopaedic department, and near the laundry. Most would take 20 people each, and were planned to shelter a total number of 191. Visitors and patients from different wards and staff from each department were allocated to certain trenches to avoid panic and overcrowding.[123] As in the rest of town, windows at the hospital were papered in black. Instructions were issued in case of a raid: patients on verandahs were to be moved to wards away from possible flying glass, the gas was to be turned off, primus stoves and hurricane lamps readied, water collected in baths and kettles, and fire fighting parties were to assemble.[124]

Although their officers were generally admitted at St John of God Hospital, both Naval and Army regular sailors and soldiers were treated in the community ward at

---

[120]   Correspondence, M. Peerless to Dr Christie, medical superintendent, 5 August 1942, FH.
[121]   O. Jones, interview.
[122]   Allen, interview. See also H. Peek (née McCall), notes, FH.
[123]   Notes, FH files.
[124]   Staff notice, FH files. See Appendix 4.

Fremantle Hospital for which the government paid ten shillings and sixpence a day each. On 13 June 1940, word was received that the old isolation ward had to be renovated overnight to take 46 convalescent soldiers. The men stayed for two months until a new ward was opened for them at Claremont, but the stock and equipment were held ready in the Fremantle ward in case it was required again. In the following year, the ward was taken over by the Army for a venereal diseases hospital and it was soon dubbed with the distinctive new title of 'Primrose Cottage'.[125] With the increased number of patients, an extra maid had to be employed, and the domestics' quarters was crowded to its limit, with three maids sharing each of the rooms.

Because servicemen had been fighting for the homeland, various auxiliaries were particularly concerned about their welfare. Red Cross volunteer, Gwendoline Trivett, recalled going to the hospital at 8 a.m. one day to visit returned soldiers and merchant seamen with a very old grocery basket containing cigarettes for the servicemen—one packet each a week, which was often not appreciated by civilians in adjoining beds when such luxuries were rationed:

> You had to go from bed to bed and check, and you had to use your own nous as to whether they were really telling you the truth because I had one man and I said to him, 'Are you a Returned Serviceman' and he said, 'Yes', and I really was very dubious ... 'Where were you serving?' He said 'I'm always serving Christ' and I looked at him and said ... 'So you are not a Returned Serviceman?' He was a member of the Salvation Army.[126]

Eventually special Red Cross quilts were placed on servicemen's beds each Monday morning to designate those who had fought. Cigarettes were not the only benefit resulting from military service. The overdue medical accounts of debtors who enlisted for military service were written off.

In almost all areas of the hospital, war took its toll. Medical supplies became scarce. Although a large shipment of 'cellona bandages' to Western Australia made some available for hospitals, doctors were still admonished to use crinoline and plaster where possible. Stocks of sulphonamide tablets were jealously meted out, and at times, the powder was unobtainable for local use.[127] Due to reduced staff, overtime was worked in all areas of the hospital. Dentists were instructed to go to hospitals to be taught how to give anaesthetics in emergencies and by 1942 doctors in civilian practice were being urged by the Medical Department to conserve their professional time and simplify their duties so that they could attend greater numbers of patients. Chemists also found their stocks limited and over-the-counter lines were often unprocurable. Agarol was one of the hardest to get and the elderly who had become dependent on it for their daily comfort clamoured for the preparation.[128]

On the wharves, work increased to a pitch unknown in even its busiest years as ships of all sizes from all parts of the world churned into the harbour and berthed,

[125] L. Allen, interview.
[126] G. Trivett, interviewed by C. Jeffery, 5 and 18 December 1984, FH. On her death in 1986, Mrs Trivett bequeathed $194,000 to Fremantle Hospital for Medical Research.
[127] Correspondence, J. G. Hislop, Director of State Civil Emergency Medical Services, to doctors, 12 June 1942, FH files.
[128] H. V. Sunderland, interviewed by L. Stevens, 27 February 1985, 13 March 1985, FCL.

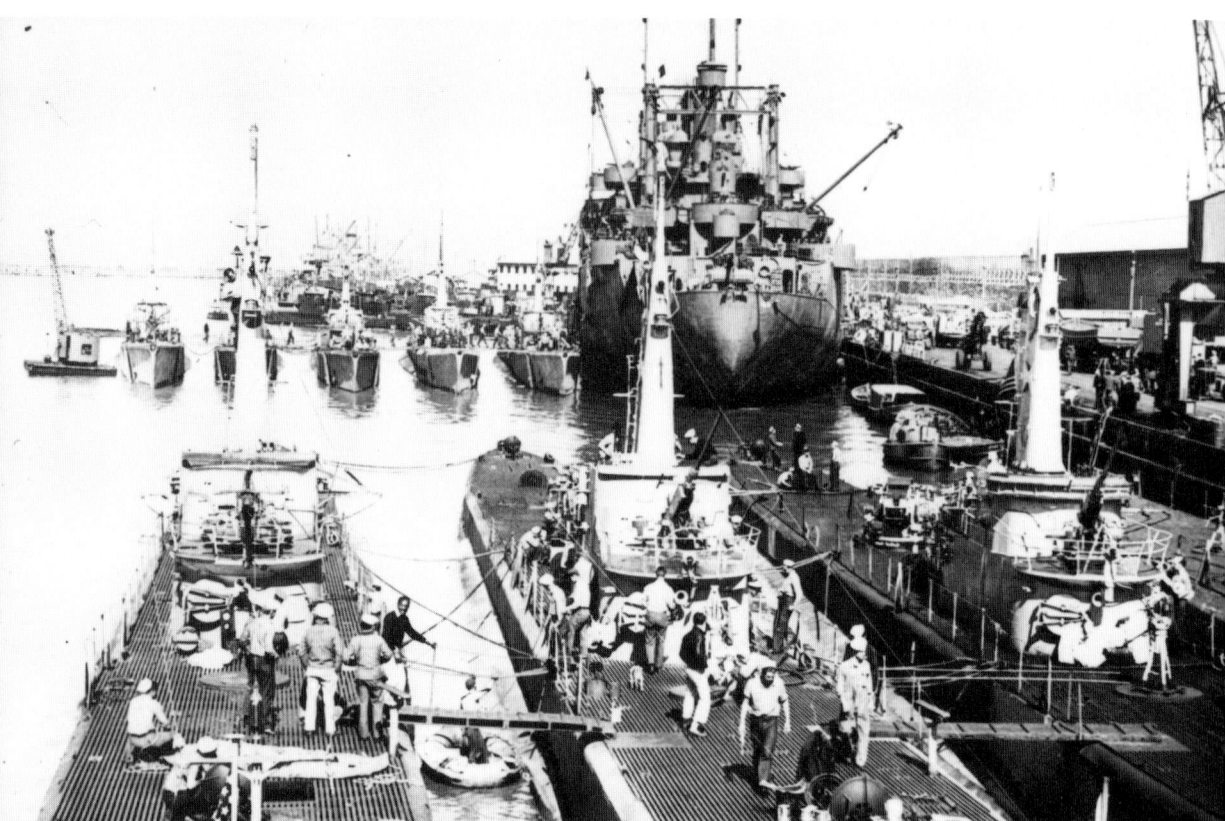

Plate 50.   Submarines berthed at Fremantle harbour during World War Two.

Fremantle was the base for many Americans and in 1943 when a convoy on its way to the Middle East called at the port, New Zealanders and U.S. forces clashed in town.

Helen Peek
Nursing Staff

double banked. Most were grey war ships: cruisers, destroyers, aircraft carriers, battle ships, troop ships and submarines, and with many of them came crews and troops of overseas forces.[129] One resident of the town recalled that:

Fremantle was really a beehive with all the various servicemen. We had Americans ... But then we also had Dutch seamen ... We had our New Zealand friends here ... as well as our army, air-force and navy. And at times there were some big mix-ups, quite serious ... But when on leave, these Americans really filled the town ... We used to see the servicemen being exercised, all in formation, with their bands. [They] would come along Marine Terrace ... from as far as the Esplanade to out of sight, past South

129   See Ewers, *The Western Gateway*, pp. 148–9.

Street, Price Street, about eight abreast and with their band playing quite loudly ... whilst they were in port.[130]

Sometimes there were conflicts over local girls between the Americans, who had stockings, lipsticks and abundant money, and the Australians, who didn't; but these were nothing to the occasional international fights with dozens involved and hundreds lending their vocal support. Heads and cafe windows were often smashed, and at the hospital, extra casualty staff were called in during a crisis. Many of the forces were determined to have as good a time as they possibly could and, at times, the line-up outside the Bannister Street brothel called The Palms, 'extended the full length of Bannister Street, down Market Street, and part the way down Collie Street'.[131]

Work in the various hospital departments continued as normally as possible under the circumstances. In John Miller's absence at war, X-ray work was carried out under the direction of Miss Malpas, who had been employed as a technician since February 1939. When she left to marry in 1940, staff nurse Veryard then carried on as the assistant, and Mr Laycock was recruited as radiographer in October 1940. There was still a problem with radiation. By May 1941, Veryard had developed a very low blood count. Staff Nurses Lindsay and then MacBride were employed, but in three months, the latter also developed a low blood count.[132] In 1941, despite the competition for funds by associations such as the Australian Red Cross Society, The Australian Comforts Fund, the Salvation Army War Time Fund, and other patriotic war funds, an appeal was launched for desperately needed new X-ray equipment. With the help of the Lotteries Commission and the Medical Department, a unit costing over £2,000, was installed with funds raised through community concerts. Later, two old transformers and a portion of the second-hand mobile X-ray unit were given to students at Fremantle Technical School for use in a pre-apprenticeship course.

The community concerts were an effective and popular means of raising funds for the hospital during and following the war. The chairman of the organising committee was William Wauhop. Fremantle youth groups assisted in setting up the Town Hall, and many of the hospital staff, including nurses as usherettes, Robert Benbow, G. Pearson, Stirling Hamersley and F. Whitton, the collector, gave their time freely.

> People ... arrived by tram and on foot and from all directions every Friday night ... Little songbooks were sold in the Music Shops, with words on all of these popular songs of the day, and people just joined in, for the majority of the night. And on occasions if you didn't have a song book in your hand, on the screen would be the words put up ...[133]

There would be two or three regular artists and three or four contestants who waited nervously in the wings until someone said 'Righto, you're on'. The Relax Amateur Trials were broadcast on radio and the winner might receive 'hankies', a box of soap

130   Silich, interview, FCL.
131   Sunderland, interview, FCL.
132   Minutes of Executive Committee, 14 May 1941, 16 July 1941, 17 November 1941.
133   Silich, interview, FCL.

or a crystal vase. To avoid the possibility of a contestant sending out a message by radio to an enemy at sea, only the item stated on the application form could be performed. In 1939 the hospital shared some of the proceeds with the Fremantle Free Milk Council, and during the years until 1950 the concerts raised hundreds of pounds towards buildings, the X-ray department, wireless equipment at the hospital, kitchen equipment, rubber mattresses for patients and furniture for the nurses' quarters, but never for the dispensary.[134]

The dispensary was one of the most neglected areas of the hospital. In 1935, when refrigeration was being introduced in some areas of the hospital, an ice chest was requested for the dispensary to house the special serums. Not until 1949 was a 'six-cubic-foot President electrical refrigerator' purchased for £100 for the department.[135] Until Stubbe intervened in 1937 the dispensary scales were defective. When the assistant dispenser, Stirling Hamersley, joined the forces in 1940 his place was taken temporarily by Mr J. E. Crimmins, until he too, enrolled with the military. In that year it was noticed that the drug register had not been kept correctly. The head dispenser was admonished, and shown how to keep the account efficiently. Next April, a considerable shortage of narcotic drugs was again noticed and, although the police were called in, their report took time to compile. A small quantity of morphine was missing in November and once more the register of drugs was unsatisfactory. Although at the subsequent hearing in the Fremantle Police Court on 24 November 1941, it was found that the shortfall was through the chief dispenser's carelessness and not impropriety, not surprisingly, Huelin, of the Medical Department, was adamant about the dispenser's dismissal. Only a short time earlier the Government Stores pharmacist in Perth had been discharged for a similar offence[136] and the Medical Department's dispensary slate was becoming increasingly difficult to keep clean. The dispenser resigned and in his place, from 22 January 1942, John Jeffery was appointed as head of the department. Jeffery was a man of forceful character and soon became well known for his uncharitable acts to nurses, especially those who might try to pull a little rank and demand some drugs or extra combine dressing for their ward. At these times, the trap door through which pharmacist and nurse communicated would be firmly slapped down. The majority of unfortunate trainees dreaded and evaded the task of a message to the dispensary.[137] Of the few who earned the dispenser's approval, some senior nurses were granted the status of:

> Dispensary Drip . . . she shall not be thrown out, kicked, sworn at, spat upon, or otherwise abused except at our discretion.[138]

The hand-wrought certificate was valued as much as the general wisdom and competency of the man who signed himself 'Grand High Abuser'. In October 1944 Prime Minister John Curtin requested the release of John Jeffery from his hospital work so that he could go to Canberra for three months to work on the proposed

134   *Ibid.*, interview. See also Manns, interview; Minutes of BM and Executive Committee, 1939-1950. The community concerts ran for over ten years.
135   Minutes of Executive Committee, 15 March 1949.
136   J. Jeffery, interviewed by C. Jeffery, 1985 and 1986, FH.
137   C. Jeffery, taped recollections, 1987, FH.
138   See Figure 16.

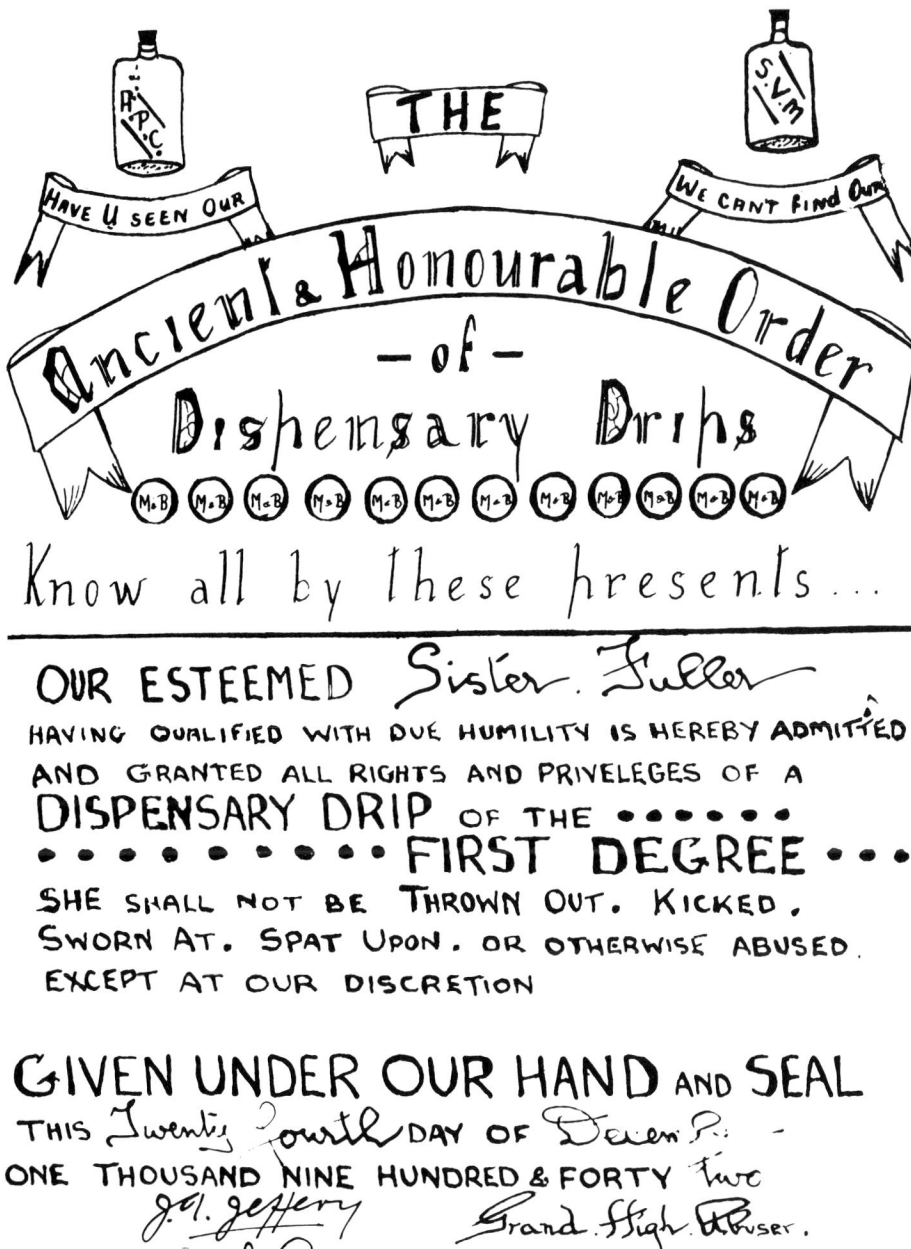

THE Ancient & Honourable Order — of — Dispensary Drips

HAVE U SEEN OUR

WE CANT FIND OUR

Know all by these presents...

OUR ESTEEMED *Sister Fuller*
HAVING QUALIFIED WITH DUE HUMILITY IS HEREBY ADMITTED
AND GRANTED ALL RIGHTS AND PRIVELEGES OF A
DISPENSARY DRIP OF THE • • • • • •
• • • • • • • • • **FIRST DEGREE** • • •
SHE SHALL NOT BE THROWN OUT. KICKED,
SWORN AT. SPAT UPON. OR OTHERWISE ABUSED.
EXCEPT AT OUR DISCRETION

GIVEN UNDER OUR HAND AND SEAL
THIS *Twenty Fourth* DAY OF *December* -
ONE THOUSAND NINE HUNDRED & FORTY *Two*

J.J. Jeffery Grand High Abuser.
Grand Chucker Out.

Fig. 16. Certificate awarding 'dispensary drip' status.
   I remember when John Jeffery retired in 1967, we had a lovely afternoon down in the Balding Home sitting room. I plucked up my courage and on behalf of the 'dispensary drips' I wished him well, and John and I were the only ones in that hospital who knew what I was talking about.

Sister Lou Allen
Nursing Staff

National Health Scheme. The three months turned to six, then 17 before his return to Fremantle in mid-April 1946, and trainee nurses were well pleased at the delay. In Jeffery's absence Mr Keys acted as dispenser until he joined the military in October 1945, and then Mrs Lorna Nicholls filled the position of chief dispenser at the welcome full male rate of pay.

The massage department suffered a similar neglect and the turnover of staff due to war was high. Mrs Ackland and Miss Richards had resigned in 1937, but with the increasing need for masseuses to treat poliomyelitis cases, it was difficult to replace them until Miss Slattery came from Adelaide in 1939 and worked at the hospital for a year. Miss Sobels, also from Adelaide, stayed for the following nine months until September 1940. Another Victorian, Miss Bell, arrived in October 1940, but was called by the military for service abroad. Her successor, Miss E. J. Liddle, worked at the hospital from only 9 a.m. to 11 a.m. each weekday. Not until 1946, straggling seven years in the wake of a decision by the Australasian Massage Department to change the name, was the department at Fremantle referred to as the physiotherapy department.[139] Following the war, the benefits of physiotherapy treatment were more widely appreciated and in the latter half of the 1940s, infra-red apparatus was purchased by the hospital. Despite this, when Margaret Cooper was brought from the Eastern States to join the staff in 1949, she decided not to accept the position of physiotherapist because of the hospital's lack of necessary equipment. To remedy the want, the board converted the billiard room into a physiotherapy department and purchased more apparatus. Mrs V. J. (Penny) Dixon, as the repatriation therapist for the Fremantle area, became the hospital's physiotherapist and was allowed to treat ex-servicemen with the hospital's equipment during office hours. Within three months, the repatriation cases had been made hospital out-patients and the government's payment for treatment was made directly to the hospital.

With the dual needs for workers at war and the home front, the Department of Manpower was organised to regulate the movement of people in and out of employment between civilian and military positions. When it seemed that the assistant secretary, James Scrymgeour, would be called up, an appeal was made to the department to retain his services. A Fremantle Hospital staff nurse wishing to resign her hospital duties and take up a position as a surgery nurse to a private doctor was denied the move by the Deputy Director-General of Manpower. The department also determined leave in special cases, and caused some heartache in 1944 when it ordered that only a week could be taken by a member of the nursing staff who wished to marry. Influenced by conditions of war, where a husband was absent overseas and a nurse was needed in the workforce, the rock of tradition that prevented a trainee returning to work after marriage, began to crack. Often

> ... during the wartime exception was made and the girls continued their training. Most of their husbands were overseas or away. Some married American soldiers and continued their training.[140]

[139] A. L. Forster, 'Physiotherapy—A Response to a Challenge', in *The Australian Journal of Physiotherapy*, Vol. 21, No. 4, December 1975, pp. 125-34; Minutes of Executive Committee, 13 August 1946.
[140] O. Jones, interview.

If a matron wanted one of her graduates to remain as a staff nurse, permission had to be granted from the manpower office, but on completion of that 12 months, the nurse was required to go to a country hospital for not less than six months and not more than a year.[141] It often seemed to the nurses 'we were just farmed out at different places'.[142] So great was the need for them at home that double-certificated nurses could not join the forces.

There was always trouble getting reliable domestic staff for the hospital:

> ... we had to ring ... and you just took what they sent you. You had no choice ... we had some very peculiar people sent to us as domestic staff. Sometimes they turned up, sometimes they didn't.[143]

A girl had to be 18 before she could work in the wards. No uniforms were issued—only a supply of wide white aprons to cover street clothes. Ann Brain started in the male surgical ward in 1946:

> ... but they were that short staffed I was always being called away here there and everywhere—doctors, cafeteria, kitchen, down the blood bank, community—anywhere. Any department that was there—I worked the whole lot.[144]

There was always washing up to be done, pantry floors to mop and others to polish. Ann's father would often be sitting in casualty until 11 p.m. at night waiting to walk her home, and on the nights when he was fishing, Maud Ryan, the night duty sister, would walk Ann to the gate and watch until she reached her home nearby. When Ann started work at 4 a.m., it was a long day. Other domestic staff were not so dedicated—especially when the fleets were in—and would not arrive for work. At these times, the nurses 'just did the wardsmaids' work as well'.[145] During the war the nurses lost the privilege of a maid to help with housework at the nurses' home: 'All we had was clean linen thrown on our bed once a week and that was that ... we had fun keeping our floors polished and nice and clean ...'[146]

Under Matron Sarah Jones there were few changes for nurses in war. However, in all respects staff learned economy, and even the nurses' annual dance was suspended for a time. Probationers were still thrust into a ward to commence training: 'I went in ... someone made a cap ... you put your uniform on and at 11 o'clock you were up in the wards and you were more or less, left to it ... someone sort of took you under the wing.'[147] Most learning was still done in the wards, but as in the First World War when there was a lack of senior sisters to instruct the newcomers, the training of nurses suffered. A junior nurse of the time recalled that:

> I only ever in all my training, was basically taught three things by anybody. I just

[141] PHD File 841/36.
[142] Allen, interview.
[143] O. Jones, interview.
[144] Ann (Honey) Brain, interviewed by J. Lancaster, April 1987, FH.
[145] *Ibid.*
[146] Allen, interview.
[147] *Ibid.*

taught myself the rest ... I was shown how to give an injection. I was shown how to do
a compress of all things, and when Mavis Yates and I were in our second year in community wards, Sister Wheatley showed us how to do a dressing. A basic dressing. Mavis
remembers the man's name. I don't remember his name but I know it was in Room 4 or
5.[148]

Sarah Jones' nursing lectures were uninspiring—'all she did was read them and we
copied them down'[149]—and there were anatomy, physiology and medical lectures by
the resident, Dr Mater. Gynaecology lectures were given by Dr Dorothea Parker; the
deputy matron, Olive Smith, taught bandaging, and Dr Gawler, the ophthalmic
surgeon, lectured on the eyes. The core of ward sisters—Gill in male surgical, Rogers
in female medical, Freeman in children's ward, McGaffin in female surgical and
Olive Jones in casualty, with Fuller in McCallum, guided and taught by example and
explanation when they could.[150] For final exams, nurses took a taxi or a parlour car
to Perth and in 1942 only passed due to extra voluntary tuition by Dr Christie, a concerned acting medical superintendent. It was always a memorable day:

> On the day we went for our finals, our A.T.N.A. [Australian Trained Nurses Associ-
> ation examination], we were right royally feted. We were allowed to choose what we
> wanted for breakfast on the fateful day ... We dressed up to the nines and had two rig-
> outs, one for each day, even down to hand-bags and gloves and different shoes each
> day ... We had our Surg and Med Exam papers in Winthrop Hall, all went up there
> and back by taxi, paid for by the Hospital. Every one off duty came down to the front
> of the Hospital, outside Casualty to see the A.T.N.A. girls off and to wish them luck
> ... Then we would sit, all dressed up in our new clothes, in unfamiliar imposing sur-
> roundings in the hallowed halls of Winthrop, along with the hundreds of other finalists
> from other hospitals ... Very imposing and unnerving ...[151]

As well as all the hospital linen, the laundry washed and ironed the nurses' uniforms. These were changed from green in first year, to pink for second- and third-
year trainees, but with economies due to war, all hospitals changed to a standard
blue uniform. Probationers still wore a frilled cap and staff nurses and sisters a full
veil. Because stock was not increased or replaced until well after the war, the supply
of clean hospital linen was meagre. Often on weekends the laundry windows would
be prised open to replenish a ward with a stolen supply of sheets, towels and draw-
sheets. 'Oh! It was a terrible problem during the war,'[152] recalled one nurse. 'Everything smelled well-cooked' from the laundry, 'a peculiar odour', recalled another.[153]
Singlets and nightgowns in children's ward were often washed out at night by the
first junior, and dried on top of the bowl sterilizer in the sterilizing room, ready for
the following morning.

Sarah Jones was a large, imposing woman who sailed through the wards with
'presence' and dignity. One of her probationers recalled:

[148] *Ibid.*
[149] *Ibid.*
[150] *Ibid.*
[151] B. Pilling (née Weedon), notes, 1987, FH.
[152] Allen, interview; J. Morrissey (née Bailey), notes, FH.
[153] Pilling, notes.

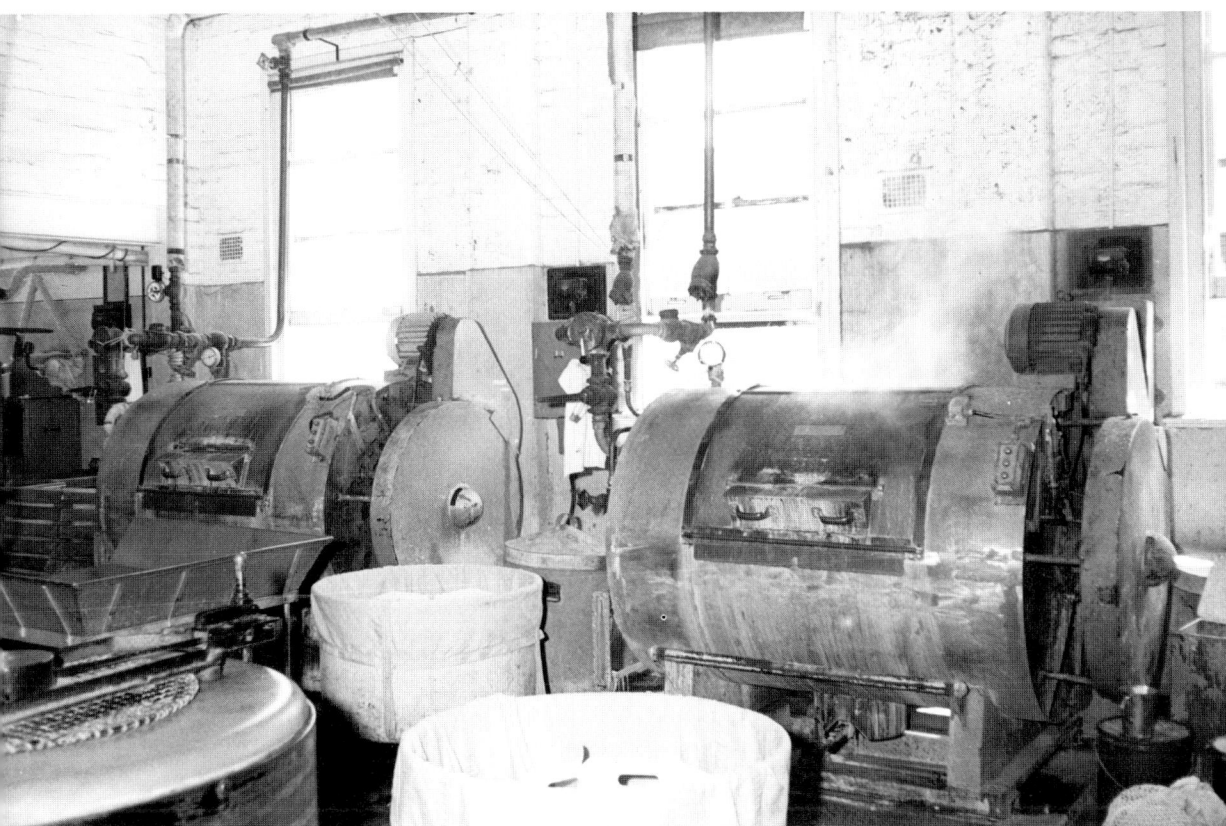

Photograph courtesy Fremantle Hospital

Plate 51.   The hospital laundry—

... and the first part of the laundry that you went into was the clean part and the other end, up the other end, was the dirty part. They had this dreadful system of sorting all the linen as soon as it came in and the infectious bags were supposed to be tied with this red thing ... But I really always felt terribly sorry for those laundry workers who were working in this really, really hot building with these machines all going and they had to sort this dreadful linen that was revoltingly dirty ...

Olga Hedemann
Director of Nursing, 1983–

I very quickly learned that you had to keep that pan room clean because Matron used to come around at about 11 o'clock every day and she would bend low and look right under every single thing for every speck of dust ... and I mean it was rather terrifying.[154]

In 1941 matron was secure in the authority of her position. When Dr Mater, the medical superintendent, demanded that a sister should be suspended for serious

[154]   H. Peek, interviewed by J. Lancaster, 1987.

neglect of duty and failure to carry out doctor's instructions, matron investigated, intervened, and disagreed. Harry Gray, the chairman, was called to arbitrate and decreed that where a medical superintendent and matron diverged in matters relating to nursing staff, he absolutely refused to carry the responsibility of suspending the sister. All involved were summoned to an executive meeting and in the light of evidence given under cross-examination, the committee supported the matron and no action was taken towards the sister.[155] Such was the authoritative word of a matron.

In 1942 Curtin spoke emotively in Forrest Place at the opening rally of the Liberty War Loan, warning that 'the enemy is coming on . . . we are defending grimly until we can take the offensive . . . the Yellow Serpent had to strike in the Pacific before all this nation realized it was in the fighting lines . . . we face what might be a death blow inside our own territory . . .'[156] When war came to the hospital's territory it was not in the shape of a Yellow Serpent but that of a medical superintendent. Under the community ward system, doctors in the town were able to admit and treat their private patients in the hospital. Initially private patients were charged for drugs and dressings, X-rays, and treatment by the masseuse through an additional flat fee. In time the system was exploited. If at times, a private patient was admitted as public, and if a doctor's patient presented prescriptions, or requests for X-rays or pathological tests and they were accepted at the hospital and filled without extra payment, both parties were content. By 1943 the hospital had become, as one employee described it, 'a milch cow'.[157] The laxity in pharmacy which led to a court hearing in 1941 was only the tip of the iceberg. As far back as 1938 the honorary medical staff had been asked to reduce the demand on increasingly costly propriety lines from the pharmacy, and had been talking about the piece work available to them through the new pathological laboratory. In 1941 the government surplus was reported as £1,768, in 1942–43 there was a deficit of over £33,000.[158] Economies such as the bulk supply of blue material for nurses' uniforms throughout government hospitals proved of little worth in the face of Fremantle Hospital's benevolence in other areas. To clean up the mess, Dr Ken Aberdeen was brought down to Fremantle from Northam.

The chance to introduce Aberdeen into Fremantle Hospital came in December 1942 when the various Fremantle honorary medical officers who were not overseas, including Drs Cook, Dermer, Radcliffe-Taylor, Parker, Muir, Bean, Hallion, Caldera and Uther-Baker, were hard-pressed with military and civilian work inside and outside the hospital. It was an opportune time to break the honorary power lock at the hospital. As a solution to the situation, Dr Hislop, the chairman of the medical co-ordination committee, suggested the appointment of Dr Aberdeen as surgeon superintendent with Dr Elphick in charge of the medical work, supported by two junior medical officers. The medical men of the town were to retain three beds each, but the main bulk of the hospital work would now be carried out by the resident staff. Assured that it was only a wartime measure the honorary staff agreed,

155 Minutes of Executive Committee, 1 September 1941.
156 *West Australian*, 21 February 1942.
157 C. Jeffery, notes.
158 *West Australian*, 16 September 1942.

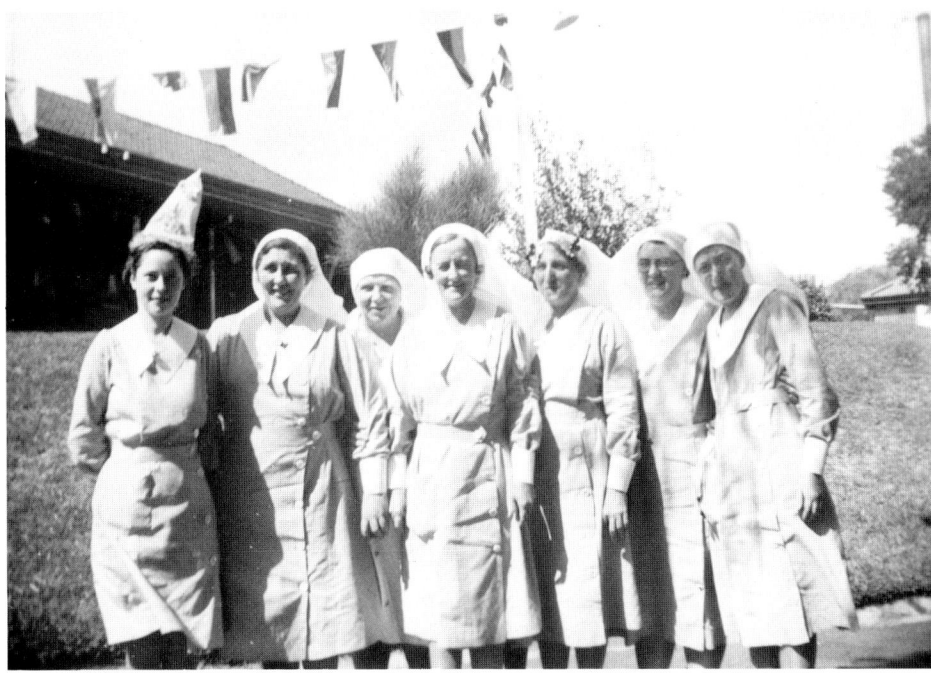

Photograph courtesy Mrs Edinger

Plate 52. *(Right to left)*: Sisters Ure, Fuller, Freeman, Ryan, Matron Sarah Jones, Sisters Smith, Kessell.

> Matron Sarah Jones, she stopped this coming in at night and checking people in. She said, her theory was that when you started a job like nursing, you did the work of adults and at least you deserved the compliment of being treated as such.
>
> Sister Lou Allen

on the condition that the new superintendent, who had conducted a lucrative and successful private practice at Northam, would not set up his plate in Fremantle at the end of his appointment. On his part, Aberdeen agreed to the appointment for a salary of £1,000 a year with an unfurnished house provided and four weeks' annual leave. He would have the right of a consulting practice, but would pay any fees received into a trust fund to buy medical books and specialties for the hospital. Most importantly, to effect his purge of the hospital, he would be in charge of all hospital administration of a professional character—including that of the nursing staff. Aberdeen was described by a contemporary as a 'unique sort of person'.[159] A natural athlete in any sport who had run professionally to earn money while he was a student, Aberdeen drove big cars 'hell for leather', often travelled 100 miles to help a new country resident with a difficult medical case and also invented several innovative splints which were made up by a fitter and turner at Northam.[160] He swept

[159] Anderson, interview, BL.
[160] *Ibid.*

into the hospital with a sharp sense of reformatory purpose and a dynamic person-
ality and could not be ignored; nor could the four efficient nurses he brought with
him from Northam to place in key positions.

It was inevitable that conflict would result in the meeting of Aberdeen and Sarah
Jones. The matron was a progressive thinker and not afraid to improve the lot of her
nurses. The Fremantle Hospital probationers were the envy of those at Perth Hospital and the Children's Hospital when she abolished the system of late night passes
believing that:

> ... when you started a job like nursing, you did the work of adults and at least you
> deserved the compliment of being treated as such. ... The only instruction there was-
> she left us on our honour to be in on time and if the night sister saw a person coming in
> repeatedly late, or especially if she knew that they were on early next morning, they
> might be chatted. If, by any chance, they weren't too sober, they might be chatted or if
> it happened again, they might be sent to the matron next day.[161]

Nor was the matron backward in confronting an annoying honorary. One surgeon
delighted in hiding small instruments to torment a nurse counting the instruments
and swabs after an operation. On one such occasion Sarah Jones entered the theatre,
summed up the situation and roared at the doctor to 'stand back from the table'. So
taken aback was the doctor that he did so, and the missing mosquito forceps tucked
between the operating table and his person clattered to the floor.[162] Being under the
direct control of Aberdeen proved insufferable to Sarah Jones, who professed that
she 'had no intention of being a matron of a hospital where she did not have the
nurses under her wing'.[163] She wrote to the board a letter of resignation:

> The reason for so doing, is that the Board have felt fit to transfer my rights as a matron
> (which were delegated to me nearly four years ago) to the incoming Medical Super-
> intendent. Apparently there is no justification whatsoever for this action as the Chair-
> man of the Board has stated definitely that the Board had no fault to find with my
> administration as the Matron. Therefore I have no alternative other than to resign my
> position.[164]

Her parting shot to Aberdeen was full of sting: 'I hope you enjoy wearing the cap
tails.'[165]

Aberdeen donned the cap tails as enthusiastically as he organised in other hospital
departments. One nurse described the period as the 'saddest time that Fremantle
Hospital has ever gone through' because the old unity and loyalty of a small number
of men and women working together through many decades was tested as the staff
took sides. 'We used to call it B.A. and A.A.—before Aberdeen and after Aberdeen. It was dreadful.'[166] The trained nursing staff from Northam were placed in
theatre, in the orthopaedic department and in the X-ray department. From the four

161   Allen, interview.
162   Hatch, notes.
163   Allen, interview.
164   Minutes of Executive Committee, 16 February 1943.
165   O. Jones, interview.
166   Allen, interview.

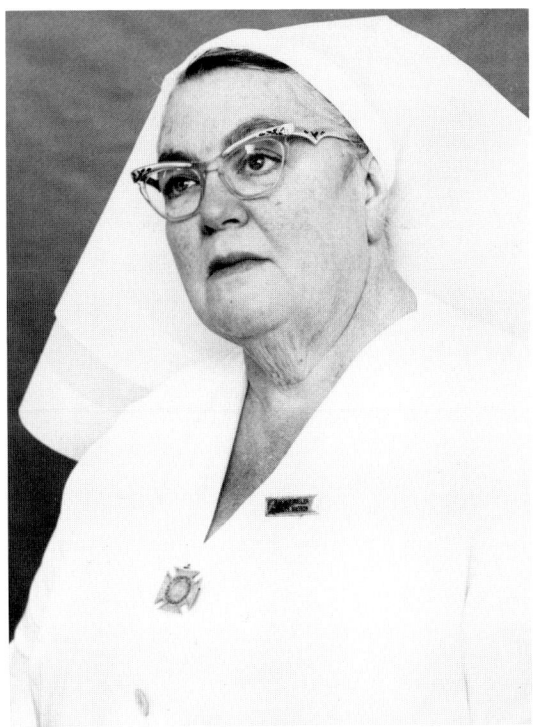

Plate 53. Mavis Fuller,
deputy matron 1959–1965 ...
nearly four decades of service at
Fremantle Hospital.

I had a lot of contact with them
(trainee nurses) and they
seemed to come to me as a
kind of mother-confessor. If
they were in trouble of any
kind, they came ... Well, we
evolved the—you knew what it
was for ... for dysmenorrhea—
'Sister Fuller's mixture'. 'Aren't
you well today]' 'No, Sister, I
have got my period.' Oh, it
became a famous mixture!

Deputy Matron Mavis Fuller

Photograph courtesy Fremantle Hospital

applications for the position of matron, Olive Jones—the hospital's quiet, slightly-
built, efficient casualty nurse and acting matron (called Skinny Jones to distinguish
her from Sarah Jones)—was recommended by the executive committee. The board
confirmed the appointment. When the position of assistant matron was advertised,
Fremantle's loved community-ward sister, Mavis Fuller, nicknamed the mighty
'Dimboola' by the doctor who named sisters after the size of boats in the harbour,
was chosen. There was a sense that medical superintendents came and medical
superintendents left, but the nursing staff endured. So it proved at Fremantle, and
for many years the matron and her assistant supervised the training of a generation
of nurses with a balance of fairness, discipline and compassion that united the nursing staff and gave them training which was recognised and sought all over the state.
Relations between Aberdeen and the new Matron Jones were brittle. Aberdeen told
the nurses, 'you needn't wear stockings'. Olive Jones said, 'I think you should wear
stockings for the health of your feet'.[167] When two applicants were considered for a
vacant charge-nurse position, the board supported the recommendation of the
medical superintendent and not that of the matron.[168] These were small skirmishes
among many. Hospital regulations were duly changed by the board to confirm
Aberdeen's new role in nursing administration; only Greenslade opposed the move.

[167] *Ibid.*
[168] Minutes of Executive Committee, 19 May 1943.

Some nurses took Aberdeen before the executive committee to complain about his language. However, the committee found only that 'the expression used was unfortunate and it is to be regretted'.[169] So different were Aberdeen's ways and so different his practices that the senior nursing staff felt themselves under great pressure. Some left. To avoid possible repercussions resulting from medical treatments, the sisters held an impromptu meeting in the nurses' home and were urged by one of their number to keep detailed ward reports—'put everything down ... to look after yourself and the girls'.[170]

The resentment of many of the nurses towards the new medical superintendent was reflected in the attitude of the honorary medical staff. They conferred in February 1943,[171] then met with the board and with Aberdeen to consider their new status as an honorary staff with a limited number of beds and diminished power. Three months later in May 1943, they considered and discussed 'the new order'[172] and the animosity which existed between themselves and the resident surgeon. Chairman Gray's reported statement at a board meeting, 'that the Honorary Staff are no longer the bosses as Dr Aberdeen is in control now and you shall take your orders from him', rankled, especially when coupled with the honorary staff's view that Aberdeen had overstepped his role as consultant.[173] Feelings ran high. Dermer claimed that in a recent case of accident Aberdeen had 'attempted to foist himself' on the doctor in his treatment of a case. While Dermer did not mind Aberdeen seeing the case as a consultant, he did not want his help, and if he did need assistance it would be from the colleagues with whom he was used to working. Parker, too, cited a compensation case where Aberdeen had intervened without cause. When Aberdeen was invited to speak he was enraged. As a respected doctor to hundreds in Northam, used to helping in difficult cases in outlying areas, and working in Fremantle only at the urging of Huelin and the Fremantle Hospital Board, he snapped a justification of his action. Hadn't he worked up a big consulting practice in Northam, and didn't he want the right of consultation with his counter-patients in Fremantle even if his fees did go to the hospital for books and equipment? And what of the hostility with which he had been met?[174] The honoraries had little recourse but to refer the matter to the B.M.A. The conflict surged on into August, with the B.M.A. Council decision that while it was contrary to their procedure for a medical superintendent of a hospital to indulge in private practice, Aberdeen's absolute power had been granted by Hislop under emergency conditions, and therefore he had the right to see any patient sent to him by a doctor.[175]

Aberdeen and his family were housed at the hospital property at 1 Stirling Street, Fremantle, and the medical superintendent settled to his task at the hospital. He nearly took over the honoraries' staff room as an office but the board, perhaps moved by the consideration that Aberdeen's stay would not be permanent and that

169   Ibid.
170   Allen, interview.
171   Minutes of the Honorary Staff, Fremantle Hospital, 3 February 1943.
172   For reference to the 'new order', see ibid., 3 February 1943, 5 February 1943.
173   Ibid., 13 May 1943. Statement was reported at this meeting but does not appear in minutes of the
      board meeting.
174   Ibid., 13 May 1943.
175   Ibid., 4 August 1943.

they would be again dependent on the goodwill of the honoraries, suggested instead the billiard room. Miss Walsh was appointed as clerk to the medical superintendent and a new shorthand typist was kept busy with work from the X-ray department, the matron and the doctor. One of Aberdeen's greatest concerns was his surgical work. It was not uncommon for theatre to start early in the morning and still be going at 7 p.m. In a forward-looking decision, Aberdeen had the traditional, bright, white operating gowns replaced with pastel green, which he believed was softer on the eyes. Those who worked with him remarked on Aberdeen's technique. At a time when most of his contemporaries used catgut for stitching, the doctor remained an advocate of cotton, suturing in rows of tiny stitches, one-sixteenth of an inch wide. Aberdeen challenged the nurses to become ambidextrous, when they came as part of their training to his theatre—an additional advantage, perhaps, when they had to thread each of the dozens of lengths of cotton thread on separate needles ready for closing a wound or incision.[176] By August 1943 he had arranged the appointment to Fremantle Hospital of tiny, efficient Sister Averill from Northam, who was expert at cutting threads close to the knots without them unravelling. Under Aberdeen's direction and to complement his work, a plaster room was built adjoining the theatre block, and the old plaster room was converted into a splint room.

Aberdeen's energies were directed to many areas of the hospital. Under the impetus for its need in 1943, the blood bank was firmly established under Sister Della Valle, one of Aberdeen's protégées. Trade unions were asked to supply donors and the Rotary Club organised recruiting committees to obtain those willing to be bled. The blood bank was officially opened two years later, on Thursday 19 April 1945, by Dr Newman Morris. When Sister Della Valle left in November 1946, Sister Horswill took her place for six months, then Sister Ure was transferred from the nursing staff to fill the vacancy. Aberdeen organised the installation of three new 150-gallon hot-water units so that the hospital was provided with hot water 24 hours a day; an air-pressure suction system was installed in five of the wards, and stainless-steel equipment bought. It was not surprising that the man who was immunizing against diphtheria before the measure was widely practiced in Perth[177] encouraged the opening of an additional immunization clinic at the hospital. Aberdeen's concern for children extended to their schooling. He arranged for a teacher to come to the hospital and bought the necessary equipment for tuition. Two cots and two cribs were also provided in a crèche next to the blood bank to assist mothers and children attending at the out-patients' department, and Sister Gjerde found herself responsible for supervising the young occupants as well as doing her social services work. As one of his last major contributions to the hospital, Aberdeen organised the building of the children's ward playground which was named after Nancy Charleston, a respected staff nurse and Dr Elphick's sister in-law, who died unexpectedly while undergoing a minor operation in theatre.

Other changes in Aberdeen's time as medical superintendent were not necessarily attributable to his influence. The first taxi service at the hospital was provided by the newly-formed Metropolitan Taxi Cabs Owners Association in 1943, which proved

---

[176] Information from Anderson, interview, BL; H. Peek, interview, FH.
[177] Anderson, interview, BL.

of great benefit to those who could afford the rates. In August 1943 the Hospital Employees Union requested permission for four of the married domestic staff to live outside the hospital. Three months later the board agreed that all domestics could live out. While the decision removed the staff from the direct control of the hospital, it also freed some accommodation, which was increasingly hard to provide, and the domestic quarters were quickly renovated for the night nurses. In another move in another department, the laundry staff were allowed to wear shorts during working hours.

Due to the financial strait-jacket of war, donations to the hospital were comparatively few. Funds were channelled enthusiastically to the immediate concern—'to help our boys at the front', although special appeals such as that in 1941 for X-ray equipment were successful. Scholars from Princess May Girls' School always gave an annual donation of £50 for the cot in their name, and the proceeds from a débutante's ball and £580 from a popular girl competition run by the Fremantle Labor Women's Organisation were ear-marked to start a community ward for women. The W.A. Rope and Twine Company and the Fremantle Virgilians, who were always reliable contributors towards the maintenance of their cots, were faithful supporters. Benbow—who was looking more and more like a 'praying mantis getting around'[178]—raised over £20 through the raffle of an electric iron. For the most part it was not a society of anonymous donors. The values of benevolence and good works were still important and a giving light was not usually hidden under a bushel. At times, donations were acknowledged over the wireless, were published in newspapers and announced on plaques on cots, and to show appreciation for outstanding giving, the board could even commission a framed photograph of a donor to be hung in the out-patients' department. These donations were essential to the hospital. Important, too, were donations in kind—such as the tram-track sleepers for firewood, from the Point Walter Tramway, delivered without cost to the hospital, and over 3,000 bottles and 1,000 jars collected for the dispensary by a pensioner named Saunders. Until 1935, when the State School Teachers' Union stopped it, this had been a task that school children often undertook.

Aberdeen was as well aware as anyone of overcrowding in the hospital and the shortage of beds, plus the fact that the Medical Department was considering an alternative site for the hospital. Without constant maintenance in the early 1940s, which was not even contemplated when it was likely that Fremantle would be invaded, the hospital was badly in need of repair. The old female medical ward in The Knowle, opened with celebration and dancing until midnight in 1919, was badly in need of attention by the 1940s. Aberdeen wanted The Knowle demolished and the government architect was commissioned to plan two new buildings, each of three storeys with accommodation for 30 beds on the first and second floors and a new laundry, kitchen, dining rooms and boilerhouse.[179] Due to the lack of finance, however, palliative measures only were taken and the verandahs of the community, female surgical and children's wards were closed in to provide extra bed space. Not surprisingly, by 1948 the hospital buildings were reported to be in a 'deplorable

---

[178]   Hatch, notes.
[179]   Minutes of Executive Committee, 27 October 1943.

state'[180] and a full-time painter was appointed and equipment purchased for the carpenters' and engineers' workshops, which were reconstructed old army huts.

By mid-1943 the concern about invasion had eased. Soldiers from the anti-aircraft battery were moved from their temporary barracks in the Adelaide Samson Children's Ward into the old isolation block, and the hospital's convalescent patients were transferred into the children's ward. Matron staggered under the weight of paperwork involved with rationing butter, sugar and other supplies to the hospital and an office assistant was employed to share the load. Rationing affected all in the community and hospital staff were not exempt. Aberdeen, however, wielded some influence and was able to provide the hospital collector, Mr Sawyer, with a much-needed car tyre so that he could continue to travel his district, and when Modess were almost unobtainable, the medical superintendent arranged a welcome supply for the nurses. At times he also offered transport to Perth, and would ring through to the Nurses' Home: 'Anybody like a lift to Perth? I've got to go to a meeting up there.'[181] But as time passed, the split between those who favoured Aberdeen and those who did not, was not appreciably eased.

Towards the end of 1944, the position at the hospital was critical, with Laycock from X-ray and Miss Boot in pathology ready to resign. Dr Caldera, after 17 years on the honorary staff, said that he was resigning on health grounds, then sent a letter to the board containing certain more pertinent reasons why he had resigned, which was greeted by the board with no comment. Aberdeen had transferred control of the dispensary from the secretary to himself, an arrangement which would have mightily pleased the chief pharmacist who, like Aberdeen, did not like anyone taking undue advantage of the hospital or its supplies. After the change, at least one family protested to the board when the dispensary would not supply medicine prescribed for them by a private doctor. Friction between Laycock and Aberdeen, however, was constant. From being a relatively autonomous head of a department, Laycock soon found that his movements, and his work were under Aberdeen's constant supervision. Even when he had legitimate cause to take time off duty, the radiographer had to seek the medical superintendent's permission. So intolerable had the position become by August that Laycock felt 'he could no longer carry on'.[182] When he left later in the month, Sister Walsh took his place. The honorary doctors Gibson and Godby also crossed swords with Aberdeen over control of the X-ray department, and Frame, the visiting radiologist, together with the Johnsons and Dr Donald Smith, supported them.[183] On Aberdeen's request, Major Long from the military department was asked for his sage advice. At a round-table conference between the protagonists, the difficulties were overcome and the Deputy Director of Manpower was approached to have Johnny Millar returned to the hospital. He came in October 1944. Only months later, in January 1945, Dr Gibson died and Dr Muir temporarily took his place on the honorary staff.

[180] *Ibid.*, 18 May 1948.
[181] Peek, interview.
[182] Minutes of Executive Committee, 29 August 1944.
[183] The Johnsons were possibly Drs Alan Syme Johnson and Maurice Johnson, and the initials incorrectly recorded in the hospital's board of management minutes as W. and S. S. Johnson. Dr Donald Smith had worked at Perth Hospital until 1932 when he lost his leg through Buerger's disease. See Bruce, 'West Coast Radiography', p. 135. Laycock worked with the Commonwealth Health Laboratories at Kalgoorlie for over ten years, X-raying miners' chests until 1936. *Ibid.*, p. 138.

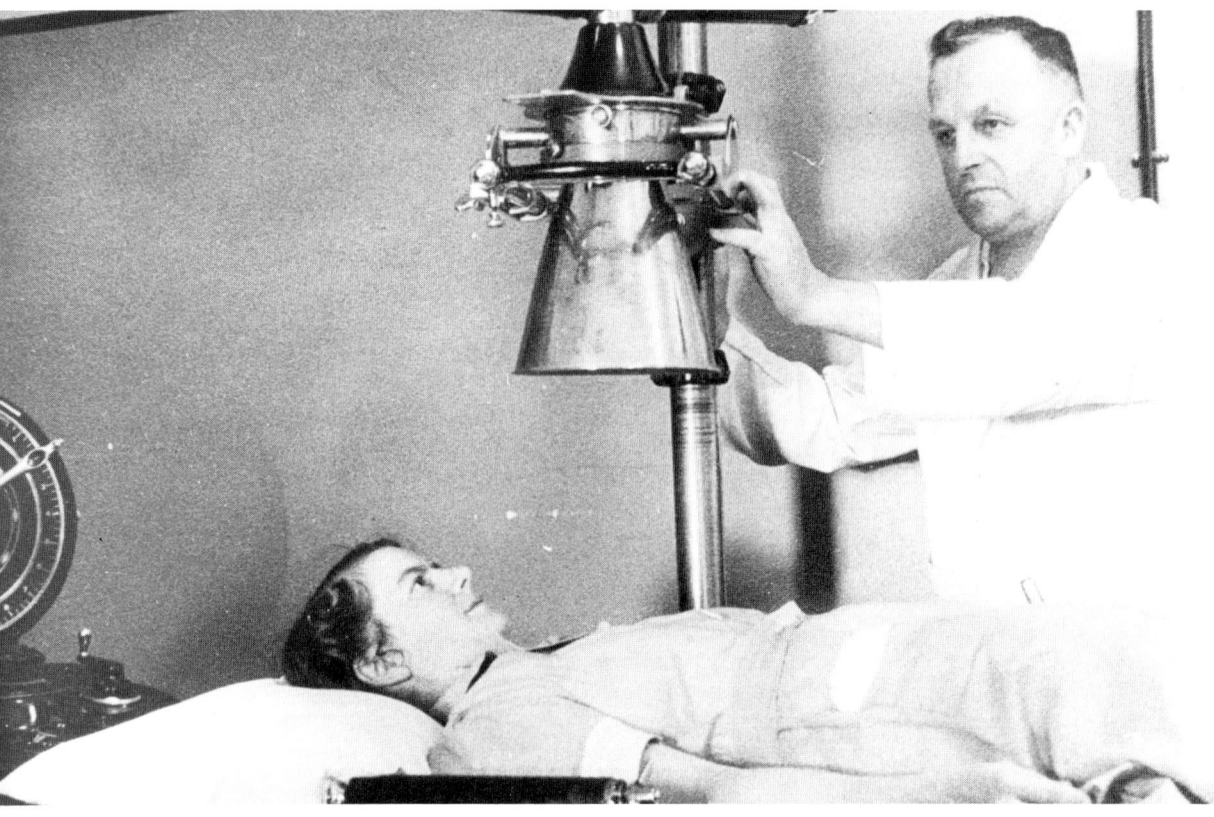

Photograph courtesy Fremantle Hospital

Plate 54. Ernie Laycock at work in the old X-ray department in The Knowle.

The original X-ray units were up to about a hundred thousand volts and the original ones had big wires and you always had to avoid these. The process involved was that when you took an X-ray everyone stopped moving in the room and therefore when you pressed the button you knew that no one was near the wires. After the war it changed to shock proof and you no longer had to worry about the electrical shock only the radiation.

John Millar
Radiographer

Dissatisfaction in the pathology department was related as much to the workload as to any conflict of authority. In 1941, a total of 3,732 tests were carried out on 1,716 patients—blood sugars and ureas, tests for tuberculosis and malaria, blood typing, cell counts, examinations of pus, faeces, smears, as well as urine microscopy and culture. Numerous tests were done on cerebro-spinal fluids after an outbreak of meningitis in the community and recurrent cycles of typhoid and amoebic dysentery increased the workload.[184] The transfer of staff and equipment to the medical

184 FH Annual Report, 30 June 1939-30 June 1940.

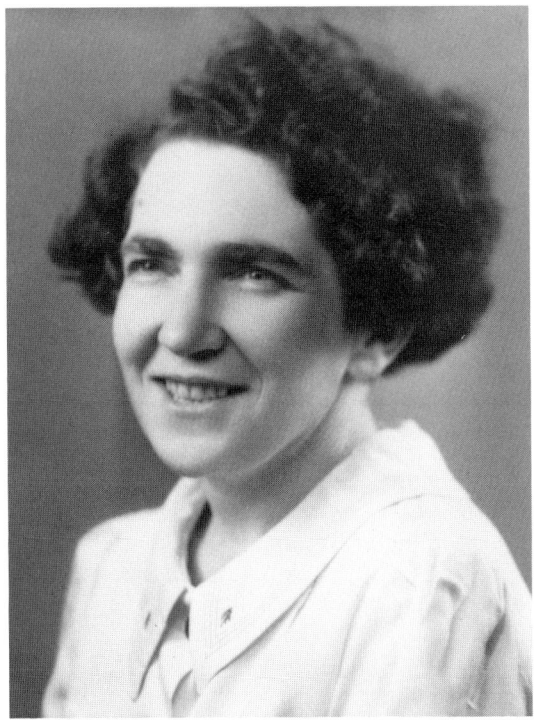

Plate 55. Miss L. L. Boot, B.Sc., from Pathology, 1940s.

Leo knew more about bugs and Biochem. than anyone could even ever hope to know ... [once] someone spilt faeces on a bench and didn't sterilise. Leo got typhoid and spent many weeks in hospital.

Ken Cole
Laboratory Assistant

Photograph courtesy Fremantle Hospital

department in Perth in 1942 when the hospital was evacuated caused some dislocation, and on its return to Fremantle, staff in the tiny laboratory were given the task of testing all local throat swabs for diphtheria. Miss Boot had to do the cleaning in the inconveniently arranged laboratory or, as she objected, 'attempt to work in an uncleaned building', for she did not think that this was the work of a laboratory assistant.[185] Compulsory blood typing of everyone in the district when it was under threat of invasion taxed the staff, who also had to locate and call donors, as well as type the blood; they went to schools to test the children there, to avoid bringing them into the city area, and 11,900 children were grouped under the scheme.[186] The establishment of the blood bank by 1944 relieved Miss Boot of the responsibility of calling blood donors and cross-typing, but that year, in an all-out effort, working eight hours a day and up to 30 hours' overtime a week with only Miss S. Anderson as a laboratory assistant, she made 4,104 reports. The able woman regretted that because of the work-load serological and bacteriological biochemical work had to be drastically reduced.[187] Miss Boot and Dr Michaels submitted protesting reports to the board about the equipment and conditions in the laboratory and Miss Boot finally requested her release from the staff. At a hastily organised special executive

185   *Ibid.*, 30 June 1941-30 June 1942.
186   *Ibid.*, 30 June 1942-30 June 1943. Ken Cole recalled that a total of 30,000 Fremantle people were tested. K. Cole, notes, FH.
187   FH Annual Report, 30 June 1943-30 June 1944.

committee meeting on 29 October 1944, the matter was considered. The assessment of public and private patients was a vital issue and this, the board pointed out 'has been and still is the responsibility of the secretary or his deputy'. Miss Boot wanted a portion of the fees which were collected for pathological examinations, directed towards new equipment which was needed, but the executive committee baulked and decided that such purchases should be considered in the annual estimates. Miss Boot raised the issue of resident medical officers using her premises and pathology equipment when she was off duty. Aberdeen suggested the purchase of an additional microscope for the residents. When the meeting broke up most of the issues had been discussed. To everyone's relief, Miss Boot stayed.

The meeting on 29 October 1944 was an important one for Aberdeen. Through it, the old hold by outside doctors was finally broken and new limits set. No longer could a patient be classified by a doctor and admitted as a public case entitled to the fiscal benefits of such status; the assessment of patients became the sole responsibility of the hospital office. Where an outside doctor recommended an admission as a 'hospital case' and the office assessed it 'private', the doctor was to be immediately informed and the patient placed under his care. Consultative cases were to be similarly assessed. The discussion did not stop there but surged on to consider Aberdeen's control of the nursing staff. In most areas, including financial matters, the matron would remain responsible through the secretary to the board. In affairs directly affecting the nursing staff, including their 'efficiency, welfare, discipline and training', matron would remain accountable.[188] But in matters of basic control—those 'of a professional nature'—Olive Jones would be responsible to Aberdeen and subject to his decisions. The committee duly altered the hospital regulations and confirmed the unusual situation.

The nurses were not intimidated by Aberdeen. Sixty-three probationers signed a petition in January 1944:

> As there has been much dissatisfaction among the Trainee-nurses of the above hospital for some time past, the Trainee-nurses wish to draw your attention to a few of the prevailing conditions causing this discord.[189]

Lack of tutoring and a shortage of staff leading to the necessity for working overtime were mentioned: 'With pressure of work they feel they are not learning to do their work efficiently, nor do the patients get sufficient attention.' Probationers pointed out that when domestic staff were absent from duty without permission, members of the nursing staff had to do their duties. Food, inedible at times due to poor cooking, was complained about: 'Meat when served in the Nurses' dining room has often been found to be bad. Breakfasts, intended to be hot, are often cold when brought to the dining room.' Years later, a laboratory worker shuddered at the memory of a typical meal: 'You had to be mighty hungry to eat it ...'[190] The nurses stressed that patients suffered the same disagreeable food, and that special diets lacked variety and quantity. Another issue of contention was night sponging. 'It is

[188]   Minutes of Executive Committee, 29 October 1944.
[189]   Copy of petition, 10 January 1944, held at FH.
[190]   Cole, notes.

necessary for the Nursing Staff to commence sponging patients at 11 p.m to enable them to cover all the ward work satisfactorily by 7 a.m.'[191] This procedure, the probationers claimed, disturbed sick people lined up on both sides of large hospital wards. The nurses argued that at Kalgoorlie and Perth hospitals night sponging had been discontinued. Could not the cessation of night sponging in this hospital be arranged? As a result, some improvements were noticed, but extra staff could not be taken on, the food was better for only a while and in time things reverted to the same unsatisfactory state. Matron did try to get a dietitian, but in 1944 there were no applicants to staff this 'whole new area'[192] and when two males applied in 1946, matron declined the offer considering the possible conflict in 'having a male in charge of the female kitchen staff'.[193] Sara Beard, the assistant dietitian from Perth Hospital, filled the position for two months in 1947, but despite advertising the position in local and eastern papers each year, there were no other applicants in the 1940s.

While they had their differences, there was one area of concern that the medical superintendent and matron shared. Fremantle Hospital was the only main hospital without a nurses' preliminary training school and, although the board raised the subject every year, the concerns of war took precedence. The nurses' examination results were often excellent, however, and few failed. In 1940 matron was commended by the board on the pleasing results of her pupils, one of whom came third in the state. In June 1941 all nurses passed the examination, but the anatomical models which Matron Balding had ordered remained locked in their box. In January 1944 Jones and Aberdeen met with the manager of the Children's Hospital to discuss a combined training school, with both contributing towards the cost of five pupils each. Negotiations were slow and Aberdeen meantime arranged for three Fremantle nurses to attend the Wooroloo Preliminary Training School. They were given 48 hours' notice before commencing. On 10 July 1944, with Sister Reedy from the Children's Hospital as tutor sister, the combined school opened and for the first time Fremantle nurses were given a course of introductory training before they entered the wards.[194] During the year, in eight different schools, each lasting six weeks, a total of 45 new probationers at Fremantle '. . . got up early, had their breakfast at seven o'clock and left at half past seven to get a bus to Princess Margaret in West Perth'.[195] It proved an unsatisfactory arrangement, especially when a good number of the Fremantle trainees failed their exams in June. The idea of private transport was discussed and then rejected, as was a proposal to use the old isolation ward as Fremantle's own training school. Collaboration between the hospitals came to an end over finances. Not unnaturally, a proposal to increase Sister Reedy's salary and appoint an assistant tutor sister was suggested by the Children's Hospital in October 1945. The Fremantle Hospital Board demurred when it was faced with a share of the increased cost because it really wanted its own school. It did approve payment for an additional tutor sister so that senior nurses could receive

[191]   Petition, 10 January 1944, FH.
[192]   Minutes of BM, 20 October 1944.
[193]   Minutes of Executive Committee, 10 December 1946.
[194]   Notebook, 'The P.T.S.', kept by O. Jones, FH.
[195]   O. Jones, interview.

more training, but as a tribunal was about to review the salaries and conditions of nurses, the board preferred to await this decision before granting a rise in Reedy's salary. It was an opportune time to establish a Fremantle Preliminary Training School. The Medical Department, the Lotteries Commission, and the board each gave £750 towards a new building.

The need to start was imperative and Sister Helen Bailey, who had trained at the Queen Elizabeth Hospital, Birmingham, in England, where the block system of nurse training was conducted, commenced with five probationers on 29 April 1946. At first lectures were held in the old dispensary and then in the nurses' small study, where the administration room was a bedroom and part of the passageway. For eight weeks the nurses were taught anatomy, physiology, hygiene, general nursing and bandaging, through the encouraging wisdom of their tutor sister. Saturday mornings they spent in the wards. Miss Alice F. Jeffrey, who had taught classes as far back as 1928, continued her instruction of invalid cookery. During the year, 63 nurses passed through the school in the new 'block system'. The experienced nurses about to take the A.T.N.A. examination worked in the wards during the busiest period of the day from 6 a.m. to 8 a.m., then went to the school until 4.45 p.m. They not only had lectures and watched films, but visited factories for specialised areas of learning and were conducted over different departments at the Perth and Children's Hospitals. The results spoke clearly in favour of the system and its tutor. Of the first graduates from the block system, three gained the top three places in the state in February 1947. In June candidates again shared top places, and in February 1948 two Fremantle trainees shared first place and one came second. Outside the hospital, the results could not be ignored and in June 1947, Helen Bailey was appointed as the organiser of nursing training in Western Australian Government Hospitals. Although the building of the preliminary training school was no further advanced, Olive Jones was content and carefully saved the good reports of her nurses published in the newspapers.[196] Sister Perryman commenced as tutor sister on 8 July 1947 and in February 1948 moved probationers and equipment into their newly completed prefabricated preliminary training school built between the nurses' home and the workshops. As assistant tutor, Sister S. Campbell worked for eight months in 1949, and was followed by Sister E. Hamersley, and later Sister McGaffin for a brief time in 1950.

The change in nursing training was timely. Olive Jones observed in 1950:

> As ward sisters are occupied with doctors most of the morning, they have very little time to supervise the training of student nurses. A clinical supervisor should be a help to the nurses and also raise the standard of nursing.[197]

Filling this position from 1951, Sister Hamersley found some resentment from ward sisters at the new appointment and at first the probationers hurried through their work to finish it before the supervisor arrived. By March 1951 she reported that it was 'now a rare occurrence and supervision [was] welcomed by most nurses'.[198]

---

[196]   Notebook, 'The P.T.S.', kept by O. Jones, FH.
[197]   *Ibid.*
[198]   Reports of Clinical Supervisor, 3 March 1951-March 1953, FH.

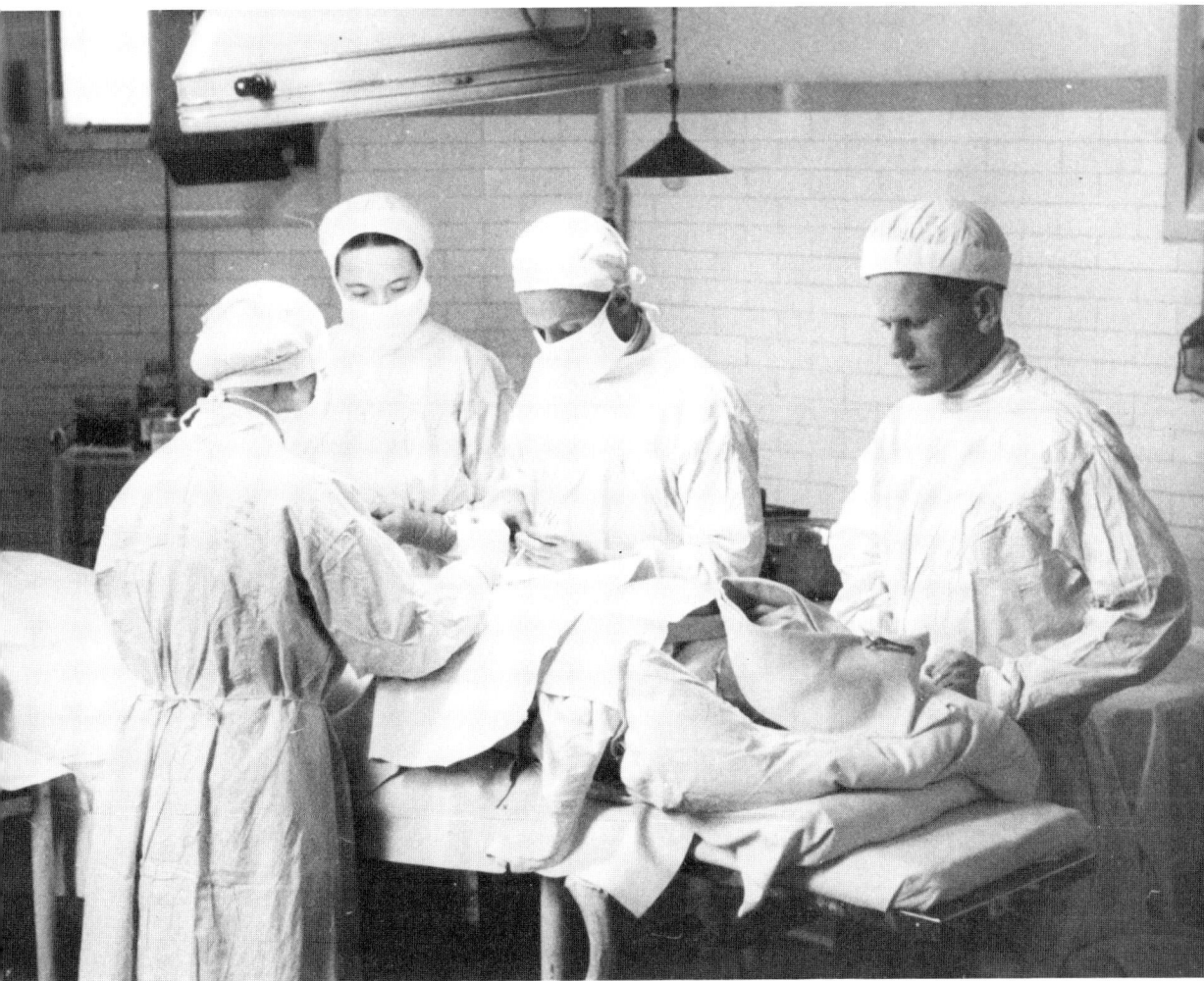

Plate 56.   In the operating theatre at The Knowle 1940–41.
(Left to right): Sister Ure, Nurse Mary Savage, Dr D. Hendrikson and Dr G. Hall.

In February 1945, Aberdeen arranged the transfer of Sister Ure from her position as theatre sister. It was a move that tested his authority and nearly split the hospital in two. Sister Ure protested at the decision. The secretary of the honorary staff and seven of its members supported her and the matter was referred to a special meeting of the newly announced board, of which Mr Bailey was the only new member and Gray had been re-elected chairman. Some preferred the easy course of passing the decision on to the medical superintendent of Perth Hospital and the acting Commissioner of Public Health. Others preferred a hospital executive committee resolution in collaboration with Matron Jones, Sister Ure and Dr Roy Muecke, the medical superintendent at Perth Hospital. Greenslade and Turton wanted Sister Ure back in the theatre until the issue was resolved, but they were outnumbered. For her part, Olive Jones conducted a quiet campaign of protest by transferring theatre staff to ward duties against Aberdeen's authority.

Matron and Sister Ure were invited to a special executive meeting at 8 p.m. on Monday, 30 April 1945. Aberdeen submitted a statement, Ure her testimonials and Muecke a special written report. Matron wanted to use the situation for an inter- pretation of her position in controlling the nursing staff but this issue was not dealt with. Gray and Wauhop supported Aberdeen's action but, in a majority decision, Turton, Greenslade and Dr Cook decided not to support Ure's transfer from theatre. The special board meeting held the following Friday was a fiery one. While most of the board upheld the executive committee decision, Gray and Wauhop still opposed it. Aberdeen wanted to speak, but Greenslade and Turton suggested that he do so in the presence of Sister Ure. When Aberdeen threatened to retire as 'his right to state a case was being made a conditional matter'[199], the board agreed instead to read his report. It was going on for 11 p.m. and the board wanted a resolution. Twice Wauhop moved that Ure should remain in her new position but twice the motion was lost. Nothing was resolved and business moved on to the installation of a 'Stay Brite' sink in the minor theatre.

Perhaps there was illness in the town, perhaps there were other demands on their time, but only five members arrived to debate the issue of the transferred theatre sister at the May board meeting, which consequently had to be cancelled. By June the issue had settled into that of authority over the movement of nursing staff. The Minister for Health had written to say that in his opinion the responsibility 'to remove the nursing staff from point to point in the hospital' rested with the medical superintendent.[200] Led by Greenslade, Matron's supporters on the board decided to write to the minister to explain the full facts of the case. In July, when the death of Prime Minister John Curtin was marked by members standing as a gesture of respect, and while they were still jubilant about Japan's surrender after the bombing of a place called Hiroshima, Aberdeen asked for and was granted two months' sick leave. Five months after her transfer, Sister Ure requested an official reply to her protest at being removed from the operating theatre. Certain members believed that the reply should have been given face to face, and Chairman Wauhop was elected to the unpleasant task. With that over, the board settled once more to the more mun- dane, agreeably uncontroversial matters of hospital administration.

By 1946 most of the honorary staff who had served in uniform had returned. They met in February 1946 and agreed to ask the board to reappoint them to the hospital on a pre-war basis and together the doctors thrashed out a recommended list of appointments.[201] The board passed the matter to the executive committee for their consideration in a move that the honoraries considered a ploy for time. They agreed in April to the return of the honoraries, but not on a pre-war basis; Dr Ken Aber-

---

[199] Minutes of BM, 4 May 1945. The original minutes of this meeting were destroyed and re-written. See also Minutes of BM, 23 March, 30 April 1945.

[200] *Ibid.*, 8 June 1945.

[201] Minutes of the Honorary Staff, 13 February 1946.

deen would retain 15 beds under his control. The honorary staff decided that their return could only be under pre-war conditions and Dunkley, Stubbe, Muir and Baker met with the Commissioner of Public Health to protest their cause. The three years of Aberdeen's appointment had passed in various degrees of conflict. In the midst of the upheaval with the honoraries, when the board decided that it—after all—had the right to vary the conditions of the medical superintendent's appointment at the end of the current period in June, Aberdeen announced his return to Northam and submitted his resignation as medical superintendent from 26 May. At the same meeting at which it was accepted, the board agreed that the honorary medical staff should resume duty on a pre-war basis from 20 May 1946. It was the end of the new order.

In May, the honoraries gathered in force in their room at the hospital to consider a different issue. On 1 January 1946, Labor's Commonwealth Hospital Benefit Scheme, on which John Jeffery had been called to work, was introduced. Under the scheme, the Commonwealth Government subsidised all occupied beds—public, private and intermediate, at a rate of six shilling a day—and it put an end to the system of interrogation about finances at the front desk before a patient's admission.[202] The scheme benefited the public patient, whose costs it covered. It benefited the intermediate and private patients who could be admitted to the hospital in a socially distinct area under their own doctor. However, it did not benefit the honorary doctors who objected to volunteering their services to other than the needy. Dr L. le Souef, president of the B.M.A., Western Australian branch, and Dr N. Stewart, a member of the B.M.A. council, with Dr H. Craig, president of Perth Hospital honorary staff, met with the Fremantle honoraries to discuss the action to be taken should the hospital honorary medical staff appointments be advertised vacant after 30 June. When, in due course, the appointments were advertised, the honorary staff was there to fill them as they always had, but there proved to be times when the doctors refused to treat a patient gratuitously if they considered that he or she was playing on their benevolence and could pay. In the following months, the honorary staff turned their attention to other matters—a donation towards a new anaesthetic machine and an electro-cardiac machine, the purchase of a haemometer for Miss Boot's use in pathology, the organisation of regular monthly meetings, lectures and clinical consultations. Dr O'Donnell donated his photograph for hanging in the staff room and arrangements were made to hang East and Gibson likewise.[203] The old order settled comfortably into the post-war society.

By mid-1946, both wars in Fremantle had ended and both left their mark. In December 1945, to everyone's delight, it was estimated that 61,000 Australian troops would leave overseas for home during the month, not 30,000 as earlier predicted.[204] Many came back to Fremantle past the new cranes and slipways built to service the American fleet, past the cafeteria for port workers, and the new visible signs of mechanisation at the harbour.[205] The *Oranje*, a hospital ship still bearing her distinctive Red Cross symbols, berthed at Fremantle with 400 Dutch civilians

[202]   See *West Australian*, 10 February 1943, 10 February 1944, 13 September 1945.
[203]   Minutes of Honorary Staff, 16 May, 13 June, 8 August 1946.
[204]   *West Australian*, 7 December 1945.
[205]   Ewers, *The Western Gateway*, pp. 147–50.

who had been interned by Japanese. In her 35 voyages as a hospital ship, the converted Dutch luxury liner had carried 30,000 wounded home.[206] Many had been landed at Fremantle.

At the hospital, Aberdeen left smarting hurts but also a hospital administratively tightened and organised. Many of the old employees, including Sister Kessell from the R.A.A.F., orderly Igglesden, G. Forbes, Drs Stubbe, Harry Hill and Percy White, applied to return to the staff. H. Mutton went back to office work, Hamersley to the dispensary, G. R. Noble, the admissions clerk, to his front desk. There were many others. John Jeffery had the dispensary back under his firm control by April 1946. Sister Wheatley from Fremantle Hospital was awarded the A.R.R.C. for devotion to duty in New Guinea.[207] However, some did not return. Louvima Bates died in Malaya as a result of enemy action; Charles Fletcher—who, as head orderly, had so often helped lift heavy patients and raced to the gate at night to let an ambulance in—died while a prisoner of war. His place at the hospital was filled by Bill Lucanas. Like an outraged echo from the past there was a letter from Sister Ure when Aberdeen left, requesting a copy of the board's decision on her transfer from theatre. Such hurts run deep.

On 18 June 1946 the Executive Committee decided to pay the hospital's next medical superintendent £750 in his first year, with a house rent-free. No beds were set aside for his patients. But the greatest change came with the restoration of matron's powers. It was agreed that:

> The Matron be responsible to the Medical Superintendent for the nursing service in all its detail. This includes not only the actual care of patients but also the government and discipline of those on her staff.
>
> In order to properly fulfill these responsibilities, she will have the authority and assume the responsibility for making the selection of the nursing staff. As a matter of courtesy and co-operation, she will consult with the Medical Superintendent with regard to selection of head nurses. But the final decision as to employment and discharge of the nursing staff will rest with her, subject to the Board's endorsement.[208]

Olive Jones privately rejoiced.

A legacy of war which was less easy to shed than a uniform on return to civilian life was that of venereal disease. In 1942 the *West Australian* was reflecting the Army's concern at a definite increase in its incidence. By 1943 the newspaper was reporting the disease as a 'scourge' and the Commonwealth Government estimated that over £112,000 would be necessary for its treatment.[209] A booklet issued by the Department of Public Health in 1942 outlined the symptoms of, and precautions to be taken against, the affliction, and urged young men in heavy print that 'sex is not essential to robust good health'.[210] In 1943 the Police Boys' Club at Fremantle was arranging lectures on social diseases for boys between 15 and 18 years accompanied by their parents, and a booklet entitled *Guide to Virile Manhood* subsequently

---

[206] *West Australian*, 3 December 1945.
[207] Minutes of Executive Committee, 14 March 1944.
[208] *Ibid.*, 18 June 1946.
[209] *West Australian*, 13 August 1942, 8 December 1943, 14 December 1943, 25 February 1944.
[210] PHD pamphlet, Acc. WC 140/1942.

became available.[211] The publication was timely. A writer to the press made an appeal to spare the sensibilities of women and children from the 'disgusting scenes to be witnessed outside the houses of ill-fame in full view of the Perth-Fremantle train service' with 'crowds of allied servicemen jostling, pushing and fighting to gain admission to those "residences" at all hours of the day'.[212]

Those at Fremantle who suspected themselves infected could be treated at the hospital clinics. The 'V.D.' department was buried on the lower floor of the Ron Doig Block and operated only at night. Patients varied in nationality and their degree of infection, and ranged in age from 18 to 51. They came individually or sometimes in groups from ships and were treated and sent on to a doctor in the next port. There were 88 men undergoing treatment in December 1943, and 84 in December 1945. The number gradually dropped: 65 at the end of 1947, 13 in 1949 and 12 in December 1951. One labourer who contracted syphilis in 1932, when he was 25 years old, was still being treated in 1957.[213]

For an extra £1 a week, John Jeffery was required to fill the prescriptions on V.D. clinic nights. It was found that patients who spoke little English, particularly Lascar seamen, would sometimes drink the lotion they were supposed to apply, apply the mixture they were supposed to take, and swallow the anal suppositories. It was distressing to see some infected crewmen from the boats that called increasingly frequently in the 1950s and which left in an explosion of exchanged coloured paper streamers that tenuously linked the traveller and those on the wharf. Some infected seamen, thinking perhaps to relieve their venereal condition, resorted to desperate measures, and at the Fremantle Hospital clinic

> ... it would be quite strange at times to see ... these coloured streamers used as bandages. So there'd be red ones and blue ones and yellow ones ... and the dye didn't do much towards the infection either.[214]

Penicillin, which replaced salvarson and bismuth and arsenic from the latter half of the 1940s, greatly improved the effectiveness of treatment.

For many individuals, for communities and the country as a whole, the period immediately following the war was one of dislocation and readjustment. The fortunate families reassembled themselves with a returned soldier at their head, but others had to come to terms with the loss of a husband, father, sister, brother or mother. The period of power restrictions, ration coupons, shortages of materials, and the regulation of employment by the Department of Manpower were lived through. In the 'war going on at home' against sickness and disease that Hookway spoke of in 1941,[215] there was an increase in 'casualties' as the population grew, and hospitals were accepted as the best places to receive treatment. The different departments—X-ray, theatre, pathology and physiotherapy—provided special services which could no longer be given at home. When Hookway retired in January 1948 after 22 years

211 *West Australian*, 3 and 14 December 1943, 25 February 1944.
212 *Ibid.*, 30 May 1945.
213 Register, 'Male V-D. 1941', FH.
214 C. Jeffery, taped recollections.
215 FH Annual Report, 30 June 1939-30 June 1941.

as secretary of the hospital and was succeeded by James Scrymgeour, he allowed himself the luxury of looking back, and observed:

> The path has not always been an easy one, but with the support of the staff, and the confidence of the Board, such difficulties have been overcome.[216]

It was a statement timeless in its relevance as the next 40 years would prove.

[216] *Ibid.*, 30 June 1946-30 June 1947.

Chapter VII

'No longer anyone's country cousin.'

Maxine Joy Keen
Sister in Charge, Operating Theatres
Fremantle Hospital, 1987.

A period of comparative well-being and economic prosperity in the 1950s and 1960s burst like sunshine after the heavy decades of Depression and war. The excitement and splendour of the young Queen Elizabeth's coronation in 1953 fostered hope for a fair future, but British atomic tests at the Montebello Islands and wars in Korea and later in Vietnam reminded that there were still shadows. Most Australians in the 1950s were heavily taxed by the Menzies' Federal Government, but many received old-age or invalid pensions, and child endowment, a widow's pension or unemployment and sickness benefits. Most workers were glad of the 1947 Federal Arbitration Court decision to introduce a 40-hour week and, unlike their parents, the young leaving school in the late 1950s were almost assured of a job. Wheat and wool production boomed and so did farmers' bank balances.[1] It seemed that an era of change, an era of challenge and possibly even one of magnificent hope had dawned.

The population of the Western State increased from 522,000 at the end of 1948, to 862,685 in December 1966, and to 1,250,000 by 1982. Not all new arrivals came crib-sized, enabling a new parent to receive the government's new maternity allowance. Nearly 70,000 immigrants arrived, just under half of whom were European survivors of war from refugee camps.[2] A handful had been prisoners of war detained in Australia, who elected to stay and bring out families. Many immigrants found their way back to Fremantle where they had first berthed, notably Italians, Yugoslavs and later Portuguese. Some turned to netting fish, prawning and crayfishing; others went to new industrial areas to make a fresh start, often taking factory work or other low-paid labour. Some found work at the hospital. Victor Poklad was Russian and as a prisoner of war had laboured for four years at an ammunition factory near Dresden. In 1950 he came to Australia from a refugee camp in Austria and after five weeks at Northam Immigration Camp he returned to Fremantle. There, at a small party, he met Bill Lucanus, the head orderly. 'You seem to be a good bloke,' the Fremantle Hospital employee mused, 'if I get some vacancies in Fremantle Hospital as an orderly, would you like to be working?' Nine months later, in 1956, the trained geological research technician, with no certificates and little knowledge of English,

---

[1] F. K. Crowley, *Australia's Western Third: A History of Western Australia from the First Settlements to Modern Times*, 1960, pp. 322–3.
[2] Crowley and De Garis, *A Short History*, p. 93.

started work as an orderly.[3] Many of the hospital's competent female domestic staff from this time also came from Europe and were regularly called upon to interpret for patients who did not speak English. Migrants also came to the hospital for treatment: 'Sicilians, Italians and Yugoslavs and Portuguese ... they all still used the Fremantle Hospital as the first consulting point before they went anywhere else,'[4] recalled a medical superintendent. Used to a different system of medical treatment in a different culture,[5] the patients often needed extra reassurance, and in time showed their appreciation by inviting some of the staff to family weddings, or giving bottles of their home-made wine.

Perth and many of its suburbs grew in the 1950s and 1960s, but perhaps nowhere more vigorously and extensively than at Fremantle. Not surprisingly, because of its location near road, sea, and rail transport, and because of its flat, open areas of market gardens and desolate dunes of sand extending past South Beach to Rockingham, the area was eyed by the government for an industrial complex.[6] By 1955 British Petroleum Limited had built a huge oil refinery. An extensive steel rolling mill was developed there and, in 1964, an alumina refinery. A fertilizer works, a large power station and a nickel refinery followed. Many other firms and industries claimed a place and started production at the Kwinana industrial complex, 15 miles south of Fremantle. Busy jetties splayed out into the sea and channels were dredged to allow the berthing of bulk carriers and oil tankers.[7] The spare but beautiful coastal strip at Cockburn became a centre for noxious trades which wrinkled the nose as even beached seaweed could not.

New housing mushroomed, as suburbs such as Medina, Calista, Orelia, and Parmelia, Coolbellup and Hamilton Hill, were strung with power and telephone lines and linked underground by drainage and water pipes. There were self-serve supermarkets in large shopping complexes and new schools and sports grounds. The population in the Fremantle area burgeoned. In 1954 it was estimated to be 84,700. In the Cockburn area alone, between 1951 and 1963, it doubled to reach 8,200; in another two years it topped 12,000 and doubled again in the five years ending 1970.[8]

The post-war years were times of other equally rapid change in most of the western world. A burst of technological knowledge and advance was channelled into medical areas, transforming methods, diagnoses and medical procedures, and demanding a different training for all staff, including the technologists who had to learn to operate the new machinery. It was not always easy for the old to keep up. At the hospital, when engineer Robert Benbow requested an increase in salary in 1948, his experience and qualifications gained 30 years earlier were considered and found wanting. The Medical Department recommended instead of a pay increase, the appointment of a qualified steam engineer with trade certificates, an electrical licence and a good knowledge of refrigeration. Bob Longstaff was taken onto the

[3] V. Poklad, interviewed by C. Jeffery, 30 August 1985, FH.
[4] J. Rowe, interviewed by C. Jeffery, October 1984-February 1985, FH. See also Smith, interview.
[5] See G. Pasquarelli, 'The General Medical and Associated Problems of the Italian Migrant Family', *The Medical Journal of Australia*, 8 January 1966.
[6] Ewers, *The Western Gateway*, pp. 161–5.
[7] M. Berson, *Cockburn: The Making of a Community*, 1978.
[8] *Ibid.*, p. 190.

staff and Benbow was made the assistant engineer. Two years later, in 1950, after 32 years of loyal service at the hospital, the original engineer retired and was presented with the wireless set which he had wished to have.

At the workshops, in X-ray, pathology, the theatres, in the wards, laboratories and at the pharmacy, new discoveries transformed old ways. In 1955 Dr Jonas Salk discovered a vaccine for poliomyelitis, which had flared in crippling epidemics from the late 1930s. During non-epidemic periods such cases were nursed at Fremantle Hospital, but most patients were transferred to the Infectious Diseases Hospital at Subiaco. Twenty-two-year-old Sister Pat Barber died with the disease after nursing an afflicted patient at Fremantle Hospital in 1943. Her death shocked workmates and other staff, some of whom worked at the clinic which was subsequently set up in 1956 to immunize children of the area against the disease.[9]

The last 40 years of the weave of the tapestry of Fremantle Hospital's history become busy and dense. Threads of concern and interest, growth and change, cross and pass around other strands of the fabric. Strands of continuity wrap the history round. Always there were shared moments of laughter: a nice hot bath run for a tired nurse by straight-faced class mates who first removed the bathroom light globe and added a handful of Condy's crystals to the water, which left the nurse distinctly blue;[10] a resident's writing on a headsheet that transformed the cause of a lumper's back injury from 'working on a difficult winch' to 'working on a difficult wench';[11] a sailor who rang the hospital looking for a date and was told to come and ask for Miss Melaena Stools.[12] There were many welcome flashes of fun. Christmas was always celebrated with the decades-old traditional decoration of wards by nurses and willing patients—sometimes based on a theme, sometimes through sheer inspiration and innovation. Always there was a staff member disguised as Father Christmas bearing toys, and when visiting the children's ward he was often accompanied by nurses dressed as fairies. The revered gentleman was almost late the year that one of the hospital cats had a litter on the red suit and Dr Dunkley understandably had it washed and sterilized before he wore it.[13] For many years it was the orderly Bob Ellis who 'ho-hoed' around the wards. Always there was the visit by the Governor and his wife a few days before Christmas to see the patients and share the festive Garden Party under marquees on the Balding Home lawns, where staff and volunteers mingled and ate dainty cakes and thinly-sliced, 'fly-away' sandwiches for which the kitchen was famous. Always too were periods of tiredness for nurses and doctors and for laboratory and departmental workers as they worked overtime or were called back in emergencies. It was not unusual for a junior resident to be 'still going at ten and eleven p.m., and the nights you were "on" you just did not get to bed and you were expected to be up all the next day'.[14]

9   Information by courtesy of the Barber family. Includes undated press clippings. In 1938 there were 47 cases of poliomyelitis reported in Western Australia, 2 in 1947, and in July alone in 1948 there were 60. 'Little is known of the disease. Medical Men admit this without reserve,' reported the *Daily News*, 17 August 1949.

10 E. Davies, notes, FH.

11 M. Hatch (née Borwick), notes.

12 A. Hanrahan, notes, FH.

13 L. Moorhouse, notes.

14 P. B. Smith, interviewed by C. Jeffery, 1985, FH.

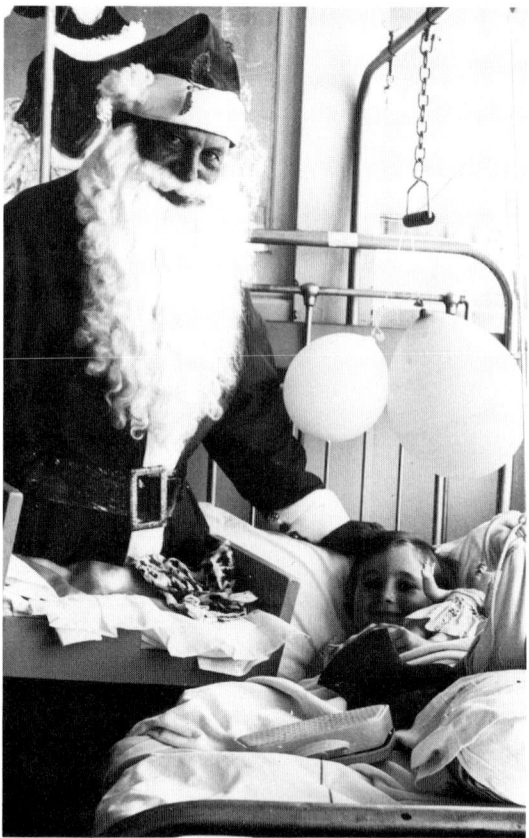

Plate 57. Father Christmas, Bert Ellis, visiting 'Samson' Ward.

One of the orderlies, Bert Ellis, dressed up as Father Christmas and the nurses dressed as fairies. In latter years they decorated an electric mobile trolley and Father Christmas would go down to the kiddies' ward. We put a big canvas cover up and hessian around the fence for the children's party. It was always a busy time around Christmas.

Len Marshall
Carpenter

Photograph courtesy Fremantle Hospital

Not always, but sometimes, there were even periods of mystery. Tales of a ghost in the nurses' quarters near Attfield Street had been aired when, during site excavations in 1918, skeletons had been unearthed there. In the 1960s there was also talk about a ghost in the children's ward. Years earlier there had been a very ill child in the small cottage attached to the ward and his mother had been allowed to visit the boy whenever she could. Wearing a long white dress and high-heeled shoes one windy, wet night, she came to the cottage to say goodnight to her son. Along the length of the Adelaide Samson Ward she walked, but when she arrived at the cottage, she found her son dead. Frantic with distress, she rang the call-bell—long, loudly and unceasingly. It was said that, overcome with grief, she then collapsed, died, and from that night haunted the ward. Some staff were sceptical, others prickled with doubt, especially when on night duty. One night in 1965, after the routine handover from evening to night staff in the children's ward and on an occasion when the cottage was empty, the ward's main entrance door banged, footsteps were heard, but no one entered the office. Then the alarm bell shrilled, and the two night staff on duty investigated, thinking more of prowlers than of spirits. The senior nurse recalled:

> When I opened the cottage door I immediately turned all the lights on and strangely enough the ringing stopped. We both checked the rooms and not one call bell was in situ. As soon as we turned the lights off and locked the door the bells started ringing again.[15]

Not until two orderlies removed the fuses from the meter box did the bells cease. Strangely enough, just a year earlier, other night duty staff in the ward had shared a similar experience. The hospital priest was called to bless the cottage, 'which he did in my presence', recalled the senior nurse.

Although Fremantle was still a place where new settlers might temporarily stay to work out a future, many of the hospital's patients lived much of their life-cycle in the area. Some were admitted as children, perhaps with a burn or for a tonsillectomy, returned after a motor bike accident or an illness in their teens or early twenties, and were treated again in their old age, frequently for an ulcer, heart problem or diabetes. Older staff members might see three generations of a family come to the hospital. One patient professed that: 'Fremantle is my home town. I even feel uncomfortable in Perth',[16] and another—a fisherman at the port like his father before him—confided that he would 'never quit Fremantle'.[17] One woman was a regular.

> Every Monday morning Mrs _____ from Hamilton Hill would come up. She had quite a number of children and there was usually something wrong with them, but if she couldn't bring one of her own, she would bring one of the neighbour's children ... Dr Dunkley would say to her, 'Well, Mrs ... who have you brought today?' And she would say—'Alma's very sick or Harry's very sick'. Doctor was very sympathetic towards her ...[18]

So much a part of the hospital was she, that when extensions were considered, someone would invariably wonder what the hospital's most regular visitor would have thought of the improvement.

Another section of the community who continued to come as patients were prisoners from the gaol. At times a warder or policeman would be posted to guard such a patient, but at others, as a medical superintendent explained, 'we had a consultation and more or less had an honour system and we didn't have many people escape at all'.[19] Occasionally an uneasy night nurse would wedge a chair under the patient's door handle until morning to prevent a possible escape. The staff often wondered what crime their patient had committed, and once, when a kitchen worker recognised a patient as the man who had raped someone in her family, they knew. But as one who nursed him rationalised, 'to me he was a patient'.[20] One inmate who was regularly admitted from the gaol scared some nurses but was greeted by others as an old friend who helped wherever he could in the ward. Nicknamed 'Dennis the Menace' by nurses, he wrapped razors blades, darning needles, nurses' hair clips and bobby-pins, or whatever sharp objects he could lay his hands on, in fresh bread, and

[15] M. Christie, notes, FH.
[16] *Daily News*, 25 July 1968.
[17] *Ibid.*, 6 June 1968.
[18] O. Jones, interview.
[19] Rowe, interview.
[20] N. Toy (née Gray), notes, FH.

swallowed. 'They did multiple operations, all over him. His stomach looked like a battle field,'[21] reflected an X-ray technician. One nurse recalled the prison cases as 'always very lonely and we were never allowed to talk much to them, as if they had leprosy'.[22] An exception was a man said to have killed a family member with a pair of scissors and who was awaiting execution at the prison:

> ... he was out in the exercise yard, apparently being given his daily limit of exercise and he ran for the wall and didn't make it over the wall. I don't know that he even wanted to. But he fell from well up the wall and he broke both arms and both legs. He came into hospital and both arms were in plaster and strung up. Both legs were in Hamilton Russell extensions and he was with us for many weeks while all of those healed ... we of course, had to feed him every meal. We had to do every single thing for him, because he was unable to do anything for himself and he then went back to the gaol.[23]

Time and dependency forged ties of friendship. Not long after his return to a cell, one fresh morning at eight o'clock the prison bell tolled the grim news of the man's hanging. It was a devastating day for those who had nursed him.

Each day, visitors came to see patients in the wards. Churchmen came regularly and so did representatives from various organisations such as lodges, the Red Cross, political groups and the Waterside Workers' Federation. Sister Alice from the Little Sisters of the Poor who organised a sewing circle for the hospital, and Curly Molyneux from the Buffalo Lodge, were constant callers for many years. The lodge erected a drinking fountain in the out-patients department to mark the many years of service by their member. Oscar Stack was an Elder from the Reorganized Church of Jesus Christ of Latter Day Saints, and well known in Fremantle as the 'lightning barber', for the speed with which he could cut a 'trammies' hair before the tram could navigate the turnabout at the terminus and return past the shop to pick him up. Stack was also welcome for his singing in the hospital wards. At first, it was as he shaved a patient or cut a head of hair, and later, for the joy of hymning.[24] Religion was not always a vital concern to a patient and one confessed to registering as Anglican, only because he could not spell 'Congregational'. Visiting hours were strictly kept and it was not until 15 December 1958, that fees were abolished and visitors no longer had to queue at the wooden gate at the bottom of the steps opposite the Lodge and purchase a ticket—a different-coloured one each night—to gain entry to the wards.[25] The income from visitors' passes was reliable and £170 a month was not an unusual total in the mid-1950s.

During the busy time of world war, much power had been granted by the board to the executive committee comprising Gray, Wauhop, Cook, Turton and Greenslade—who consequently made most of the decisions affecting the hospital. As the community struggled to regain order in peace-time, Chairman Gray found his

[21]   J. Millar, interviewed by C. Jeffery, 26 January 1987. See also J. Morrissey, notes, FH.
[22]   Pilling, notes, FH.
[23]   O. Hedemann, interviewed by C. Jeffery, 11 October 1985; 11, 19 April 1986, FH.
[24]   O. Stack, interviewed by L. Stevens, 1 May 1981, FCL.
[25]   A. Smith, interviewed by C. Jeffery, June to July 1985, FH. The board did resolve to discontinue the charge to visitors in October 1949, but rescinded the decision at the following board meeting in November.

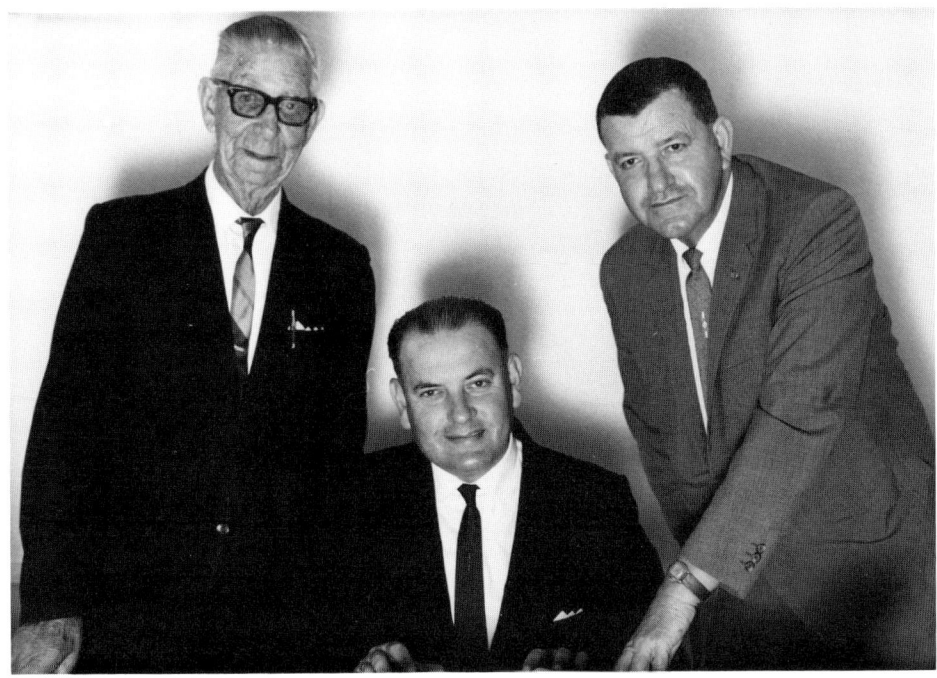

Photograph courtesy West Australian Newspapers

Plate 58.   The appointment of Mr A. J. Smith as Administrator.

(Left to right): Mr W. Wauhop, Chairman of the Board, Mr A. J. Smith, Mr J. M. Scrymgeour, retiring Administrator.

William Wauhop, M.B.E., J.P., was elected to the East Fremantle Town Council in 1922, was Mayor of East Fremantle 1944–1964, President of the Fremantle A.L.P. 1942, and Chairman of the State Licensing Court 1949–1958. He joined the Fremantle Hospital Board in 1933 and was Chairman from 1947 to 1970.

> People do care about their bills and they get to the stage where they are almost destitute and they're worried and frightened to go and see someone or do something about it. I think Jamie Scrymgeour was a good bloke in this way, he had an attitude towards the people as well as the administrative attitude of being a secretary of a hospital.

> Dr John Rowe
> Medical Superintendent

pressure of work so great, that he announced his retirement from the board in August, 1946. No board or executive meetings were held in September, and in October, William Wauhop was elected chairman by a small majority. In November the board meeting was cancelled. Appointments to the board were late in 1947 and as a result, meetings were not held in either February or March. There were no new faces at the April gathering after the appointments were announced. Meetings had to be abandoned in May 1947 and in July and September 1948 when there were insufficient members to constitute a quorum, and often business was rushed through. Increasingly the executive committee made the vital decisions. In February 1949, when

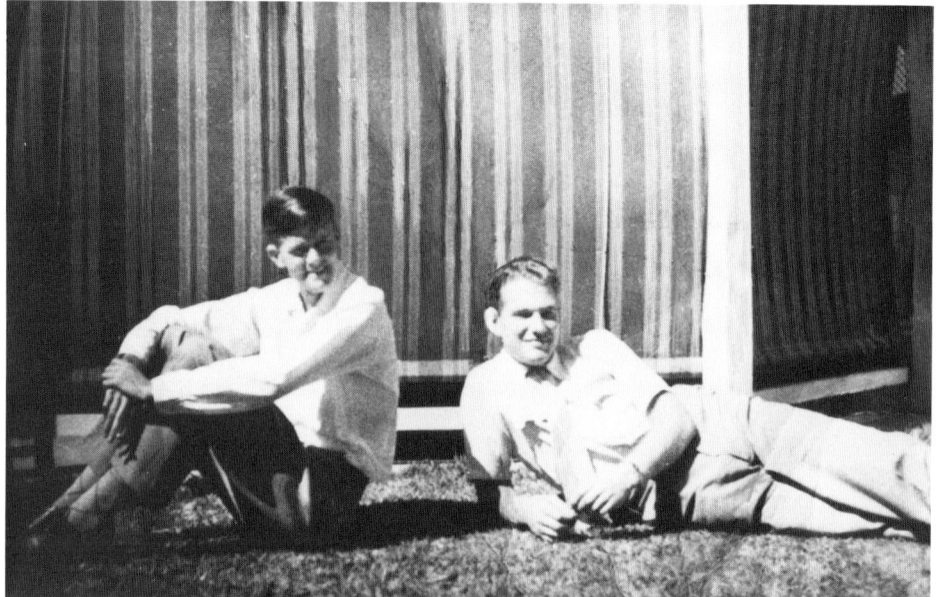

Photograph courtesy Fremantle Hospital

Plate 59.   Dr Peter Smith and Dr William Cook, two of 'Rowie's boys'.

I had good teachers and I would like to emphasise here, that the teachers that we had, were not only the honoraries but they were the ward sisters and you know, I had my ears boxed by Fitz [Sister Fitzgerald] and I was jumped on by Bette Needle and I was manoevred by Dot Daly. And Backie [Sister Backshall] of course, in kids' ward taught me more about children in a week, than I had learnt at med. school, and they definitely taught you.

Dr Peter Smith
Medical Superintendent

the board appointments were due, the Medical Department requested the executive committee of William Wauhop, A. L. Priest, the Honorable E. M. Davies, J. R. N. Greenslade and W. S. Cook from the honorary staff, to continue to administer the hospital's affairs until arrangements were made for a new board. When the new board was announced in August, the old executive committee was retained and only three new members joined them. They were teacher and South Fremantle footballer Ross Hutchinson, who would become Minister for Health in 1965, the principal medical officer Dr C. E. Cook or his deputy, and H. T. Stitfold, the under-secretary. They administered the hospital into the 1950s with fully restored powers as a Board of Management. Through the reorganisation there was greater government knowledge about the hospital's immediate needs, and also a greater potential for government intervention in Fremantle's health services. The trend for an all-male board was set, which was not broken for 34 years. By 1958 C. C. Bennett of Fremantle, had joined the board and Mr A. Daly-Smith was the honoraries' representative, replacing Dr D. R. Gawler.

Following Aberdeen as medical superintendent, doctors Charles Price, W. Scott and then the English surgeon Murray Drew served at the hospital until 1952, and Dr John Rowe was appointed in 1953. Educated on the goldfields and with experience as an Army doctor, more interested in medicine than surgery and therefore less prone to compete with the surgeons for beds, his coming was a breath of fresh air to the hospital.

'Rowies' boys', as the young doctors coming under his direction for experience in hospital training were called, were given a good grounding in both medical learning and common sense, which was often dealt out at the residents' dining-room table as the medical superintendent at its head, carved the roast. The young doctors were taught to take a medical history, do an examination, sit back and think, make a diagnosis, then verify it with a chest X-ray and blood picture. They were also advised that if they really wanted to learn about medicine they should listen to the long-serving ward sisters. If Rowe was strict he was fair, if he was forthright he was compassionate. Coming as he did, when the hospital was set to expand, Rowe was influential in planning new buildings. For nine years while he was medical superintendent, each of Rowies' boys worked long hours and was encouraged to act independently. Tiredness and the stress of new practical learning, somewhat different in practice than when learning in medical school, occasionally had its compensations:

> You saw your patients post-operatively. One of the reasons you did that of course, is that being a small hospital there was an expectation of the public of the doctor. You turned it on a bit. We had a theatre garb which was a pair of white strides and the top of it was like a sailor top. You had a theatre cap which you left on and you had a mask which you left hanging around your neck. You put your white coat on top of that with your stethoscope and of course your face was white and you had marks from the mask on your face, and you swept into the ward in the middle of visitors. The reason you did it of course, was because you had been working so hard, you had to work out little techniques to bolster the old ego, and then you saw all the rellies ... sometimes ether and ethyl chlor anaesthetics were used and of course, a slight spray of the ethyl chlor around the place really carried the message.[26]

The local doctors, including Leigh Cook, Uther Baker, Ebell, Dunkley and Bean, still served on the honorary staff. They were also entitled to admit their own patients, who were X-rayed, obtained medicine from the pharmacy, and benefited through the pathology services of the hospital without cost, unlike those who chose to be admitted to a private hospital. At Perth and at the Children's Hospitals, an honorary staff of specialists had been serving for a number of years, and in 1949 the decision was made to adopt the system at Fremantle Hospital. The Commissioner of Public Health, Dr C. E. Cook, addressed a meeting of the honorary staff on 26 October 1949. Carefully dissociating the board as the source of his remarks, he stated that:

> ... he believed the shortage of RMOs at the Hospital might he relieved if the Hospital were to be recognized as a teaching hospital by medical faculties, notably at Sydney and

---

[26] P. B. Smith, interview.

> Adelaide. This could only be brought about by staffing the honorary appointments
> with recognized specialists ...[27]

on the voluntary termination of staff appointments on the 31 December 1949. The
discussion which followed during the next months was divided for and against the
proposition. Some long-serving general practitioners who had met the needs of the
hospital and the community in an honorary capacity for much of their working
lives, smarted at the seeming rejection of their services. However, the new system
was adopted and at a meeting on 5 April 1950 the honoraries decided that members
should retire at 60 years of age, that senior honorary physicians, surgeons, and
gynaecologists should retire after 15 years in their appointment, and others after 20
years. When the list of appointments to the honorary medical staff was issued in
1950, besides in- and out-patient physicians and surgeons, it included a cardiologist,
dermatologist, allergist, ophthalmic and orthopaedic surgeons, a paediatrician,
radiologist, psychiatrist and various assistants. The expanded list was due in part to
the need to staff the new cardiology and neurology units.

The decision to change to an honorary specialist staff was prompted and generally
supported by the people of Fremantle:

> ... it was a case of the community talking to one another and gradually accepting that
> this was the type of medicine and surgery that they wanted. And it was by evolution and
> not by resolution that this occurred and it was by the people themselves and this is how
> the system of specialists really came down to Fremantle and also how the specialists
> then resided in Fremantle and conducted their practices from Fremantle.[28]

The move not only benefited Fremantle patients through their access to treatment by
specialists at Fremantle, it also extended the learning of young resident medical
officers through the 'passing on of things by the oral tradition'.[29] To the hospital's
advantage, local doctors could no longer use the hospital's beds and facilities without payment by their private patients.

The ethic of honorary service was still strong in 1951. A suggestion that the honorary specialist anaesthetist be paid on a sessional basis was turned down as 'contra to
the Honorary System'[30] and the honorary doctors recommended the appointment of
a full-time salaried anaesthetist—to teach the junior medical officers, to supervise
anaesthetic records and apparatus, and to act as a resuscitation officer. Like contemporaries at Perth and the Children's Hospitals, there was some tension felt by
doctors about offering honorary service to those who could pay, and they categorically stated that no section of the community could claim free treatment as a right—
only as 'an act of grace'—and that the honorary medical staff had the right to state
whom they would serve without cost.

> The principle should be true charity to those who cannot afford treatment they require.

[27] Minutes of the Honorary Staff, 26 October 1949, FH.
[28] Rowe, interview.
[29] Daly-Smith, interview.
[30] Minutes of Honorary Staff, 7 February 1951, FH. Sessional payments for doctors were commenced at
      FH in 1976.

Nowadays people do not consider 'indigenous'—or the reception of charity—to be a stigma. True honesty is disappearing.[31]

At the time, 52 per cent of taxable wage earners were on or under the basic wage. Just over 62 per cent were eligible to receive honorary treatment under the combined decision by the metropolitan hospitals to base honorary service on a basic wage plus 25 per cent.

In the years following the war it became increasingly obvious that the hospital needed extra beds for those who sought treatment. In the twelve months to mid-1951, the number of patients admitted to the wards totalled 4,898, and increased a year later to 5,160.[32] With the cancellation of the free hospitals' treatment scheme which hit sensitive wallets in 1952–53, the demand for beds dropped slightly. It was observed that parents were nursing children at home rather than face a minimum payment of 30 shillings a day, and even adults received medical attendance at home rather than pay the daily charge of 35 shillings, which could cause great hardship in a carefully calculated family budget.[33] However, with the increasing acceptance of medical benefit cover, the number of patients again rose, until between mid-1956 and 1957 admissions totalled over 6,000.[34] As a temporary measure to overcome the bed shortage, the board proposed erecting prefabricated wards in the hospital grounds to accommodate 50 patients, but the medical department rejected the plan because of costs. Ward verandahs were still closed in, but now with louvre or aluminium draught-controlled windows. New, necessary but minor alterations which could not be put off any longer were undertaken in the early 1950s—to the kitchens so that staff could cope with the greater number of meals, an oil burner in the boiler house to supplement the three wood boilers and provide more steam, a new lift in the Ron Doig Block to replace the old one which was positively dangerous, and in mid-1955, extensions to the laundry to provide sewing, linen and storage rooms. But the number of patients at Fremantle Hospital continued to increase and although the board envisaged a 500-bed hospital, built to an integrated plan over a decade or so, a new ward could not be constructed until the government decided whether or not it would change the hospital's site to land it had already reserved at Hilton Park.

Many who came to the hospital were community patients. In 1950 there were 1,601, nearly 300 of whom were workers' compensation cases, with another 187 coming from ships.[35] Most were just ill or injured men seeking the best treatment available, for private hospitals in Fremantle were few and small in size, and with modern diagnostic techniques and treatments, it was now difficult to treat a patient conveniently in a private home. The number of patients increased yearly and beds for private patients were rarely free for long. Women and children community patients were also accepted, but there was no separate accommodation and they were nursed in the general wards. In 1955 there were over 2,300 private patients and the hospital's capacity to accept such cases was reached.

[31] *Ibid.*
[32] FH Annual Reports, 1951, 1952.
[33] *Ibid.*, 1953.
[34] *Ibid.*, 1957.
[35] FH Annual Report, 1950.

When it came to major improvements, the first area to receive attention was the old operating theatre. 'You couldn't still smell the chloroform but you knew that chloroform had been used there,'[36] recalled a surgeon. Although it was insufferably hot in summer and uncomfortably cold in winter, the old theatre had a questionable advantage. Cramped conditions meant that '. . . everything was close at hand. You could just about reach out and get it.'[37] There was not a great deal of lining in the roof[38] and a theatre nurse related:

> . . . we had to wash the walls as far up as we could, and with the sun coming through in the morning, you could stand at the door and see the dust motes coming down and I can remember thinking to myself—'Thank God they have found penicillin'.[39]

Mr Price evolved the idea of wearing a sweat band on his forehead to prevent perspiration dripping into a patient's wound, an idea which was adopted by others, and Mr Max Minchin had a fan directing air up the skirts of his operating gown to cool him down. There was surprisingly little post-operative infection. All manner of surgery was done:

> If a head injury came in, we had to deal with that. We dealt with stove-in chests, we dealt with everything that presented. We never transferred anything to Perth. Not in those days . . . I had to open skulls and chests and abdomens and deal with leg trauma and so forth.[40]

Mr Harry Hill treated the orthopaedic cases and was later joined by Mr Frank Bell.

There were inevitable emergencies. A surgeon was operating in the old theatre one afternoon when a two-year-old Italian child, admitted earlier with a head injury, became unconscious. When told, the doctor ran up to the old Samson Ward and

> . . . saw this child, absolutely limp on the bed . . . So, I gathered the child up in my arms and ran down two flights of stairs and then down the corridor and dumped the kid on the theatre table, screamed for antiseptic which I washed in and washed the child's head and a knife, and then—in a thrice we had the flap turned back . . . peeled the skull back . . . evacuated about a tablespoon of clot, and undersewed the bleeding middle meningeal artery. Then we had to give the child an anaesthetic . . . because he woke up in the theatre . . . The child was out of hospital within a week and all healed up and I'm sure nobody had any idea of the drama that had been.[41]

Work on a prefabricated theatre block imported from England was slow due to a shortage of labour, but when it was ready for use in May 1953, the two air-conditioned theatres and a sterilizing room in which stock was autoclaved for the whole hospital, the doctors' lounge, a plaster room, an anaesthetic room and change rooms were a great improvement. The number of major operations done in the first

---

[36] Daly-Smith, interview.
[37] *Ibid.*
[38] M. Minchin, interviewed by C. Jeffery, 15 August 1985, FH.
[39] C. Jeffery, theatre staff nurse, interview.
[40] Minchin, interview.
[41] *Ibid.*

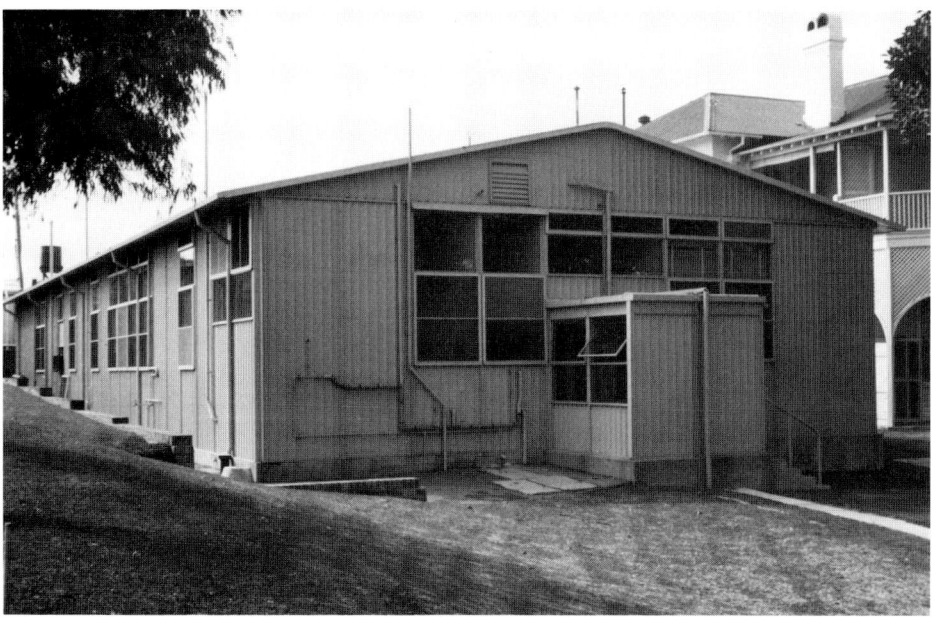

Photograph courtesy Fremantle Hospital

Plate 60.   The new prefabricated theatre, 1953.

> It was just so hot because it wasn't air-conditioned and it was aluminium—and we recorded the temperature at something like a hundred and twenty or a hundred and thirty at one stage in the autoclaving room. But then of course at night, as night came on, after that extreme heat and the place cooled down ... it creaked and cracked at night and there were great stories that used to go around about the theatre being spooked.
>
> Olga Hedemann
> Director of Nursing 1983–

year almost doubled from 1,122 in mid-1953, to 2,162 in mid-1954, and each year the number increased. By 1957 there had been 3,223.[42] Sisters Olga Hedemann, Aileen Bush and Peg Stevens were theatre sisters at different times and doctors Max Minchin, Lou Daly-Smith, Charlie Price, Ralph Cato, Frank Bell, Doug Gawler, Christian Wilson and Frank Farmer were among the many surgeons who operated there. Some of the old plated instruments and the improvised ones—a few made from old levers—were replaced with stainless steel, but nothing, as one junior resident medical officer recalled, was ever wasted:

> ... shortly after I arrived, I learned very quickly that if an instrument was of no further use to the theatre, and a new one was bought, that instrument was handed to the casualty department. When that instrument was of no further use to the casualty department, it went to the wards. When it was no further use to the wards, it went to the post-mortem room and we had scalpels that were the old thick scalpels ... and in

---

[42]   FH Annual Reports, 1953, 1954, 1957.

the post-mortem room was an emery wheel and they used to be sharpened again and again and again.[43]

Any expansion in hospital facilities was tightly related to, or reflected in the expansion of other areas. The increased number of patients for surgery added to the overcrowding in the wards and stretched the laundry, kitchen, pharmacy, X-ray and pathology departments to their limits. A cardiological unit and an intensive-care area added to the strain. Although new ward accommodation was desperately needed, it could not even be considered without increasing the nursing staff which, however, was impossible in quarters already overcrowded, despite the acquisition in 1950 of Warwick House, in nearby Solomon Street as extra nurses quarters. Nevertheless, Sister Kenny, in the department for many years, was pleased at the transfer of X-ray to the old theatre, giving this department two X-ray rooms, a dark room and even change areas, so that patients no longer had to undress in cubicles across the hall, and sit in the busy main Knowle corridor awaiting their turn in a slip-on white gown, slit down the back. There was still a place for improvisation in the X-ray department. Films would be taken dripping from the developer, washed and then hung up to dry, at times on a clothes line strung up on The Knowle's verandah.[44] Unlike earlier years, when reductions and removals of foreign objects were done under X-ray in Johnny Millar's X-ray room, leaving it a mess of plaster, it was usual to do portable X-ray work in the theatre while an operation was in progress.

> And it had to be viewed while the operation was going on . . . so it was in the theatre, take your pictures and out of the theatre . . . The gowns stayed on while we did a sprint down to the X-ray and processed the films in rapid developer—and back . . . with wet films dripping all the way . . . As far as I remember the time that sticks in my memory, was two and a half minutes. That was the best any of us ever did.[45]

The problem of limited space and facilities at the hospital was addressed soon after another small project had been undertaken in 1952—the construction of a lavatory for Asiatic seamen, who often felt distress at the strange pedestal facility which they were expected to use when they were admitted to the hospital.[46] Although the board envisaged hospital expansion in an ordered sequential plan on the main site, when patients from Bundi Kudja Maternity Hospital in Hampton Road were transferred to Woodside Private Hospital in 1956, the board eagerly accepted from the government the beautiful old building adjoining the Warwick Home in Solomon Street, as extra accommodation for nurses.[47]

As a result of the volume of patients coming to the hospital, and the technological changes and new knowledge which were bringing science and medicine closer, the staff in pathology, X-ray and pharmacy were working to capacity. The 'advent of the new antibiotics' seemed miraculous. However, they had their drawbacks:

> I well remember that early penicillin—made for us by the CSL. It came into our Phar-

[43] P. B. Smith, interview.
[44] Millar, interview.
[45] J. Pugh, interviewed by C. Jeffery, 2 September 1985, FH.
[46] FH File 20, 'Lavatory for Asiatic Seamen', March 1950 to 24 October 1952.
[47] For brief sketch of annexes and nurses homes, see *Fremantle Gazette*, 24 September 1980.

macy as a brick-red powder, sterile, and in 10 or 20 cc glass amps. It had a very persistent, unpleasant smell—to me, anyhow, reminiscent of onions. If you were making it into a cream or an ointment, despite being extra careful, you could not avoid getting traces of it on your hand or even on your clothes, and believe you me, you took the onion-like smell home with you. Petrol being rationed, most of us had to use public transport and when I got on the bus at the end of the day, the passengers in my proximity were soon sniffing and looking round for the culprit! ... At that time no commercial firm in Australia was making pen-in-oil ... if you wanted a particular pen prep you just got down to the job and, reading what information you could collect and employing what apparatus you could either scrounge or improvise, you just 'Did-it-yourself'.[48]

By 1951 it was noted by the pharmacist that 'penicillin therapy is now well established'.[49] A nurse recalled:

> ... the excitement of nursing in an era when antibiotic drugs were starting to be used; the recovery of seriously ill patients who before the advent of sulphas and penicillin would have died—pneumonia, septicaemia, gangrene. I remember especially the recovery of a sub-acute bacterial endocarditis patient, the joy of being involved in the recovery of a small boy with tetanus, [and] the young boy who had fallen from the roof of the Fremantle Town Hall and fractured his skull. I was present at the first signs of his becoming conscious after twelve days unconsciousness, after an operation to have a plate inserted in his skull—there were a few tears shed.[50]

John Jeffery and his staff in pharmacy had less time to be excited, as each year the number of prescriptions submitted and drugs dispensed, increased. In pathology, the increase was felt perhaps more than in any other department. Each year the volume and variety of work grew, and the department's expansion was bounded only by its cramped quarters. Early in May 1956 the blood bank ceased to function as a donor panel, and a new scheme was inaugurated, with the blood bank in Perth supplying the hospital's needs. In the first year of the scheme, 345 pint bottles were received from Perth and in the following year it increased to 1,801 bottles.

Overcrowding due to the number of patients was so great by the mid-1950s that something had to be done. The use of old lounges as emergency accommodation had become routine. On the Knowle verandah, staff 'squashed all the patients up against the wall' as some protection against 'any breeze, wind, rain, storm or otherwise'. In the wards, continued one of Rowie's boys:

> ... we would do a ward round in the morning and we would discharge say, ten or fifteen patients and we would look at others for discharge and we would say they weren't well enough. And at one o'clock we would do another ward round, because of the demand of patients coming in, and we would discharge the patients we thought weren't well enough at nine o'clock. We would then do another ward round at five, and you would then discharge those patients that you thought weren't ready for discharge in the

---

[48]   J. Jeffery, notes, FH. CSL—Commonweatlth Serum Laboratories.
[49]   FH Annual Report, 1951.
[50]   Joan Curran (née Strange), notes, FH.

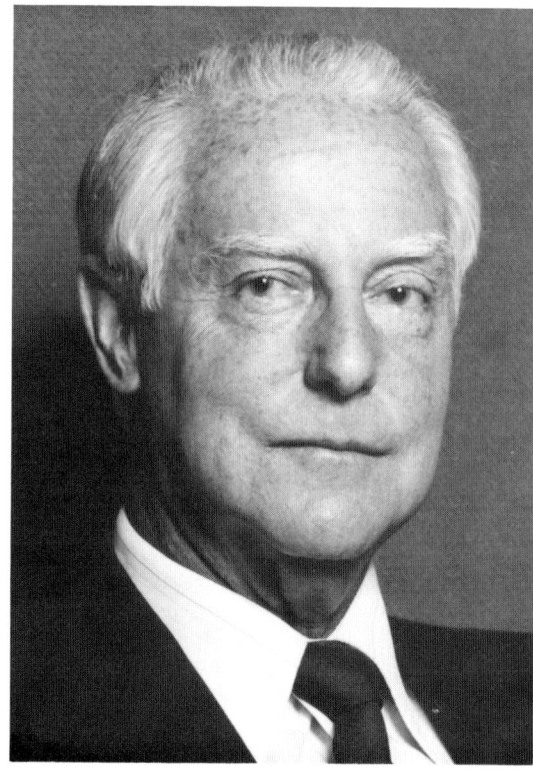

Plate 61. Neville Lane, Chief Technologist, 1945–1985.

I think I should pay tribute to Mr Lane who had joined the laboratory shortly after its creation in the early years of the 1940s who was, when he retired from the hospital in 1985, a member of the staff who had been there for forty years. Mr Lane was always most enthusiastic and hard working and very responsible. He carried much of the laboratory work on his shoulders in the early days and subsequently became the chief technician of the pathology department. He started with Miss Boot. He was at one stage the laboratory boy.

Dr John Holme

Photograph courtesy Neville Lane

morning or the lunch time rounds, and you would end up with two empty beds, having moved about forty people.[51]

Conditions in out-patients were little better:

> Some mornings it was so busy you couldn't get in through the door, you went in through the window ... and indeed, my first attendance at the casualty department at Fremantle Hospital as a junior resident medical officer, I was dragged through the window. The crowd was so great. They would all hand in their prescriptions and there would be up to a hundred people—a hundred, a hundred and twenty people—waiting. Standing room only. Crying children, you know. The lot.[52]

There was one way to increase the number of patients treated in a hospital which had only limited beds, and that was to discharge patients earlier and more frequently. With the opening of the theatre, which almost coincided with the use of antibiotics, the bed-stay decreased from an average of 12.15 days to 10.68 days. Seventeen beds were required daily for new admissions in 1956, and the average patient-stay was 10.52 days. In 1958 it was 11.3, compared to 19.5 at Perth Hospital.

[51] P. B. Smith, interview. Patients were not coddled during their hospital stay. See Appendix 8.
[52] *Ibid.*

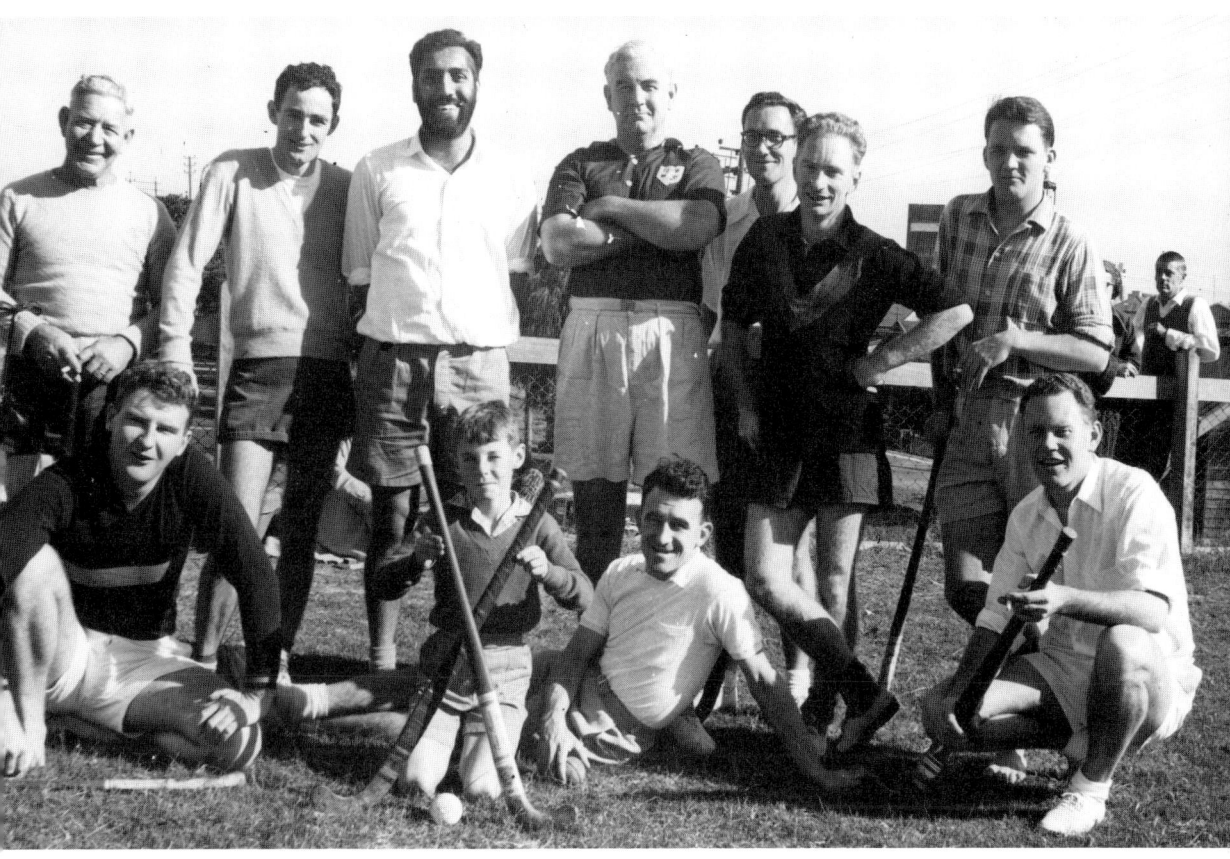

Plate 62.   Recreation at Fremantle Hospital, 1959.
Back row (left to right): Bunny Armfield, Ambulance Driver, Dr Joe Parry, Dr Prithee-Singh, Dr Geoff Leyland, Dr Peter Burvill, Dr Vic White, Dr John Olden.
Front row: Dr Bill Dawson, Guy Leyland, Dr Russell Bisset, Dr Ian Miller.

By 1971–72 at Fremantle there was a new average low of 9.29 days.[53] On occasion, no beds were available, and urgent admissions had to be transferred to Royal Perth Hospital.

The elderly and the chronic sick averaged a longer stay and proved the greatest of all the social service sister's worries, for it often fell to the almoner to free needed beds. Sometimes such patients were sent home with a relative, but most endured a wait of many months for a vacancy at a home for the aged. The position worsened in the early 1950s when many such homes closed. In 1951 Edith May Watters replaced I. M. Gjerde as the social service sister. Daily, since 1941, Gjerde had contacted homes for the elderly and helpless who had to stay in Fremantle Hospital until a bed

---

[53] Figures from Annual Reports, FH.

became available. Men could be admitted to the Sunset Men's Home but women were more difficult to place. In the year 1953–54, nine from Fremantle Hospital were accepted at the Ministering Children's League and Convalescent Home at Cottesloe, six went to Royal Perth Hospital, eight to Mount Henry, Woodside, Knutsford or the Grosvenor, and another eight to the Sunset Men's Home. Two men and two women were admitted at Salvation Army Homes, and 33 at mental hospitals.[54] Admissions to mental hospitals sometimes distressed almoners. One recalled:

> ... These dear old people, who just because they'd come into hospital and become disoriented, were deemed to be senile and were certified to Claremont Hospital ... I think in the second fortnight, eight people came through and it nearly broke my heart ... there was nowhere else to send them ...[55]

Extensions at Mount Henry Hospital improved conditions, but only marginally.

In 1956–57, of the 198 patients at the hospital, 79 were receiving an old-age pension.[56] The opening of a new ward at the Home of Peace between 1957 and 1958, and the Wooroloo Home for the Aged, relieved the shortage somewhat. By the end of the 1950s there were more 'C' class hospitals in the metropolitan area for the aged and infirm which meant that with the Commonwealth benefit and a pension, more could be admitted. The elderly were not the only patients who occupied beds needed for incoming acute cases. Convalescent accident victims were supplied with walking sticks, invalid chairs, crutches and surgical appliances to help them to mobility and prepare them for discharge, and when the hospital ran short of crutches, the waterside workers loaned theirs.

One who was eventually transferred from the hospital to a home was a 52-year-old woman. Discharged from hospital after treatment for hypertension in 1951, she had attended the out-patients' department for eleven months, receiving treatment for high blood pressure. On Christmas Eve, 1952, while having dinner, she began to cry and gradually became unable to move. A doctor referred her to the hospital on Christmas Day, where she was diagnosed as having a cerebral thrombosis. For six weeks the woman was tested and treated. A neurogram and chest X-rays, pathology tests and an electrocardiogram were carried out, her temperature, pulse and respiration were charted, and fluid input and output recorded. A plaster night boot was made to correct foot drop. But as the weeks dragged on, the patient was still unable to speak or respond intelligently. Nothing more could be done. On her papers the final directive to the almoner: 'please inquire about disposal', sounded harsh, but the woman's bed could better serve another with burns or pneumonia, asthma, tetanus, or someone with a broken but healing body.[57]

Between 1951 and 1952 the title of the department of social services was changed to 'almoner's department', and again in 1964–65 to the 'department of medical social work'. Until 1961, when Miss M. Porter was appointed, there were no available trained social workers so senior nursing sisters filled the position. Whatever its

---

[54] FH Annual Report, 1954.
[55] N. Seadon, interviewed by C. Jeffery, 21, 23, 28 August 1985, FH.
[56] FH Annual Report, 1957.
[57] Patient Records, FH.

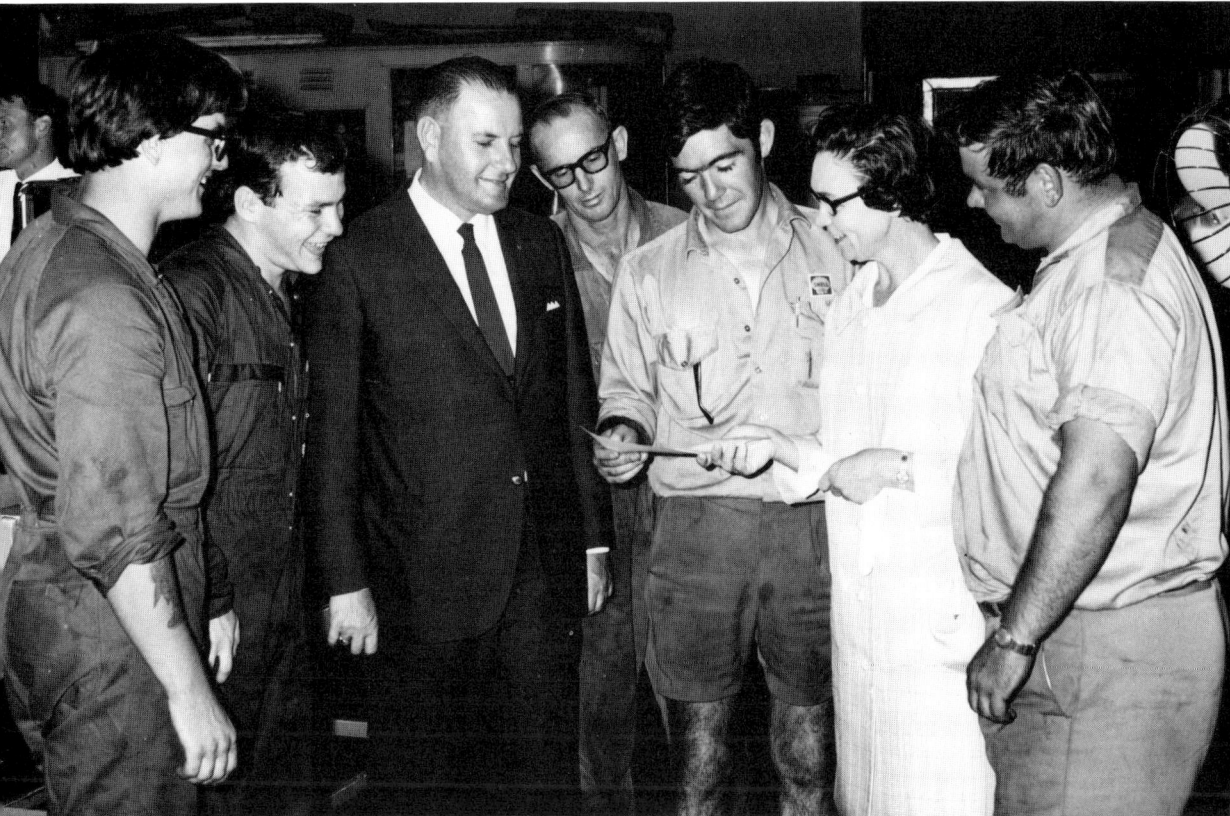

Photograph courtesy Derek T. Large

Plate 63. In 1969 the administrator, Arthur Smith, and almoner, Sister Nora Seadon, received a donation from the Shell Company, North Fremantle, towards the Mayor's Samaritan Fund.

title, the work was the same. In the early 1950s over 2,000 patients were interviewed on admission in a year. Each of the sisters in charge—Edith Watters, Esme Fletcher and Nora Seadon—was aware of old-aged pensioners who needed accommodation to help them stay out of homes for the aged, or who required advice on how to make a pension stretch to provide a reasonable standard of living. The almoner made home visits, often travelling by foot and tram. Not all those in need were elderly, for despite the growth of industry, there was poverty. In 1957 Esme Fletcher wrote that 'the amount of hardship in the community is surprisingly great, due to the large number of unemployed',[58] and each succeeding year there were reports of men with young families experiencing a difficult time, or men 50 to 60 years old, unfit and unable to work. The almoner's department, the Red Cross and the Fremantle Rotary Club were constantly helping with clothing and necessary nourishment, and

[58] FH Annual Report, 1957.

business people in Fremantle often provided the almoner with needed goods. Through the hospital, individual help of a different kind was sometimes given:

> ... we had people coming through that needed jobs ... and the hospital used a lot of these people ... I would go and see someone who ran the kitchen or someone who ran the domestic staff, the housekeeper, the engineer, the carpenter—when patients came through who needed jobs ... they were very generous in putting them on because many of them—had been ill and had to go slowly.[59]

Assistance in the form of employment continued until at least 1970. So busy was the almoner that she was given the help of a runner in the mid-1950s, and a clerk-interpreter a few years later, to help with routine work, and communication with the increasing number of new-Australian patients following the war. Fluent Italian was a necessity, but Miss Pierina spoke Dutch and German as well. In an average month in 1961, 40 interpretations were needed; two years later the number totalled 56 in Spanish and Italian alone. Another of the almoner's important responsibilities was the distribution of insulin to the hospital's diabetic patients.

In 1956 plans were made for a new three-storied block linked to the Ron Doig Block. There would be pathology and laboratory services in the basement, pharmacy and physiotherapy departments, and a blood bank. A new ambulance entry was incorporated—away from work areas, so that casualty cases in all stages of distress would no longer have to be carried through the out-patients' waiting area. Often when a patient died in casualty, out-patients had to vacate the waiting room while the body was removed. In the proposed building, there would be a new casualty department and a new out-patients' room, a casualty theatre and recovery room, and on the floor above, a much-needed ward for women. A nurses' training school was planned for the top floor. Site work was started in January 1957. To immediately ease the accommodation crisis, when the Ministering Children's League Convalescent Home became available for lease, with its rolling green lawns and deep-shaded verandahs overlooking the sea at Cottesloe, the board was glad to take it over with its complement of staff in November 1956. Known as the Mosman Park Annexe, it was used as a pre-discharge ward for post-operative and medical cases. The home proved useful to the hospital. Between 1957 and 1958 alone, 677 patients were nursed at varying times in the 35-bed building.

By 1951 moves to establish a medical school in Western Australia were under way at last. In 1952 land was set aside by the university senate for a chest hospital at Hollywood, and in 1955 a clinical research unit was established at Royal Perth Hospital. Like the Perth, the Children's and King Edward Hospitals, Fremantle Hospital, with its 201-bed capacity, was approved as a teaching hospital for clinical training. The Perth Chest Hospital (which in 1963 was renamed the Sir Charles Gairdner Hospital) was opened late in 1958.[60] Funds for the medical school were enthusiastically gleaned and given from all quarters, and as part of its contribution, Fremantle Hospital organised a boxing match on the South Fremantle Oval, with a proper ring and seating. The undertaking was fraught with difficulties. On the night,

---

[59] Seadon, interview.
[60] N. Stanley (ed.), *The First Quarter Century (1957–1982)*, 1982.

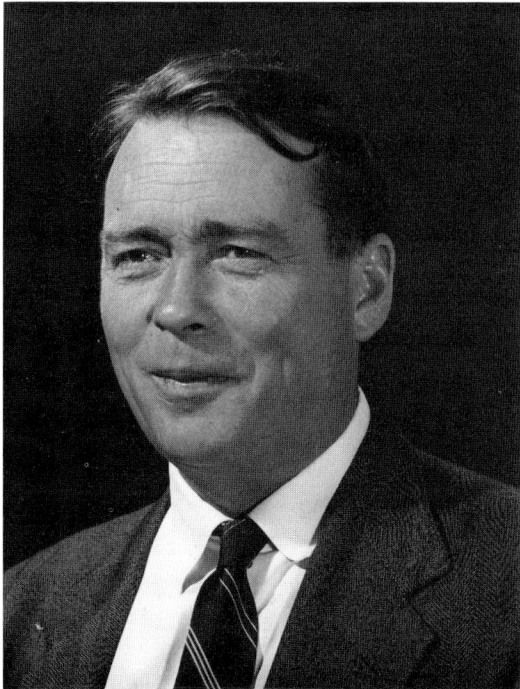

Plate 64. Dr H. J. Rowe, Medical Superintendent, 1952–1962.

We sailed along fairly well with the local doctors, although they regarded every bed as their own and they wouldn't discharge one without making sure they had another patient to come in but I found out that the law said, 'That the medical super-intendent could discharge patients', and I investigated this and from time to time I would walk around the wards and discharge people.

Dr H. J. Rowe

Photograph courtesy Fremantle Hospital

the first fighter billed could not appear, as he was in gaol for robbery. Then it was found that the local professional fighters had a tendency merely 'to strike a blow and lie down';[61] young boxers from the Police Boys' Club proved worthier opponents and were recruited to extend the preliminaries and entertain the crowd. Just before the main match, the West Australian boxer who had been set to fight an opponent from the Eastern States, came in with a badly cut finger and it seemed that the fight would have to be called off. Fast talking and an anaesthetic block in his hand delivered by Medical Superintendent Rowe convinced the man to go on. The eastern competitor was asked to hold his opponent up, at least until the fourth round. It was a magnificent effort 'and everyone saved their faces and everyone had a jolly good night out ... but we raised quite a few quid from this and other methods, and we were actually involved in the medical school because of this,' recalled John Rowe.[62]

Fremantle Hospital's involvement with the medical school did not stop at fund raising. With the ensuing organisation of the school, which naturally centred on the Royal Perth Hospital rather than other metropolitan hospitals, there was a good deal of discussion. The decision in 1955 to place one person nominated by the university on each of the boards of the participating hospitals was not universally welcomed. At Fremantle, Rowe explained the move as:

[61] Rowe, interview.
[62] *Ibid.*

... like having someone on the board of every football team ... on the South Fremantle and the East Fremantle—the whole lot.[63]

The board understood. Jealous of the Fremantle's entity as a community hospital, it united with Rowe in resistance to the proposed new board member's appointment. While happy to offer the facilities of the hospital with its unique potential in the metropolitan area for localised clinical experience from babies to the elderly, and with its shipping cases including tropical and other diseases not usually seen in Western Australia, the board did not want Fremantle Hospital's identity and integrity made subservient to possible empire building by the medical school. If a new representative was to be appointed to the board, the hospital wanted the right of recommendation which they believed was theirs under the *Hospitals Act*—preferably someone with a Fremantle background, with business acumen, with Fremantle interests at heart:

> ... someone that *they* would like to sit on their board, rather than to have one person with the ear to the ground in every hospital in the metropolitan area. We thought it was healthier ...[64]

Few major decisions by organisations are made exclusively over a board table, and while the university held gatherings to work out its aims and directions, impromptu meetings of the Fremantle Hospital board were sometimes held on Sundays over 'a bit of malt'[65] in an old shed among the cabbages and cauliflowers behind Bill Wauhop's house. The potential power of the university in the hospital's affairs was discussed many times and, finally,

> ... it was determined ... that the university would come down there as a group, [only] to run a clinic ... not the whole of the hospital and all of the staff ... Otherwise [the hospital] wasn't going to become part of the university hospital system, and that was really the final say-so.[66]

At a meeting held at Perth Hospital to discuss the position of the university and its influence in the state's hospital system, Rowe strongly voiced the Fremantle Hospital board's reservations and the 'meeting ended in chaos'.[67]

When the medical school was officially opened at the University of Western Australia on 10 April 1958, there was no university representative on the Fremantle Hospital board. Nor was one appointed by 1960, and although the two interest groups co-operated, it was with a certain tension. The decision to create a third surgical clinic for the use of the university at the hospital, and to equally share the new cases, coincided with a down-turn in patients and, as the two existing clinics continued the

---

[63] Daly-Smith, interview.
[64] *Ibid.* Daly-Smith commenced as the honorary medical staff's representative on the board, in April 1957.
[65] Rowe, interview.
[66] *Ibid.* For conditions of training, see University Medical School, *Teaching Hospitals' Act 1955*, 4 Elizabeth II No 31 of 1955.
[67] Rowe, interview.

treatment of patients already under their supervision, it seemed that the hospital was commanding the lion's share of new work. The university

> ... reckoned for a long time that we somehow or other had engineered that we got all the work. That we got all the acute ops. and everything. So they weren't too happy ...[68]

In September 1962, and again in August 1963, the university senate requested representation on the hospital's board, but nothing further was done.

After studying precedents of university representation in hospitals in the Eastern States, the board in January 1964 received an imposing deputation. Sir Alex Reid (the Chancellor), Professor Clews (the Deputy Vice-Chancellor) Sir Laurence Jackson, Dr H. Stewart and Mr Crawley (the Registrar of the Faculty of Medicine) pointed out that their involvement on the board would benefit the hospital in the planning and development of teaching facilities, and would prove a financial advantage through the provision of funds for required facilities. When the deputation left, the board agreed to nominate a member of the senate to the hospital board—but only from a list provided by the university. The decision was not agreeable to the senate who wanted a representative of their own choice. For three years the matter remained in abeyance. At the end of 1966 Dr Geoff Leyland, who had succeeded Rowe as medical superintendent in 1962, received word from one of Fremantle Hospital's honorary physicians, Dr Robert Leedman:

> It is a pity that the differences between the Board and the university are still so unsolved. With this in mind I feel you must develop the hospital on a post-graduate level ...[69]

Leedman recommended the provision of senior registrars, the employment of a full-time radiologist and a radiological registrar, and encouraged access to the medical physics department at Royal Perth Hospital. Although the Dean of the Faculty of Medicine, Professor Rolf ten Seldam, was anxious to resolve the rift between the hospital and the university, it was another year before the question was again broached. The senate remained unmoved in its view that the university's representative should be a person of its own choice and not necessarily a member of the senate.[70] As its representative, they recommended Professor G. G. Lennon, the permanent Dean of the Faculty of Medicine. This time, the board's attitude softened. Coincidentally, John Rowe was not in his chair at the meeting when the board agreed to the university's proposal. With Lennon's appointment, a greater correlation between the board and clinical training at the hospital was forged.

Building of the new block, under architect Ben Clifton of the Public Works Department, was not without difficulties. Hospital routines were interrupted and there was noise and dust as walls tumbled, ceilings were brought down, concrete mixers churned and pneumatic drills gnawed at concrete and people's patience. In the pharmacy:

---

[68] Minchin, interview.
[69] Minutes of BM, 23 January 1967, FH.
[70] *Ibid.*, 22 January 1968.

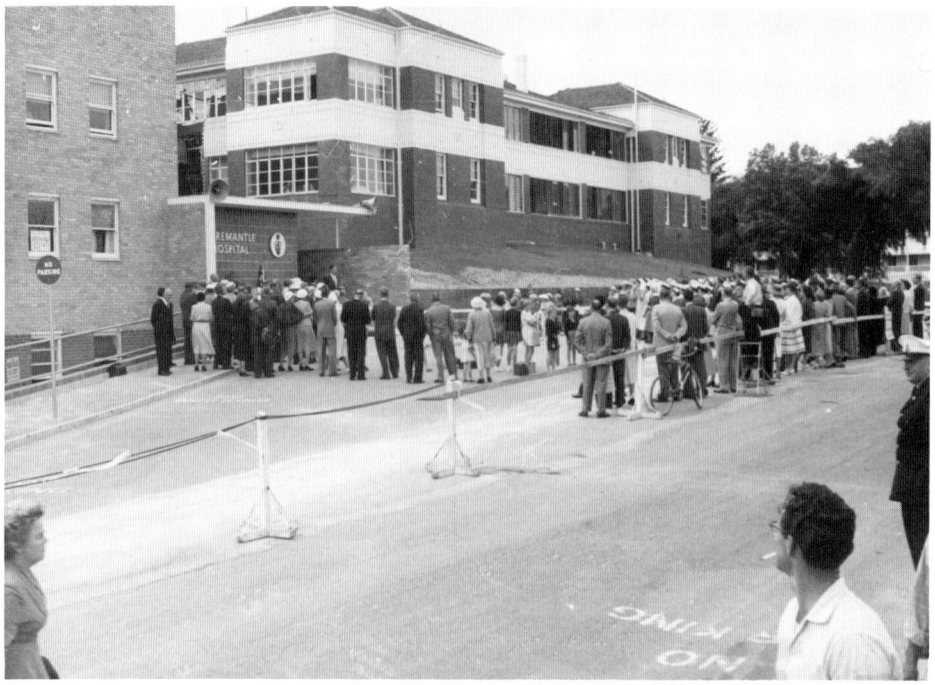

Photograph courtesy Fremantle Hospital

Plate 65. Official opening of the William Wauhop Wing, 22 April 1960. McCallum Block can be seen on the right.

> I think they [the wards in the McCallum Block] started with about twenty-two beds, but after a while in the male community [the downstairs ward], the alcoves were used for beds and then the back verandah was enclosed with canvas blinds ... sometimes they had thirty-six patients there. It was a very busy ward.
>
> Matron Olive Jones

... for days on end the staff carried out their duties surrounded by a haze of fine plaster dust and in a condition of mind closely akin to a state of suspended animation.[71]

The trip to the pharmacy bulk storerooms in the old Ron Doig Block basement was frequently hazardous, with building rubble from above rattling down with spent mortar. Other departments were similarly affected.

William Wauhop had been on the board since 1933 and had been a wise administrator and co-ordinator, and straight and honest in his dealings as the chairman since 1947. It was said, tongue-in-cheek, that 'even if he barracked for East Fremantle, he would do things for South Fremantle or anyone else',[72] and many recognise that he 'was prepared to do anything, go anywhere, be available at any time for

---

71 J. Jeffery, FH Annual Report, 1960.
72 Daly-Smith, interview.

the hospital'.[73] It was decided to name the new wing in his honour. At the official opening on Friday, 22 April 1960, many people from all sections of the community attended as Ross Hutchinson, M.L.C., the Minister for Health, declared the William Wauhop Wing open. The enthusiastic public flocked through the building on tours of inspection when it was opened on the following Saturday and Sunday. Perhaps only nurses were disappointed. So great was the need for beds that the plans for their training school had to be sacrificed for ward space.

When the pharmacy transferred into its rooms in the William Wauhop Wing, which Jeffery had designed, there was room for the pharmacist to indulge in his crusade to cut costs. Dressings and drugs were bought in greater bulk, including cotton wool by the hundredweight bale, and other necessities such as methylated spirits—in 44-gallon drums. In 1966, however, the department had to buy cotton balls, because the cotton fluff released in the tedious making of the balls by the nursing staff, choked the air conditioners. Great demijohns of senega and ammonia and morphia and aspirin were mixed ready for issue; nothing was bought that could be made. Work in pharmacy increased and diversified. With the introduction of the *National Pharmaceutical Benefit Act*, all drugs dispensed had to be carefully listed in order to claim the government's subsidy. Advertisements for new drugs which proliferated from the mid-1950s took time to study, and until 1957, when Bob Willetts from Watson Victor took over their responsibility, surgical instruments had to be ordered, repaired and distributed through the pharmacy department. A drug register had to be kept, and occasionally, Jeffery had to admonish young residents for nipping the pure alcohol to spice a punch. The cost of drugs changed continually. In 1967 when the patent right to produce them expired and Australia was involved in their production, the cost of antibiotics began to drop, but it seemed that other drugs rose in compensation. This prompted the formation of the Tender Board. Rowe, Jeffery, the honorary doctors, and the chief pharmacists of the other metropolitan hospitals listed basic effective pills and potions which were ordered in bulk through the Government Stores. Drug companies undercut each other for the orders, and private doctors at the hospitals were issued with a basic list of the stock which would be available through the hospital. As a result, pharmaceutical costs were reduced—both through the supply of cheaper drugs to the hospital, and the issue of tried, effective medications, the supply of which cost less than almost identical newly-released ones, high in price because of added vitamins and minerals. When John Jeffery retired in 1967, after 25 years at the hospital, Wally Slaven took both his place and his task of keeping up with the increasing number of out-patients' prescriptions, with costs and ward supplies.

In 1958, before the move to the new wing, Dr John Holme, the full-time pathologist, noted 'the world-wide tendency for laboratory procedures to play a more important part in diagnoses and management of patients'.[74] Some new equipment was bought for the department, but very reluctantly, and when Holme requested a new microtome he offered to loan the board £100 if it would agree to contribute to the purchase. The offer was not taken up, but the board did order the microtome.

[73] A. Smith, interview
[74] FH Annual Report, 1958.

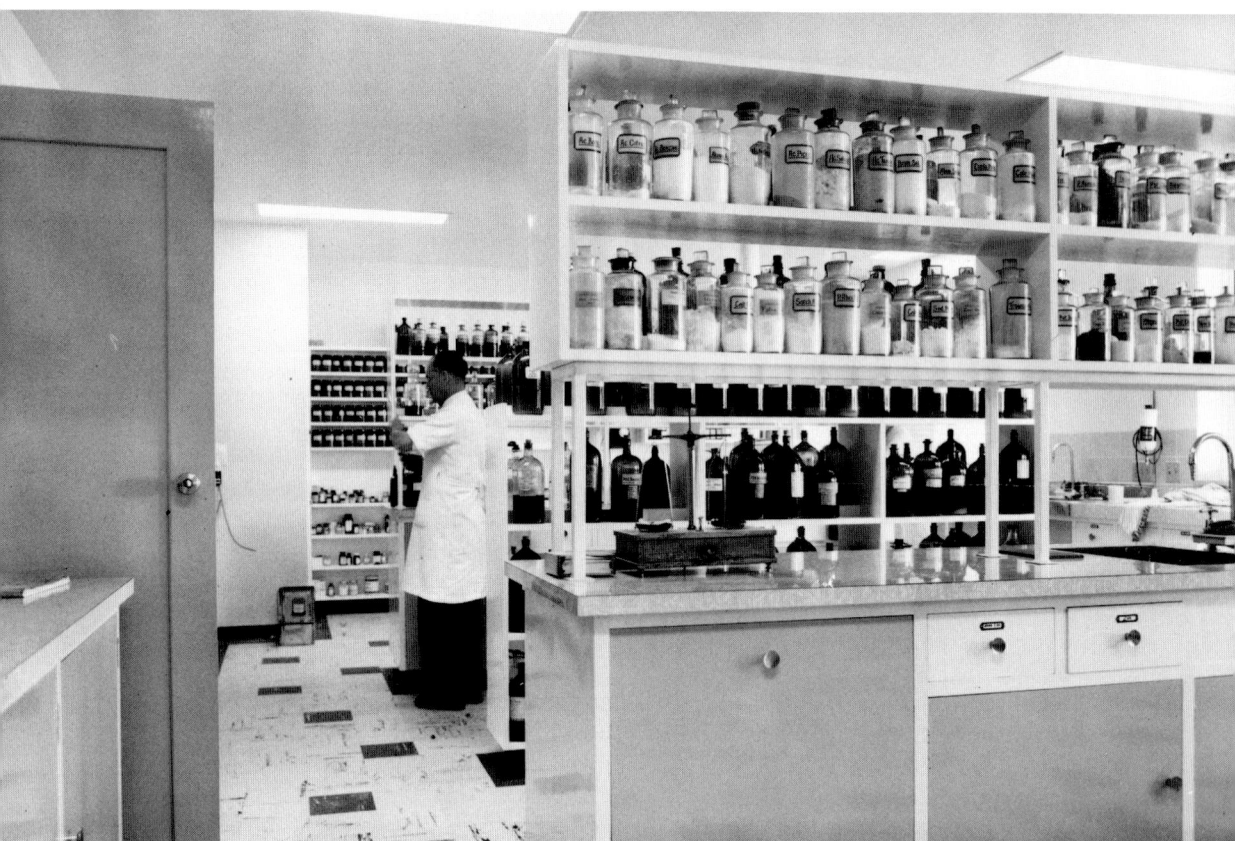

Photograph courtesy Fremantle Hospital

Plate 66. Les Cooper in the new pharmacy. In June 1960 the pharmacy department was moved from a cramped room in the Ron Doig Block to a spacious new area in the William Wauhop Wing.

> From Pharmacy, you were only allowed one roll of cotton wool and one roll of combine per week. Now, it didn't matter if you had six suprapubic prostatectomies that were all pouring fluid from their suprapubic wound, you were still only allowed one roll of combine per week. It was absolutely impossible at times to do this, so the person who got on well with the staff was sent physically by the sister, to go down and wheedle out of them whatever else she needed.
>
> Olga Hedemann
> Director of Nursing

Although in 1956, when the number of autopsies increased, and a new pathologist, Dr P. B. Nicholl, was appointed in charge of morbid anatomy and histopathology, separate departments of morbid anatomy, surgical pathology and haemapathology were not immediately established within the pathology department. These came in 1968. With the move to the William Wauhop Wing, the work of the pathology department increased. The blood bank, which was incorporated into pathology's

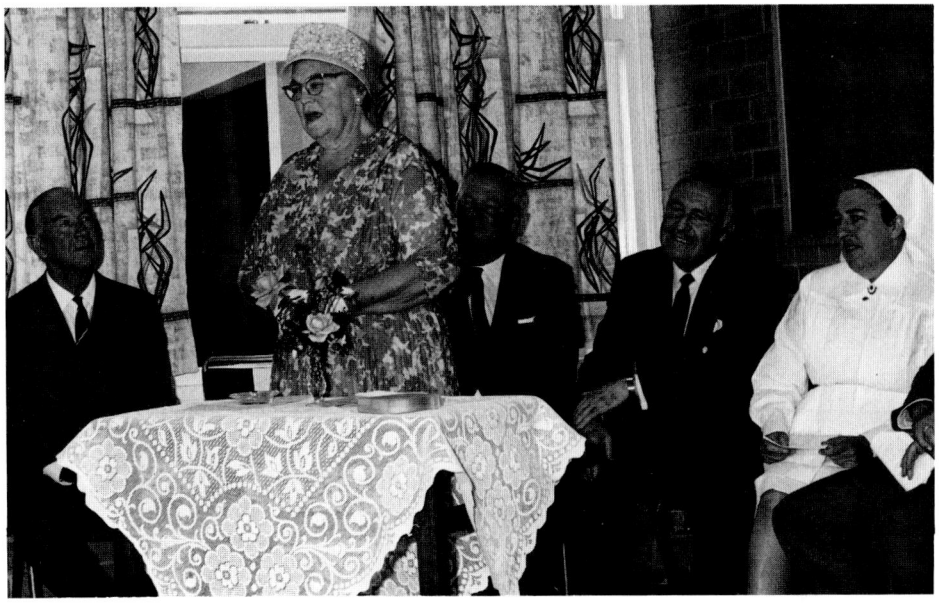

Photograph courtesy Fremantle Hospital

Plate 67. Official opening of the Mavis Fuller Wing of the Olive Jones Nurses' Home, by Honourable G. C. MacKinnon, M.L.C., 18 February, 1971.

(Left to right): Dr G. Leyland, Medical Superintendent; Sister Mavis Fuller; Mr C. C. Bennett, Chairman of the Board; Hon. G. C. McKinnon; Matron M. Leworthy.

haematology department from September 1968, changed from glass bottles to plastic packs in 1965 and although the sisters still worked in the blood bank, they also helped the Fremantle council in its poliomyelitis and triple-antigen immunization programme at the Birmingham Infant Health Centre in Fremantle.

Despite the need for a nurses' training school to replace the small prefabricated building erected in 1948, there was an even greater need for nurses' accommodation. In 1958 there were five separate nurses' homes. The senior home in the hospital grounds accommodated 114, and there were 21 beds in the junior section of Balding Home. Nine nurses lived at number 1 Stirling Street, and there were 26 living in Warwick House and 36 at the adjoining Bundi Kudja property.[75] To accommodate the nurses needed to staff the new William Wauhop Wing, a new nurses' home was envisaged, and when a property in Solomon Street, adjacent to Warwick House came onto the market early in 1958, the board formed a deputation to appeal for its purchase. Costing £13,500 the property was named Atwell House after its previous owners. The next expansion on the site was the new nurses' home. Built with views over Fremantle and the Indian Ocean to Rottnest, the new, multi-storied home accommodating 101 nurses, was opened on 20 July 1962 and named the Olive Jones Nurses' Home in honour of the retiring matron. One last time the quarters for

[75] *Ibid.*

nurses were extended, and in 1970 the Mavis Fuller Wing was named in remembrance of the deputy matron.

Olive Jones and Mavis Fuller with Sylvia Gill as third in command of nursing at the hospital, proved a rare blend of compassion and competence. The slightly-built matron was a fine administrator and nurse, and expected the same high standards in her staff. It was usually only in times of distress that a nurse realized the depths of Olive Jones' concern. Many years later a nurse observed: '. . . She always knew everything about you—more than you thought!'[76] Twice a day matron would visit sick nurses in their special ward to quietly inquire about their well-being. Although she was reserved, it was obvious that Olive Jones 'really cared' and would even wait in the quarters to 'seek out anyone missing from meals' to ask: 'what have you had for lunch today nurse?'[77] Far from being reserved, it was said of Mavis Fuller that 'she was our other mum',[78] and the extent of her compassion for patients and nurses alike was boundless. It was understood by nurses that the wharf was taboo to them, unless there was an occasional officers' party to which senior nurses, through matron, were invited. Not all followed this dictum. Sailors coming to port would often ring the various metropolitan nurses' quarters in the hope of finding an escort, and it was well known on the wharves that in order of availability, the main hospitals were named and ranked as Bulk Store No. 1—Children's Hospital; Bulk Store No. 2—Perth Hospital; Bulk Store No. 3—the less likely Fremantle Hospital. But some nurses did go to parties on ships and it was not unknown for a wharf worker to ring Sister Fuller with the advice. She recalled on one occasion, a wharf night supervisor's call:

> He said, the police have been notified . . . but my daughter is training with you and we know down here what you stand for—and the hospital. And you're the only one who can solve it. So I said to [Mildred] Murray . . . Come down . . . I put my dressing gown over my night dress and went down, and he [the supervisor] put her [the nurse] into a little cubicle place that was attached to an office, and as soon as he saw us coming—see—we were able to take her and put her in a taxi and take her away and we'd only just got out of one portion of the wharf when the police came . . .[79]

Such was her presence that few admonished by the deputy matron repeated a misdemeanour. Sister Gill (Gilly) was respected and regarded by nurses and medical staff alike, as a sympathetic nurse who 'comes on duty and at the end of time of duty, the work is done'.[80]

Between 1945 and 1987 there were many changes for nurses. In those first years they still slept on horse-hair mattresses in rows of iron beds along the Balding Home verandah:

> We slept out on the verandah. Two to a room, but that only held the wardrobes and dressing tables. The beds were all lined up like a barracks on the verandah, not en-

[76] K. Grimshaw, notes, FH.
[77] Pilling, notes.
[78] M. Christie, notes, FH.
[79] Fuller, interview.
[80] P. B. Smith, interview.

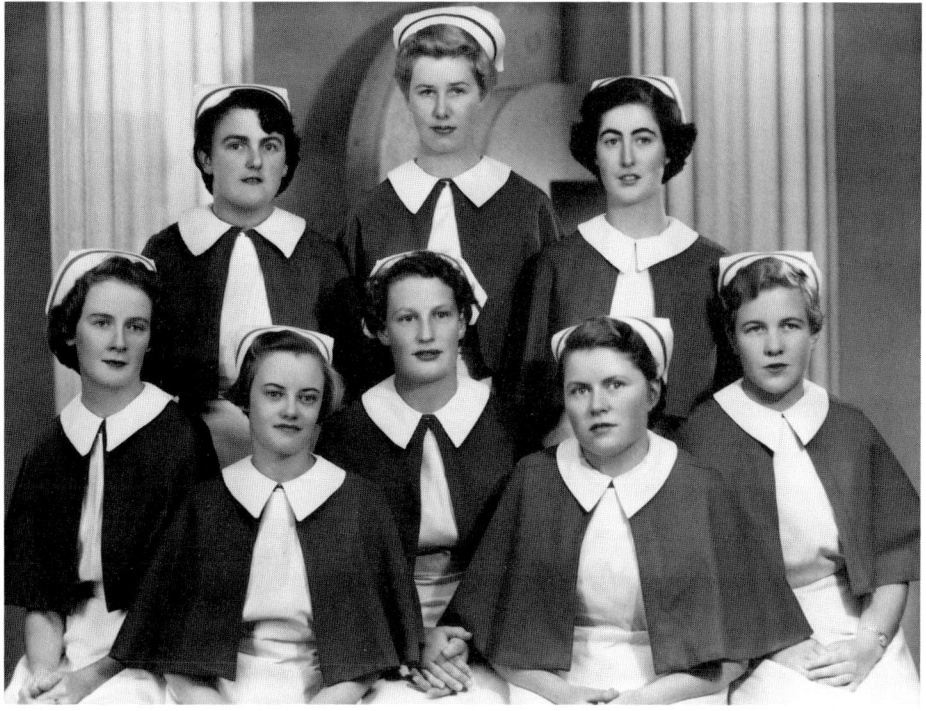

Photograph courtesy Fremantle Hospital

Plate 68. The preliminary training school class, February 1952.

Back (left to right): Olga Hedemann, Lois Wroth, Joan Mulloy.
Front: Noreen Wolfe, Rhonda Gillon, Olive Doran, Jean Hamblett, Joan Newling.

> Well, in that first preliminary training school, which as I recall it, it lasted for ten weeks, we had anatomy and physiology and that was always the first lecture of the day, because it was the hardest and you were supposed to be more alert at that time. We were a very innocent lot. I had come through a very protective family, but I found out sitting in that classroom, that other people had come through more protected or non-communicative type of families than I had, because when we got to some of the anatomy lectures we found out about our own bodies, it was quite a scream—the little we knew about what was there.

Olga Hedemann
Director of Nursing

closed, canvas blinds that flapped and leaked the rain in the winter. There were two bathrooms for the ground floor, which meant you were sharing two baths—no showers—two baths with probably about thirty people.[81]

There were snores and muttered sleep-talk, and no privacy until a senior year when sometimes rooms were shared between two, or a single room was allocated. It was difficult not to stir when the junior night nurse came around to rouse those on early

[81] D. Western, interviewed by C. Jeffery, 23 March and 4 April 1987, FH.

shift. Shared rooms at Bundi and Atwell, outside the hospital precinct, meant greater freedom, and while the Olive Jones Home promised the privacy of a single room it 'lacked the homeliness of the others'.[82] Nevertheless, in the early 1960s when the music was played there, it seemed that everyone would leap into the corridor and dance the 'slosh'.[83] Many nurses heard the comforting words 'you'll be alright honey' from a special domestic; 'I looked after those girls from the time they came in to train,' said Ann Brain proudly.[84] Cooking at the nurses' homes sometimes showed initiative: eggs boiled in an electric kettle or fried on the sole plate of a hot iron. One nurse summed up her training as 'friendships and mateship, hard work, but happy days, living together. Pride in being a nurse at Fremantle.'[85] With the training of nurses at W.A.I.T. (later Curtin University), hospital-based living-in and training was phased out, but many ex-trainees regretted the change.

In the 1950s there was a lack of basic ward equipment. Nurses often started early, just to obtain bowls for washing their patients:

> You're on duty at 6 a.m. but we always were on the wards by twenty to six, for two reasons: because you had to go to breakfast at quarter to seven, but before you go to breakfast at quarter to seven, you had to do two full sponges, and two bowls . . . Before you could do your two full sponges and your two bowls, you had to procure the bowls with which to work, and if you had a mate on the evening before, she would tell you when she came off where she had hidden two bowls.[86]

There were only 12 bowls in male medical for 31 patients. 'We worked and we worked—but a great deal of satisfaction was had,' recalled one nurse.[87] Nurses under the Columbo Plan came in July 1956; runners—girls too young to start training but who worked for a year doing messages and helping where they could, and enrolled nurses, were introduced to supplement the basic nursing staff.

In the 1960s there were the Beatles, the Bay of Pigs scare, the assassination of John Kennedy and the landing of men on the moon. Closer to home, the Meckering earthquake shook wards and quarters. There was staff member John Gerovich, a footballer and local heart-throb. There was an end to testing urines with methylated burners, the introduction of steam sterilizers and a change to ampoules for injections, replacing the tablets dissolved in a teaspoon of water. Throw-away packs from C.S.D. ended days and nights of 'cutting square pieces of gauze and combines . . .'[88] With the use of vitamin B12 in treating pernicious anaemia, there was even an end to the old treatment:

> Take a fresh animal liver, place it in your hand-operated mincer and macerate it, being careful to catch and preserve the turgid blood which oozes from it during mincing.
>   Place this blood in a glass and top with orange juice. Put the mangled liver between

[82] R. Morgan (née Hood), notes, FH.
[83] L. Gaughin (née Hamilton), notes, FH.
[84] Brain, interview.
[85] Pilling, notes.
[86] Western, interview. A 'bowl' was the term used for a patient who was given a bowl of warm water with which to wash. Backs had to be washed by the nurse.
[87] J. Morrissey, notes.
[88] Western, interview. C.S.D.—Central Sterilising Department.

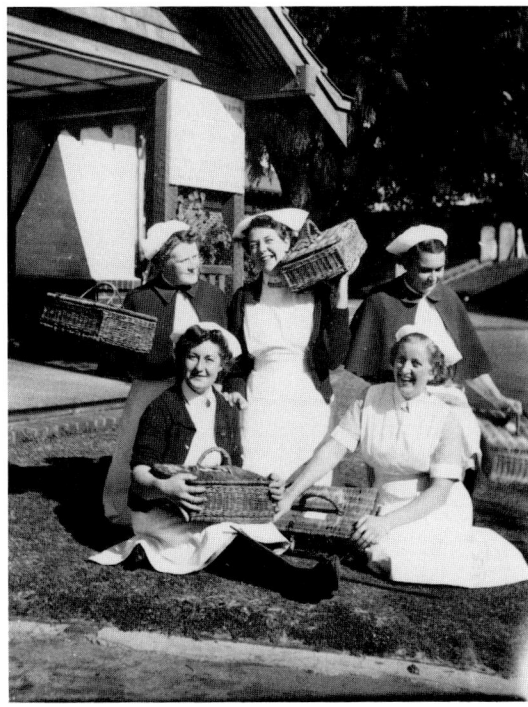

Plate 69. Nursing night staff. They shared the decades-old practice of concocting a meal from the contents of the night staff baskets.

(Left to right): Pat Giles, L. Bennett, C. Lardi, M. Yates, C. Craig, *c.* 1950s.

As far as the night staff meals went [in 1930–33], we had five cane baskets put out for us, with one tin of salmon or half a dozen eggs as the case might be, between all of us—eight on night duty and a night sister or staff nurse in charge.

Hilda Heath
Nursing Staff

Photograph courtesy Fremantle Hospital

bread and butter to make a sandwich then take it, with the bloody orange cocktail, to the patient. Persuade him that it is both beneficial and palatable before the bewildered person begins gagging and retching and you may safely leave.[89]

Most nurses still learned to bolt their food, to queue to use the telephone, to come in undetected without a late pass. Sometimes young residents were sympathetic:

... there was the gate to the hospital and it was locked at night, barbed wire fences ... you'd pull your car up in Alma Street, open the four doors of your car. There would be cars around with nurses and their boyfriends and you would hear click-click, click-click of their heels on the road, and you just sat there. Somebody would get in beside you and then there would be two more who would get in the back and then another one would get into the back and then you would drive up to the right, turn your lights on, and drive up to the gate. The orderly would come out, turn the torch onto your number plate, and then he would open the gate and you would drive right into the hospital. Then you would pull up at a point near the old Moreton Bay fig and the nurses would dive out and race up to the back of the hospital ... everybody knew it went on, but nobody sort of said anything. And Fuller knew about it.[90]

All nurses learned never to say 'Isn't the hospital quiet?'[91]

[89] J. Lancaster, notes, FH.
[90] P. B. Smith, interview.
[91] Garswell, notes, FH.

The rigid ranking of nurses in the 1950s seemed as set as concrete. In the first year it was 'standing hands behind the back and waiting to be noticed by a senior nurse'.[92] In the second year it was still 'bowing and kowtowing'.[93] Except for night-duty staff, even the dining-room tables were allocated according to seniority. But by the 1980s, with increased familiarity between senior and junior staff, with the re-organisation of nurse training, and changes both in the perception of their duties and the status of nurses, the old hierachical system has been largely undermined.

Although in the 1980s a reduced staff serves the hospital at night when patients sleep and wards are quiet, there was a dearth of night staff in the mid-1950s and 1960s. Usually a third-year and a first- or second-year nurse were allocated to each ward, with a staff nurse in charge of the whole hospital. The junior on each ward was still responsible for collecting the night staff's food in the large old wicker baskets. When routine work was finished there were always swabs to make from an open roll of cotton wool which 'fluffed up' to make better balls when placed on top of the little floor radiators, but which had to be carefully watched as they could catch fire. 'The doctors prowled around all night, always hungry, looking for a feed,' remembered one nurse.[94] Some nights were exhausting and nurses shared experiences well outside those in other areas of paid employment such as teaching, domestic or factory work. One staff nurse recalled a night when

> ... there was an operation going on in theatre and the other staff nurse was in theatre doing the operation ... I was looking after casualty and the rest of the hospital and I only had student nurses on. So I had to check every drug, everything, myself ... While all this was happening, a patient with myocardial infarct comes into emergency—in the casualty department. So, I diagnosed this and left him in casualty while I ran up to the theatre and ... I put my head inside the door there to the doctors, who were both in theatre ... I tell them that I have got a patient down in the emergency department or down in casualty with a heart attack. So they tell me to go back and give him some morphia and admit him. I go back and I give him some morphia and I admit him and I get that done, but while I'm in the middle of doing this, they ring me from female medical to tell me that a patient up there has gone absolutely berserk. I get up to see her and tell them to get the strongroom ready over in female surg for this woman that's gone berserk. I got an orderly to come and help me to get her over into the strongroom and still I have got no help, because the doctors are still fiddling around trying to get an appendix out or something, you see. So I get her over in there and we lock her into the strongroom. In the morning, I go and see how she is going in the strongroom, because I looked in through the hole in the door and she seemed to be quieter. I went in and she attacked me and she pulled off my two pockets and ripped my uniform down the front and it's just before I have to go and see Matron Jones. I go off and see Matron Jones who is sitting up in bed with her long tresses, brushing her hair and she asked me, What on earth have I been doing? most disapprovingly. So, I give her the report and I go back to the wards to check the insulins and things, because all of the seven o'clock drugs have to be checked, and I'm racing around like a hairy goat. I'm in female medical checking the insulins and I look across and I see the window of the strongroom is open. I drop the insulin and I rush across to female surgical to the strongroom, and

[92] M. Davis (née Mawson), notes, FH.
[93] Peek, notes.
[94] Pilling, notes.

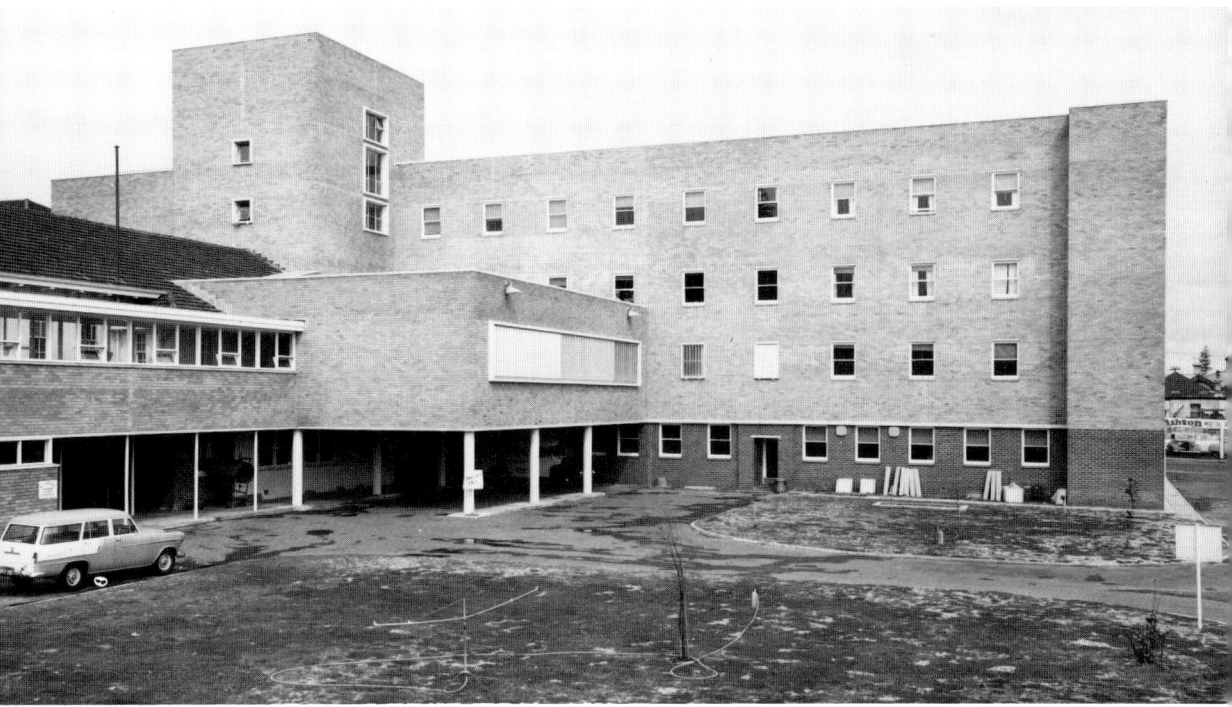

Photograph courtesy Fremantle Hospital

Plate 70. Fremantle Hospital William Wauhop Wing, north-western section. The pharmacy department is in the basement on the left, with the pathology department to the right, casualty on the ground floor, then male community and female community wards on the first and second floors respectively.

there is no woman. There's a roof outside, a bit of roof, and she's got out of the window onto the roof and jumped to the ground below. And you can see her lying face down on the ground below. So with heart in mouth and everything, I race around there and find that, yes, she's still alive. However, she has fractured her femur. We had to get her back up and into bed and you can imagine what time I got off that morning![95]

Such nights were unforgettable.

Some learning gained from experience was also unforgettable. There was one sensitive area of concern that Olive Jones, understandably, never overcame in her administrative career, even by 1960. Casualty in the William Wauhop Wing contained an eight-bed, two-room observation ward for post-minor surgery with a minor theatre attached. The sister in casualty supervised the whole area, but there was a staff nurse in charge of the theatre. A sister of lesser rank who was to be employed in charge of the observation ward in 1960, was interviewed by both matron and the medical superintendent. Rowe claimed that as the observation ward

[95] Hedemann, interview.

was outside the main-stream, it was therefore under his jurisdiction. Jones did not outwardly disagree, but the new sister found after a while

> ... that there was a fair amount of obstruction. I couldn't get the things done that I wanted to, and it just wasn't working well at all. Dear old Dot Daly took me aside one day and explained in words of one syllable, and she said it was because I was actually on the staff of the medical superintendent and not the matron.[96]

The echoes of dispute between medical superintendent and matron over the control of nurses was familiar, and while the parties were amicable, the principle remained unchanged. This time there was little contention, and the sister was transferred to a position under Matron Jones.

Two years later, in 1962, just before she left her flat, the matron propped a note on the telephone:

> Welcome to Fremantle Hospital. I hope you are as happy there over the years as I have been and I will pick you up at eight o'clock in the morning to take you down to introduce you to the hospital.[97]

Like Matron Balding before her, Matron Jones had seen changes and made changes and with Rowe, had been part of a formidable team in administering the hospital. When she retired, she had been matron of Fremantle Hospital for nineteen years. Ex-trainees, when they gathered as they had since the late 1930s, invited the new Matron, Mavis Leworthy, to their next meeting, and as usual they recalled old times. Many Fremantle ex-trainees retained a strong loyalty to the hospital, and often kept up the friendships of their training years. Each year a reunion dinner or celebration was held. Cake stalls to raise money for the Eleanor Harvey House for retired nurses were also well supported. In 1966 Mrs Parker, the secretary of 28 years, resigned. Mavis Leworthy worked well with the ex-trainees and encouraged graduating nurses to join the association. She was adopted by Sister Fuller and professed to finding 'a warmth in that hospital which I don't think I have ever felt before'.[98] The new matron also worked well with Medical Superintendent Geoff Leyland but was not so keen on monthly board meetings, when she had to stand outside the boardroom door until summoned to give her report, 'which was most embarrassing and that happened until the day I retired'.[99] She was however, a member of the building committee and influential in planning new wards and buildings at the hospital.

The growth in population and industry at Fremantle continued in the late 1950s, and in December 1959 the government finally decided the hospital's future. To meet the needs of people south of the river, extensions to the hospital in Alma Street were planned, and the land at Hilton Park was retained for a future hospital but not immediately developed. The board looked to the built-up school area to the west, and approached the Medical Department about the possibility of securing the infants' school site for future expansion. In December 1959 it took over the private hospital

[96] C. Jeffery, interview.
[97] M. Leworthy, interviewed by C. Jeffery, 3 and 17 April 1985.
[98] *Ibid.* 'Ex-trainees': members of the FH Ex-trainee Nurses' Association.
[99] *Ibid.*.

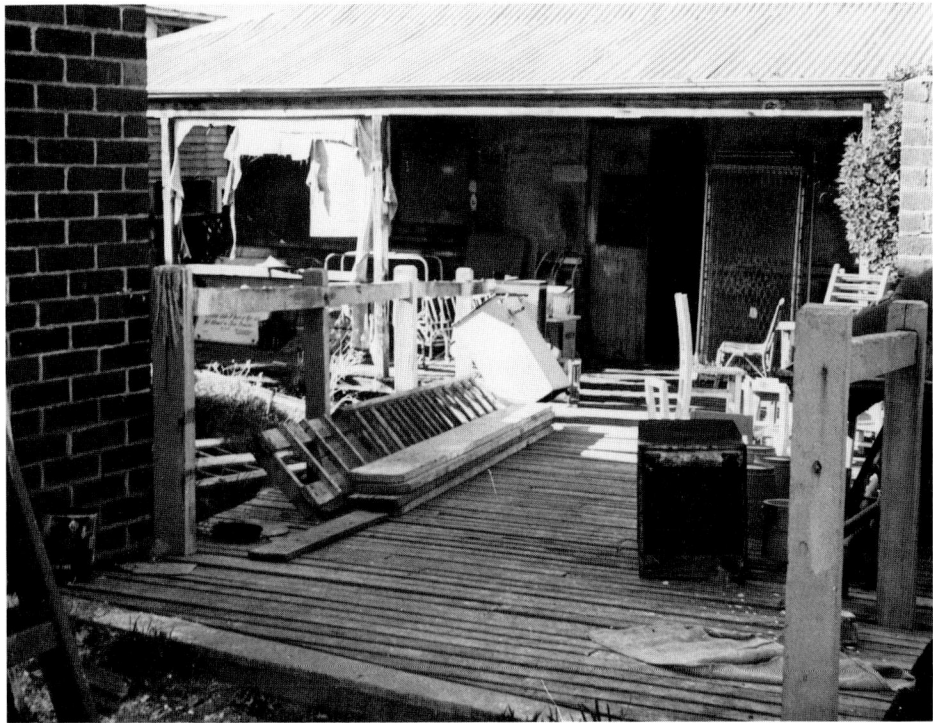

Plate 71. Looking down towards the painters' old shop, 1960. The maintenance staff—electricians, painters, carpenters, refrigeration mechanics and plumbers were increased in number from eleven in 1958 to 70 twenty-six years later.

named St Helen's at 33 Moss Street, and called it the East Fremantle Annexe. The elegant old home which had been built in 1912 for John Bateman's widow,[100] was first used by the hospital as a residence and training school for new probationer nurses before they entered the wards. This left the old female medical ward free for the block training of other nurses who had been using the Mosman Park Annexe as a temporary training school since early 1959. Not before time, plans were also made to replace the cramped, converted army huts which served as the workshops and stores departments. So old and dilapidated were they that in 1958 the stumps of the painters' workshop were reported as three to four inches 'out of plumb and the building appeared to have removed bodily downhill'.[101] The old, prefabricated nurses' training school was demolished, and on the site, new workships were erected. By 1962, the maintenance staff had taken their tools and equipment and set them up in the new buildings.

The eleven employees on the maintenance staff were pleased at the overdue move.

[100]   See *Fremantle Gazette*, 24 September 1980.
[101]   Minutes of BM, 21 April 1958, FH.

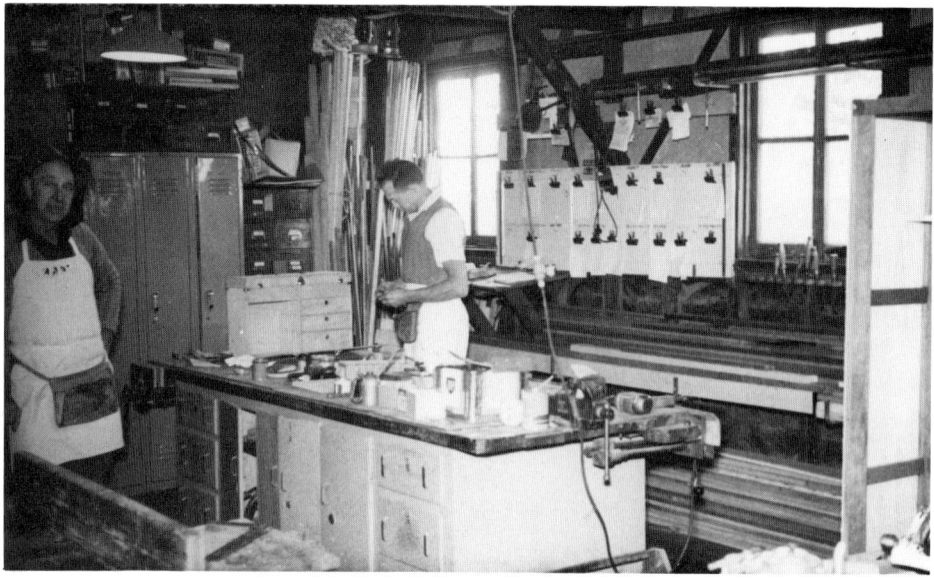

Photograph courtesy Fremantle Hospital

Plate 72.   The carpenters' old workshop.
(Left to right): Norm Christie and Len Marshall.

> ... it was very small, approximately about twenty by fifteen with only one work bench, one band saw and ... a shadow board with one set of tools ... And they were always wanting alterations or repairs ... I suppose our biggest percentage of work was new work, but there was always the maintenance to do as well in the old wards and they were always up-dating the old wards or they'd shift them around, so you were making something the whole time.

> Len Marshall
> Hospital Carpenter, 1958–1984

The previous carpenters' shop had been very small, 'approximately about twenty by fifteen, with only one work bench, one bandsaw and just a buzzer there'.[102] Lockers, storage boxes, a sliding rack on which to hang a skeleton for teaching—all manner of things were made in the shop:

> People would just, you know, say they wanted something and we'd go back and work something out ... but there were no drawings or anything. If they wanted ... things, they would go and tell us what they wanted and wave their arms around and I'd come back with the ideas and work out something.[103]

Repairs and new work at the annexes and the nurses' homes as well as at the main hospital had to be done by the different maintenance departments. The thick-set engineer, Bob 'Shorty' Longstaff, co-ordinated the work of plumbing, painting,

[102]   L. Marshall, interviewed by C. Jeffery, 4 February 1986, FH.
[103]   *Ibid.*

carpentry and electrical repairs. When George Schneider, the plumber, investigated a blockage in the medical ward plumbing, there were no sewerage plans to go by, and when he located the course of the plumbing with his spade, he found the earthenware pipes cracked with age, sediment and tree roots, and it took three weeks of digging and replacing before things were back to normal.[104] It was quite an event when new tools and supplies were provided. To transport the hospital's timber and equipment, Marshall, the carpenter, used his 1937 Chev tabletop truck with runners down each side. The hospital gave him mileage, built a cover on the truck, and fitted indicators. Supplies of timber were supplemented by car dealers in Fremantle who gave the hospital the solid, wooden packing cases in which new vehicles had been crated. From a small storage room, Bob Willetts ordered and repaired the hospital's instruments. Gordon Hunt ran the general store with its gaol-like door, while Eric Cox supervised the provisions store and discouraged intruders, but anyone was welcome at the boiler house where six-foot logs fueled the fires, nearby which it was good to stand and warm up on cold mornings. Bill Fellowes, the painter, coloured the old brick, asbestos and timber walls of the hospital, and painted lockers and cupboards. But with a smaller brush and a creative hand, in beautiful script he identified and decorated each of the nurses' graduation certificates with her name, and drew up carefully lettered and coloured charts when they were needed, and made special cards for long-term employees when they left the staff. Such work was always treasured.

Negotiations to obtain the school site to extend hospital perimeters proved successful in 1962 and in a mutually acceptable three-way exchange the hospital gained the school site, the Education Department a new school on land on the Alma Street reserve, and the council some land it required between the gaol and the rear of the Fremantle Police Station.[105] In May, the former Alma Street Infants School was used for the first time as a nurses' training centre: 'a large lecture hall ... two rooms we had as blocks, and a practical area and a pantry ... it functioned very well really,' remembered Alice Harris, the tutor sister.[106] When nurses were moved from the temporary training school at the East Fremantle Annexe, it was converted into a ward for geriatric patients, the use for which it had been originally intended.

Since 1961, real estate agents had advised the board about private houses adjacent to the hospital which were for purchase. None were bought. However, in 1965, the board looked east to Attfield Street and determined on a policy to acquire all the properties there between Alma and Fothergill Streets adjacent to the hospital. It was not a project which could be carried out speedily but, in time, negotiations were made and the houses were bought above market prices, and only one was obtained by threat of resumption. One elderly lady was allowed to remain in her home 'for her lifetime' but she lived on for years, holding up the development of the land.[107] When building was eventually commenced on the Attfield Street site, another resident came to the hospital claiming that the construction was on their family's land. A horrified board found that in error, titles had originally been issued for two Lot 2s

104   G. Schneider, interviewed by C. Jeffery, 5 April 1987, FH.
105   Minutes of BM, 19 January 1959, FH.
106   A. Harris, interviewed by C. Jeffery, 24 November, 1 December 1984, FH.
107   R. Marshall, interviewed by C. Jeffery, 20, 28 February 1987; 6 March 1987, FH.

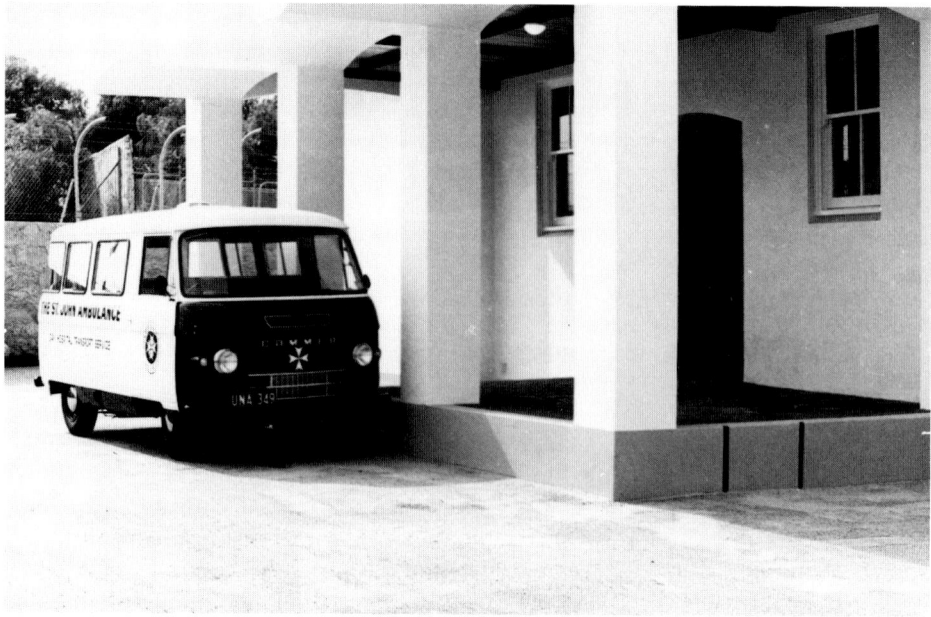

Photograph courtesy Fremantle Hospital

Plate 73.   Fremantle Hospital Day Centre.
The Day Centre was opened in 1964. That had previously been the South Terrace Infants'
School and there was a deal done. A private firm of architects was commissioned to
redevelop the building and to enlarge it, and it was the first Day Hospital ever established
in Australia in a public hospital. So that was a first for Fremantle.

Arthur Smith
Administrator

on Gordon Street, and the second purchase was quickly arranged.[108] Of the existing
houses on the block between Attfield Street and Hampton Road, one was retained
and renovated and is used by the Red Cross Blood Transfusion Service as a blood
donor clinic.

The urgency to transfer aged patients from acute hospital beds, prompted the
establishment of the Day Hospital in the second of the school buildings to the west
of the hospital. On 4 September 1964, Ross Hutchinson, whose wife had earlier been
a pupil and he a teacher at the school, declared the Day Centre open. It was a
rehabilitation concept unique to a public hospital, not only in the west but throughout Australia. Basically, as the administrator explained, 'it enabled some people to
be discharged earlier [and] enabled us to maintain them at home'.[109] Most of the
patients who came to the centre between 10 a.m. and 4 p.m. received speech therapy,
physiotherapy or occupational therapy, and a hot midday meal.[110] Most were seen

---

[108]   *Ibid.*
[109]   A. Smith, interview.
[110]   *West Australian*, 11 March 1962, 31 March 1964; *Daily News*, 24 January 1963; FH File, 'Day

by a nurse, a doctor and the almoner. Most were aged over 60 years. Many were helped to live with impaired health in their own homes on which modifications were carried out. Relatives who took an aged person into their care were given the respite which enabled them to continue the arrangement, and the lonely were able to meet together and share interests. The Silver Chain Nursing Association was essential in the Day Care concept, carrying on the work that it had started in 1951—encouraging a patient to be self-reliant, and changing dressings which were supplied by the almoners' department. 'Gradually we built this bridge,' explained Dr Peter Smith, who had been one of the hard-working team who organised the centre:

> Patients started in the acute hospital bed ... but then transferred to East Fremantle Annexe where they stayed for weeks. As they got better there, we used to bring them in by bus from East Fremantle Annexe to the Day Centre—a couple of times a week, and then three times a week, and then four times a week, and then we sent them home, having gone into their homes and constructed the ramps and bits and pieces, and taught them how to dress, and taken them into the kitchen in the Day Centre. We showed them how to use all these sorts of things, and how to bathe ... the lot. And we continued to bring them from their home every day to the Day Centre. We gradually decreased that to three a week, then two a week, then one a week, then one a fortnight, then one a month, and then told them 'OK, you're on your own at home now ...' Some of them were children with tumours, some of them with head injuries—young head injuries ... or they had unusual diseases ... We took everything that everybody sent to us because we were trying to provide a different dimension— a different dimension, you know, to medicine in Fremantle, and I think we did.[111]

One woman who had literally lived in a night dress for five years was regularly brought to the centre by ambulance, and in six months was up, fully dressed and taking care of herself. Another gained enough confidence after one day in the centre's kitchen to cook a meal for her husband.[112] In its first five months, 159 people attended the centre; six years later during 1970 there were 7,018 attendances.[113] The liaison between the Day Centre and the Fremantle Social Centre for Elderly People which organised Meals on Wheels, was strong. On 29 July 1976, the Stan Reilly Social Centre and Frail-Aged Lodge was opened on the area adjacent to the Day Centre on South Terrace, on the cleared Base Hospital site, linking the two in location, as well as in interest.

The need to transport elderly or incapacitated patients increased as the number of hospital patients grew, and the Volkswagen Kombi van bought in 1955, which had been used to convey patients between the annexes and which was often driven by orderly George Ferguson, could no longer cope. In March 1960, the Fremantle Hospital Voluntary Car Transport Organisation was established. Members took patients from Fremantle to the Perth and to other hospitals, to surgical bootmakers, to the Dental Hospital and to the Day Centre, often detouring to picnic areas or points of

Centre'; G. Leyland, 'The Day Centre in the Geriatric Rehabilitation Programme in Fremantle Hospital, *The Medical Journal of Australia*, 1966, 1: 1114 (June 25).

111 P. B. Smith, interview.
112 Undated newspaper clipping, FH Files.
113 FH Annual Report, 1970.

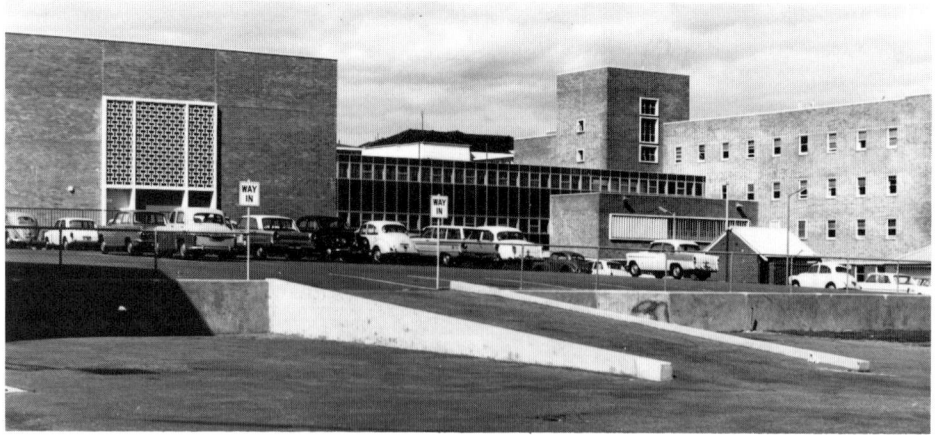

Photograph courtesy Fremantle Hospital

Plate 74.   The new operating theatre and X-ray block, opened on 25 January 1966.

interest on the way. Fifty-seven cars were rostered in the first three months, making 211 trips in all.[114] In the following year, 80 drivers were enrolled. They travelled from as far as Rockingham, Safety Bay and Mandurah, and none received payment for their services. However, one Fremantle garage offered volunteer drivers a re-duced price for a tank of petrol. By March 1964, through the organisation of presi-dent Olive Scrymgeour, 3,580 patients had been transported with 3,032[115] drivers. With the opening of the Day Centre, the need for transport increased, and the two vans bought by the hospital were supplemented by two St John's ambulances.

The next building in the hospital development plan was a new £500,000 X-ray and theatre block on the northern side of the Ron Doig Block. Hospital staff members—surgeons, theatre staff, engineers, nurses, radiographers and pathologists, all under the direction of Rowe—collaborated and contributed in planning the three-storied structure. A mechanical plant, autopsy rooms and auxiliary power plant were designed for the basement.[116] An X-ray and central supply station were planned for the ground floor, and on the first, a completely sterile operating area, sealed off from the rest of the building by air-locks to minimise infection, with plans for closed-circuit television and a wall of observation windows down one side. Path-ologists were enthusiastic about the new mortuary. The old 'morgue' had been reno-vated and refrigeration installed in 1955 but little real improvement could be made in the old shed-like room. As work continued, a separate staff amenities building with change and rest rooms for non-resident staff was designed. The high land known as Scotsman's Hill, where generations had come to watch football games outside the reach of a gate collector, was levelled for the building of the amenities block and the excavated earth used to form embankments for the new railway bridge over the

114   *Ibid.*, 1960.
115   *Ibid.*, 1964.
116   *West Australian*, 30 January 1963; *Daily News*, 16 April 1964, 17 September 1964.

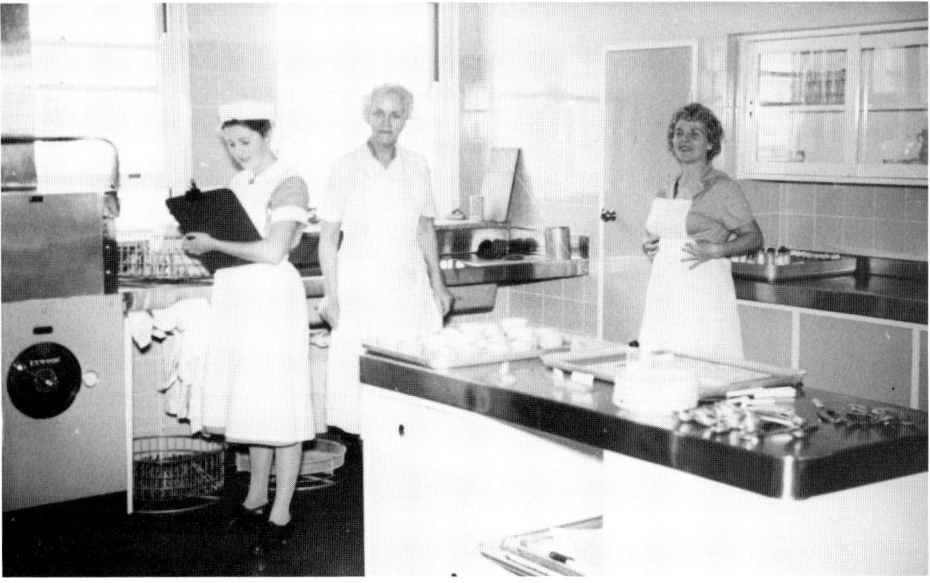

Photograph courtesy Fremantle Hospital

Plate 75.   Male community ward kitchen, 1961.

The 'mod cons' were a benefit to domestic and nursing staff alike. The latter learned on night duty 'how to make meringues in the hot box ... you had to beat them up immediately you got on duty and get on duty a bit early, so that you didn't wake the patients with the beating with the hand beater. It made meringues beautifully!

Olga Hedemann
Director of Nursing 1983–

river.[117] Despite the fact that the newly-flattened area was used for parking, regular Scotsman's Hill patrons came and sat on the parked cars to obtain their usual free view. Two years later, on 25 January 1966, both of the new hospital buildings were opened.

Although pleased to have their own area, some orderlies and domestics were possibly disappointed that their new block was so far from the main hospital. Ward-maids, however, had no regrets when electric polishers were bought for use on floors that continually needed buffing. Despite the installation of modern conveniences, kitchen work was still heavy, and it was not unusual to lose half a stone after starting work there. Those who worked in the wards were often indirectly involved with a patient's healing. One confided:

> I liked to make people laugh and I think laughter is one of the most healthy, healing things ... Now we had a very sick sailor. He'd been badly injured and he was an American and when he first came to us he was so down and depressed and his blind was closed and his door was shut. I'd go in of a morning and I would pull the blind up and

---

[117] *Daily News*, 9 January 1964. See also L. Marshall, notes.

I'd say 'Now, come on. This beautiful view', I said, 'and you have got that blind down. You mustn't. It will help you to get better to look out that window.' And then the door would be shut and I'd say 'You can't have this door shut.' I said 'You can't hear anything'. We bullied him—and would you know, he didn't want to go to America. He wanted to stay here to get over his injuries, but of course the Navy took him back. It was lovely to see him starting to laugh and take an interest.[118]

Orderlies opened the gate at night for the ambulance. They helped in the kitchen early in the morning and delivered food trolleys to the wards. They accompanied a nurse taking a patient to the theatre, and again on the return to a ward. They took patients to X-ray. When the hospital bought a Kombi van some orderlies were appointed as drivers, others worked in the central sterilising department. They also accompanied nurses taking the dead to the mortuary and a nurse was usually taught by those who had gone before her, never to go inside the mortuary door in case it was slammed behind her. Like domestics, orderlies were concerned about patients. Vic Poklad would say to his junior orderlies:

> ... it's only one reason all of us here, from administrator to the orderlies—to help for the sick person because the sick person if he didn't need our help, he wouldn't be here.[119]

Mr Scrymgeour was at the official opening of the X-ray and theatre block, and he continued as administrator of the hospital for another two years before his retirement on 4 March 1968.[120] Despite his 32 years of careful financial management, a credit balance in the hospital books was as much of a challenge as ever, as costs constantly escalated. Each basic-wage increase, each account for drugs, each building constructed, each equipment break-down, each industrial award cut more deeply into hospital funds. Of the £44,134 rise in costs in 1951, over £17,000 was due to increases in salaries and wages among the 270 employees.[121] In 1954 the fuel and light bill was an unprecedented £4,700, attributable largely to the electric ranges and ovens in the kitchen, the air conditioner in the new theatre and the steam sterilizer there. With the opening of the annexes there was an increased need for drugs and dressings, and by 1958 it was costing £1,000 a day to run the hospital.[122] The government did increase the subsidy, but it was never enough for what needed to be done, and it certainly didn't increase in proportion to hospital costs, which rose by over 400 per cent in the decade to 1960.[123]

During the 1950s contributions to the hospital faltered. Each Monday morning, however, the teachers at Fremantle's Princess May Girls' School still collected threepence from each girl or family towards the maintenance of the school cot at the hospital[124] and the W.A. Rope and Twine Company still regularly gave, inspired by the enthusiasm of their employer F. Briggs, who was later appointed to the hospital

[118] J. Purdy, interviewed by C. Jeffery, 5 September 1985, FH.
[119] Poklad, interview.
[120] *Daily News*, 29 February 1968; *West Australian*, 1 March 1968.
[121] FH Annual Report, 1951.
[122] *Ibid.*, 1958.
[123] *Ibid.*, 1961.
[124] D. McCarthy, notes, FH.

board, so great was his interest in the institution. The Trotting Club's substantial donations were welcome, and the administrator was sorry to see the last cheque from the community concerts in 1954, after 15 years of regular donations. In comparison with contributions, the response to the equipment and building appeals—for the William Wauhop Wing, the children's wards and at Christmas—the community responded magnificently.

In the mid- to late 1960s, however, donations to the hospital once more increased, and to such an extent that the secretary reported the benevolence as 'evidence . . . of the interest displayed in this Hospital by . . . a wide cross section of the community'.[125] Perhaps the interest was fostered through regular features about patients in the hospital, published by the *Daily News*, which kept the needs of the hospital in the public eye. As prices continued to rise in 1963, partly due to higher wages which had to be paid to the increasingly qualified and trained personnel who were employed, James Scrymgeour reasoned sagely: 'Yet in the final analysis what value can be set on the restoration of people to health? These things, surely, cannot be measured in the currency of the realm'.[126] A volunteer's time, and goods in kind were still important. For over 20 years the Ladies Guild of the Beaconsfield Congregational Church sewed and repaired hospital linen. Members of the Thirsty Thirties [the East Fremantle Bowling Club] always managed a substantial donation from the amount collected each year in fines for each swear word that passed their members' lips, and volunteers from the Fremantle Hospital Ladies' Auxilliary faithfully served in the hospital canteen through which they raised magnificent sums for many hospital needs.

There were still debtors as well as donors to the hospital and many cases of genuine hardship. The secretary received a letter from a man concerned about his account in 1966:

> . . . in regard to your letter on the 27th Jan. aboutt my account of £29.11.2. for my hospital benefit card, which I lost it between sept and oct last year, when we shifted back to our mother inlaws. we had to go back because she is on the pension and she took a heart attach, in that time I contacted hospital benefit fund and told them what had happened, but heard nothing, so I do not know what to do, please let me know if I will get summond.[127]

The board resolved to write off the account if the debtor maintained membership in a health fund for 12 months. Because it was a small community, the board still knew many of the hospital's debtors and each month at the board meeting, one or another would find that he was acquainted with a debtor, and would offer to visit or contact the person about an outstanding account. Often the arrangement to join a health benefit fund for 12 months would be made, and the account written off.

When Arthur Smith took Scrymgeour's place as administrator, he shared the same tight concern about the accounts. He would

> . . . go to Perth on the first working day of the month and to the Treasury Department

[125] FH Annual Report, 1967.
[126] *Ibid.*, 1963.
[127] Minutes of BM, 28 February 1966, FH.

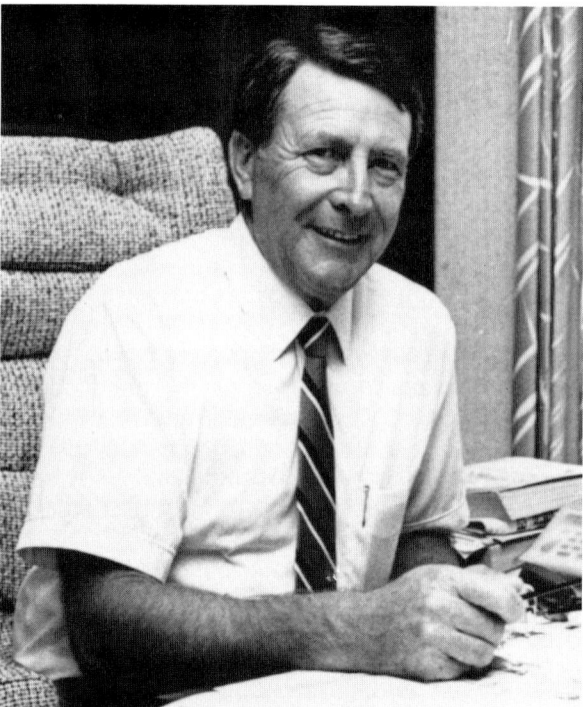

Plate 76. R. J. Marshall, Administrator, Fremantle Hospital, 1974–

Things seemed to be simpler in those days. We had—I remember seeing the big cash books in which the accounts were written up and it seemed a lot simpler.

R. J. Marshall, Administrator

Photograph courtesy Fremantle Hospital

and get the cheque and get it down to Fremantle in a hurry and into the bank so that there would be money in the account to keep us fluid ... and then we would have to decide which one of them [accounts] could be paid immediately and which ones would have to wait a few days or weeks before they could be paid.[128]

Community response to the children's ward appeal in 1970 was as enthusiastic as that for the William Wauhop Wing had been:

> We decided how many rooms there were and then we decided what a figure would be for each room and so we said to donors, 'if you would like to give us 'x' dollars we will put a plaque over the door indicating that you have furnished this particular room' ... When the appeal was nearing its finality it suddenly dawned upon me that more rooms had been promised to donors than we had to give ... I remember driving around to see all these donors and saying to them 'look you know, we said to you if you gave "x" dollars we would put a plaque up in your name ... did you really want a plaque?' And most of them said 'look we are not worried about it. We gave you the money for the children ...'[129]

When Arthur Smith left the hospital in 1975, and Roy Marshall took his place, the introduction of Medibank under the Whitlam Government solved the problem of

---

[128]   A. Smith, interview.
[129]   *Ibid.*

bad debts for public patients, and deficits were usually but grudgingly met by the Medical Department. The decade of the 1980s brought leaner times and with it 'more control . . . now over the amount of money that's given to us'.[130]

With the next burst of building activity at the hospital, the original nurses' quarters to the west of The Knowle, which were in use as quarters for the young resident medical officers, were demolished to make way for a new, two-storied, 60-bed children's ward to the north of the X-ray and theatre block. The uprooting of the giant gnarled Moreton Bay fig tree which dwarfed the residents' quarters was a loss felt by many of the staff, but when the new Adelaide Samson Children's Ward was opened by the Honorable G. C. McKinnon on 6 November 1970, most agreed that the new gain outweighed the loss. The new ward had mother-and-child units, a burns unit, class and playrooms. The new infectious diseases ward was envisaged more for infants with bowel infections than for patients suffering the old diseases which vaccination had checked. A feature was the special ward for teenagers, a concept new to general hospitals in Australia.[131] It was noted that on Saturday afternoons when the big League matches were played the number of visitors to the children's ward overlooking the oval increased appreciably.

Children often came to the hospital. In 1966 alone, 364 under the age of 14 were admitted. As a result of falls, 125 were treated; 20 came with cuts; 59 after taking poison; 40 suffered burns; another 20 were injured by falling or thrown objects, and the remaining hundred were admitted due to other causes.[132] If they came expecting a holiday from schoolwork the children were disappointed. Prior to 1955 a child's concerned schoolteacher might supply work to be done. There was also a teacher attached to the correspondence school who walked and travelled by bus and train to visit the hospitalised and home-bound students. On her retirement, the Boordaak School[133] was established at the hospital under the guidance of the Special Education Branch of the Education Department, as a base for the new travelling schoolteacher, Miss Rae Loney. With the opening of the children's ward and its colourful schoolroom in 1970, a teacher conducted a class there for all grades between one and twelve, each weekday morning, and visited her home-bound scholars in the afternoon. Sometimes these visits would be to pregnant teenagers at their home, or at the Ngala Mothercraft Home, or St Anne's Maternity Hospital annexe, until schools were established there. Many students were helped through to their important final examinations, which were also supervised by the Boordaak teacher. In one class, held in a private house, 'the group was mixed indeed, including pregnant-at-homes, a haemophiliac, an epileptic, and a boy with severe heart disease'.[134] At the new Adelaide Samson Ward's schoolroom, students walked or came in wheelchairs, and others were pushed—bed-and-all—into the classroom. At different times the patients were taught by Daisy Mahoney, Betty Marshall, Monica O'Keefe and Sylvia Torvaldsen.

130 R. Marshall, interview.
131 *West Australian*, 25 October 1967; *Daily News*, 17 July 1969, 11 September 1969; *Fremantle Gazette*, 19 August 1981.
132 *Daily News*, 13 July 1967.
133 Notes from Boordaak School, FH, 1983. See also *W.A. Parent*, Vol. 2, No. 1, 1980.
134 Boordaak notes, 1983. Boordaak is an Aboriginal word meaning 'the place where they trace' or 'tracing in the sand'.

The prospect of a new and larger children's ward for which so much clean linen was required, daunted laundry workers in the old building which was difficult to modernise and extend. In 1949 when laundry equipment faltered, washing was hung to dry on fences, spread out on lawns and draped over verandahs, but by 1968 such measures were useless when a million pounds of clothing were laundered annually by a department working to capacity. Rather than repair or replace old equipment, the board consulted the Fremantle Steam Laundry Company, which was already laundering the nurses' uniforms, and it agreed to extend its premises and undertake the hospital's washing. The old, unused laundry building near The Knowle was converted into a linen storage and issue room. In March 1975, when the contract with the Fremantle laundry expired, the hospital transferred its washing to the Central Hospitals' Laundry and Linen Service on the proposed Lakes Hospital site, and had to outlay $108,000 for the extra linen required for it to become a part of this scheme.

Despite the expansion of Fremantle Hospital to the late 1960s, the availability of beds remained a constant daily problem. The strong link between the hospital and the North, initially forged by Medical Superintendent Rowe, remained strong. Young resident medical officers were encouraged to go to towns such as Broome, Leonora, Wyndham, as well as Esperance and other centres when they left Fremantle. 'We used to try and supply resident service to help out in these areas,' reflected Rowe, 'plus the nurses we used to encourage to go to the country after they had graduated. We had a good rapport with the country and remote areas.'[135] Country doctors had only to ring a Fremantle specialist to book one of their patients into the hospital. In the late 1960s there were injured rodeo riders, victims of car accidents, a man hurt while branding a bull, and patients coming for check-ups. They arrived from many areas, including Port Hedland, Halls Creek, Wyndham, country areas to the south and from the Kalgoorlie mines.[136]

One patient in the hospital during August 1961, was an 84-year-old drover from Mt Magnet. Hospital was strange to the old man, and he fretted at the enforced separation from his eleven-year-old kelpie dog with whom he had shared over a decade of shearing, mustering and companionship. So concerned were his nurses, that they organised a collection amongst themselves, to reunite Bonnie and her master. Theirs was not the only gesture of concern. When MacRobertson Miller Airlines subsequently heard of the plan they transported the dog to Perth without cost.[137] There was little that medical treatment could do for the old man, but with his dog beside him, the man was content when he died a week later. Among Aborigines nursed at Fremantle Hospital in the 1960s, one was admitted from the Forrest River Mission with a poisoned foot after he accidentally walked on some glass. Another, who broke in brumbies, was slashed when a tightly stretched fencing wire for a steel post snapped and recoiled, and a young Aboriginal with meningitis was flown down from Wyndham.[138]

Men injured in industrial accidents at Kwinana were often admitted as patients. A

[135] Rowe, interview.
[136] Newspaper cuttings, FH scrapbook. See particularly *Daily News*, 22 September 1966, 13 June 1967, 31 August 1967, 9 November 1967.
[137] F. Dunn, *Speck in the Sky: A History of Airlines of Western Australia*, 1984, p. 167.
[138] *Daily News*, 7 November 1963, 19 May 1966, 4 December 1966.

painter with a foot crushed by a jetty pile which was dropped by a crane, a foundry worker hurt when machinery toppled onto his leg, a boilermaker who fell 56 feet through a grating, an electrician who had his leg caught in machinery, were not exceptional cases.[139] When in 1965, an explosion erupted in the BP Refinery's lubricating oil section, hurling flames 60 feet into the air, four men suffering third-degree burns were rushed to the hospital's casualty department where staff had been called from their homes to assist in the emergency. Two of the less seriously injured were later transferred to the burns ward at Royal Perth Hospital, and one of the two men at Fremantle Hospital, too ill to be moved, died before morning.[140] Shipping cases—both crew and passengers—were admitted at times, often after spending over a week with only the medical attention that those on board ship could provide. An engineer who broke his leg while working on a Norwegian tanker had only one sleeping pill to dull his pain in the six days before he was landed.[141]

In 1967 the press reported the burden of patients that Fremantle Hospital was carrying, and spoke hopefully about new hospitals at Rockingham and Bull Creek.[142] By September 1969, the board was again pointing out to the Medical Department, the urgency of its need for accommodation and suggesting the building of a multi-storied ward with 150 beds and an out-patients' block. Patients were not the only ones who needed new accommodation. One of the social workers had to use the general office because there was nowhere else she could go; the speech therapist took clinics in a living room used by resident medical officers; the medical superintendent's typists had little room to move and could barely carry on telephone conversations, such was the noise from the typewriters and talk around them. Residents had to write their reports in the cramped office of the deputy medical superintendent, and the nursing administration staff often spoke of their lack of space.[143] When the Medical Department finally agreed to the idea of a new building, the board was elated. After counselling with representatives from each department, final drawings were eventually made: the multi-storied block was an exciting plan, an ambitious plan, and well suited to the site adjacent to the Day Centre facing South Terrace. In its early stages, however, obstructions seemed to come as naturally as the winter rain.

Long before the new block took shape in concrete and brick, immediate needs had to be met—an office for the medical social workers in September 1971, a patients' clothing store, an emergency department, a medical library and university department of medicine. In May 1974, a prefabricated building for the blood bank was set up between the theatre block and the Ron Doig Block. Due to overcrowding, the pathology department was also moved into temporary prefabricated buildings. Clinics and a clerks' office were opened. With plans for the new ward underway, a new kitchen and cafeteria block had to be built to serve the new patients. These were finished in July 1975. The plans for the multi-storied ward block were nurtured and not forgotten.

139 Newspaper cuttings, FH. See particularly *Daily News*, 15 February 1968, 26 September 1968, 13 March 1969.
140 *West Australian*, 11 December 1965, 13 December 1965; *Weekend News*, 11 December 1965.
141 *Daily News*, 25 January 1968.
142 *Daily News*, 21 November 1967.
143 Minutes of Building Committee, 13 April 1970, FH.

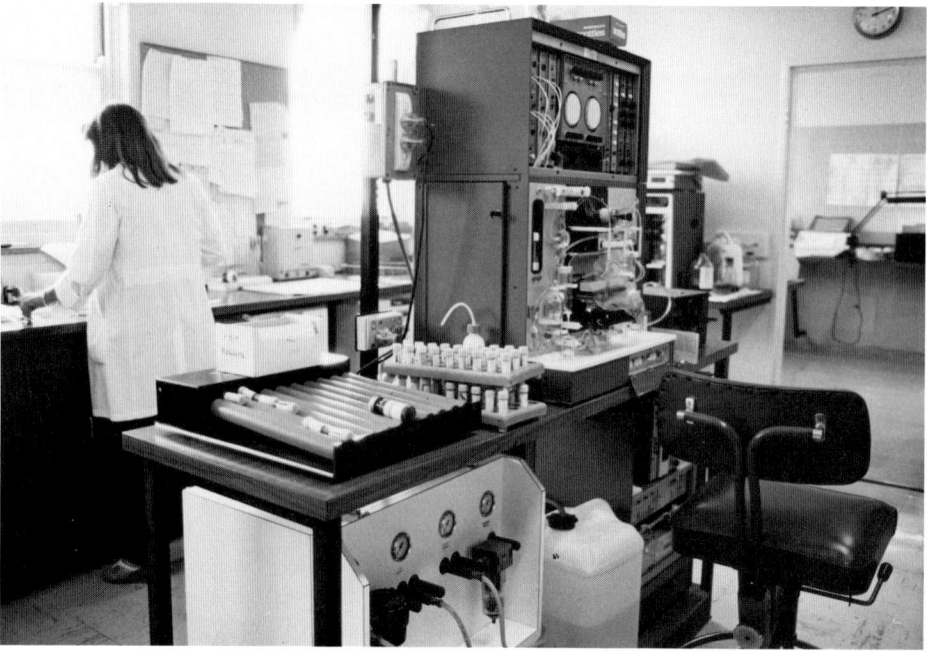

Plate 77.   The Coulter Particle Counter, situated in the haematology section of the pathology department in the William Wauhop Wing.

> The equipment improved considerably, however, when we moved into the William Wauhop Wing which was completed at the end of 1959. The laboratories in the new wing were very nicely built and at that time we thought that they had plenty of room in them which would last us for all time. This of course, was something that didn't happen because it wasn't many years later that we were bursting out of them.
>
> Dr John Holme
> Pathologist

In 1973, the clinical staff, led by doctors R. Whitford, S. Cooke, J. Woods, I. Miller, A. Fortune and T. Stack, protested to the board and the press about facilities at the hospital being 'inadequate to provide to the community served by it, the standards of medical care at present available to residents of other parts of the metropolitan area'.[144] The acquisition of Bicton Medicentre, which was promptly renamed the 'Bicton Annexe' in line with the other annexes, provided only a little relief to the need for more beds. That year, plans for a small ward block in Attfield Street were made. Although it was designed as a slow-pace geriatric ward, when the $3,130,000 wing was opened in 1976, with physiotherapy and speech therapy departments, a popular hydrotherapy pool, and a department for nuclear medicine, so great was the need for beds, that 58 acute cases were immediately admitted there.[145]

[144]   Minutes of BM, 22 October 1973, FH; *West Australian*, 13 October 1973.
[145]   FH File, 'Greenslade Wing'. See also *Daily News*, 2 March 1977; *West Australian*, 3 June 1976.

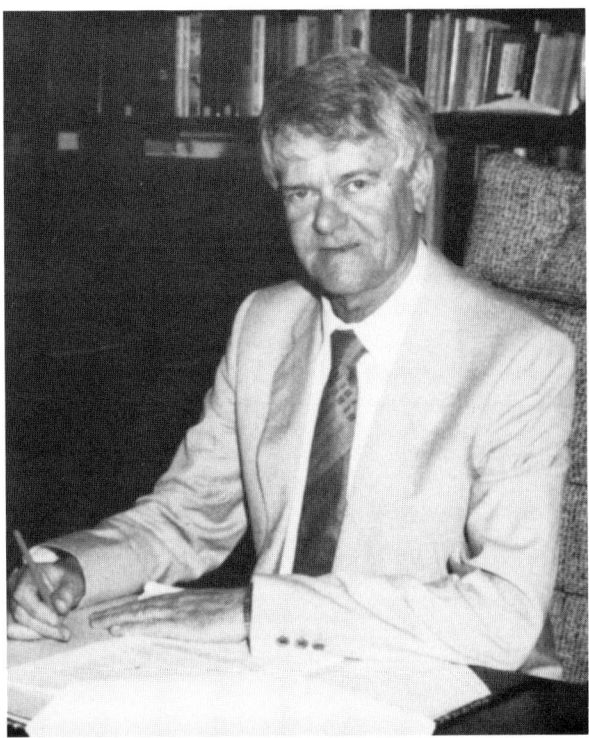

Plate 78. Doctor Peter Smith.

Peter I had a lot of time for. He really did a tremendous amount of work for the hospital and really cared very much for the place. He devoted his life to it ... Once he had ideas he was prepared to fight for them and push for them ... He was for Fremantle and he was prepared to fight for it, and he did.

Dr N. Marinovich
Honorary Physician

Photograph courtesy Fremantle Hospital

The block was fittingly named as a tribute to a board member who had walked the hospital corridors in all the years between 1930 and 1971, speaking to workers and seeing for himself where help was most needed. As the member influential in raising funds for the original almoners' department, J. R. N. Greenslade was always concerned about those in need and would have been pleased with the Greenslade Wing named in his honour, two years after his death at the age of 90.

No one in the community objected to the building of the new school of nursing and the beautiful lecture theatre adjacent, with its sensitive acoustics.[146] When they were opened on 16 September 1977, the nursing staff felt that 'we really had a house of our own'.[147] The theatre was named after Cliff Bennett, the retiring chairman who had spent twenty years as a board member; the new library in the school of nursing was named in recognition of Alice Harris, who had done so much for nursing at Fremantle and for nurses' training in Western Australia. No one objected to the new multi-level car park, of which the first floor was commissioned in 1975, and the second floor completed in 1978.[148] Not a pen was raised against the building of the new communications centre and the electrical distribution building late in 1979, but the planned multi-level ward block was a different matter.

---

[146] *Daily News*, 21 September 1977.
[147] Leworthy, interview.
[148] *Daily News*, 9 November 1977.

Fremantle was still a relatively architecturally unexploited town of old houses and shops, many of which had seen little change since the turn of the century. Many residents were fiercely protective of the environment that was 'Freo' and when it was learned that the multi-ward block at the Fremantle Hospital would be a T-shaped tower 17 storeys high, with a twin tower planned for a later date, there was some discontent.[149] Fremantle city councillors debated the environmental impact, the adequacy of parking, and the increased traffic patterns which would develop in the area.[150] Many in the town also shared the council's concern about the visual environment. The Fremantle Society in particular, objected to the height of the towers and were not without their supporters. Those who favoured the hospital plans considered that the basis of objection to the building might be political. The board and the building committee at the hospital pondered, but only briefly. An appreciable delay in construction would not only increase building costs, but postpone the provision of needed beds. Based on the environmental study which was ordered by the Fremantle City Council, and on the Llewelyn Davies Kinhill Pty Ltd plan for metropolitan Perth, which supported the development of the Lakes Hospital as the major teaching hospital south of the river, moves were made to build only the first section of the 'South Terrace' additions. Plans were made revising and reducing the original draft to a smaller, chunkier building of eleven levels.[151] By 1976, the nurses' training school on the old school site had been demolished and the new work commenced. On 1 October 1981, the Public Works Department's Principal Architect, Mr W. E. Bateman, delivered a letter to Mr C. C. Bennett, the Chairman of the Board, advising that additions had 'reached a stage of practical completion'.[152] It was only just in time. A week later, on 7 October, the building was due to be officially opened by Her Majesty Queen Elizabeth II.[153]

With the construction only barely completed, hurried preparations were made to clean up and dress up the building for the occasion. Security measures were tight. Unauthorised people were asked to leave the building, ducts were checked for explosives, stickers were placed over cupboards—'so that we were aware if they were opened after that time, that somebody had interfered with them'[154]—and security staff with weapons were posted on the hospital roof and in the flats opposite. Despite the tight security it was a tense Queen who arrived. That day, the press ran black headlines about another world leader, in its coverage of the assassination of President Sadat of Egypt. In declaring the new block open, the Queen unveiled a plaque and gave her consent for the new building to be known as the Princess of Wales Wing. As this was the first time that a public building had been named after the Queen's new daughter-in-law, the board and the community were well pleased.

---

[149] *Independent Review*, 9 July 1976. *West Australian*, 4 and 18 December 1975; 17 February, 12 March, 1 and 22 April, 5 and 17 June, 23 October 1976. *Daily News*, 3 September 1975, 12 March 1976.

[150] City of Fremantle Report Book, January-December 1975. See also Minutes of FMC, 15 March 1976 to 12 April 1976. See also *Fremantle Gazette*, 26 April 1979.

[151] Fremantle Hospital, South Terrace Additions Official Opening, 7 October 1981 Booklet. See also R. Marshall, interview; C. Bennett, interviewed by C. Jeffery, 23 March, 3 April and 1 May 1985, FH.

[152] Minutes of BC, 5 November 1981, FH. See also *Fremantle Gazette*, 7 October 1981.

[153] FH Annual Report, 1982.

[154] R. Marshall, interview.

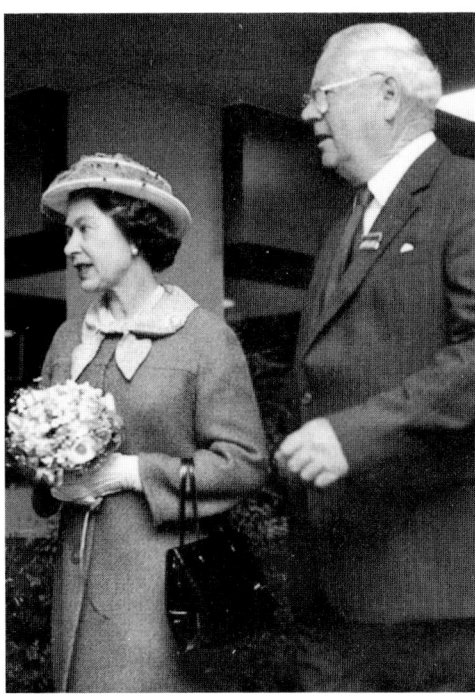

Plate 79. Official opening of the
Princess of Wales Wing, 7 October 1981,
by Her Majesty Queen Elizabeth II.
With Mr C.C. Bennett, Chairman of the
Board, Her Majesty inspected the
building.

Photograph courtesy of Fremantle Hospital

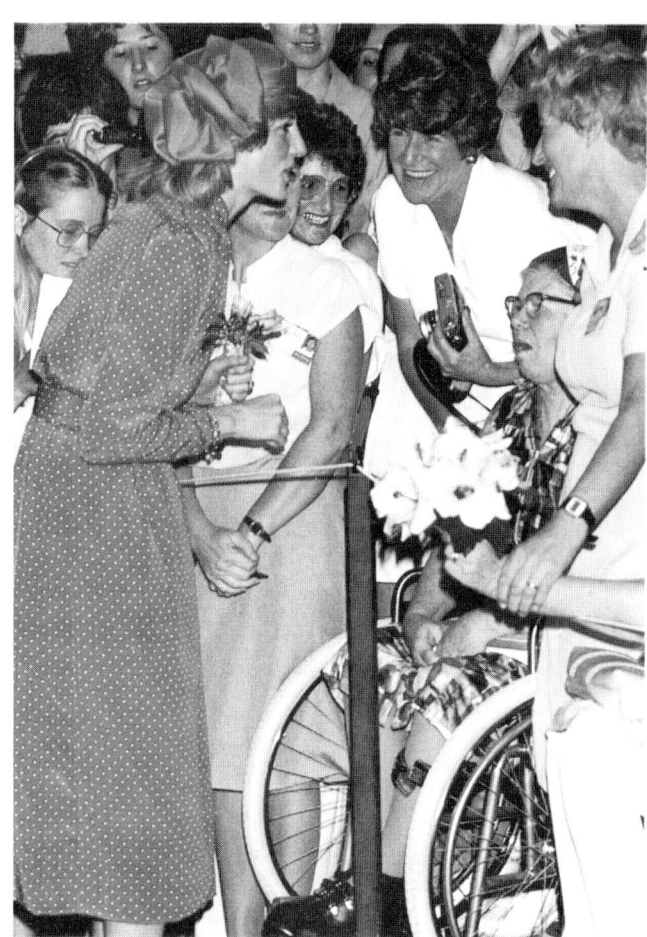

Plate 80. H.R.H. The
Princess of Wales visited the
building named in her honour,
on 7 April 1983.

Photograph courtesy Fremantle Hospital

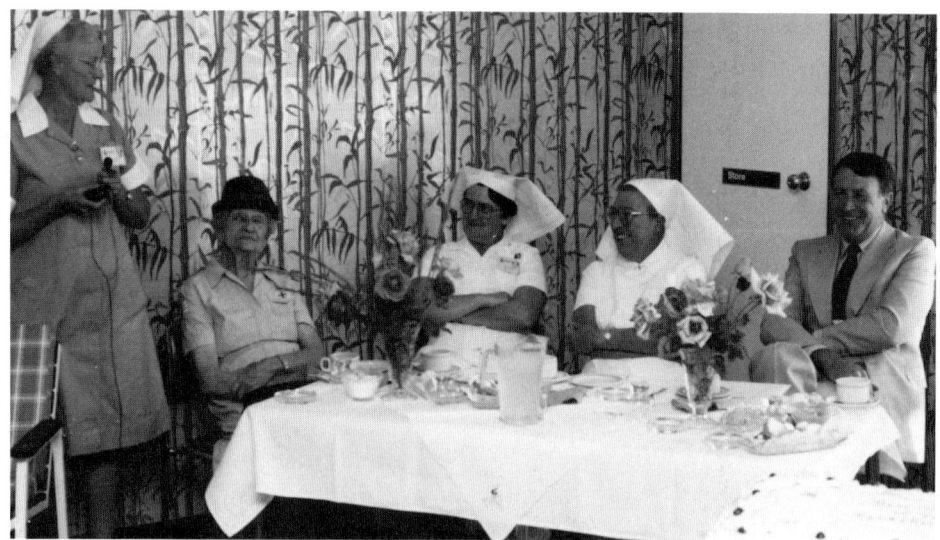

Photograph courtesy Fremantle Hospital

Plate 81. Matron M. Leworthy retired in 1983 after 21 years' service at Fremantle Hospital.

(Left to right): Sister Bette Needle, Sister in Charge, Samson Ward; Mrs Gwendoline Trivett, Red Cross representative, Fremantle; Miss Olga Hedemann, Director of Nursing; Matron Mavis Leworthy; Mr Roy Marshall, Administrator.

I have many highlights really with people. I have never regretted going to Fremantle. In fact I think I was very lucky indeed to have the opportunity to work in that hospital. But everybody has been so helpful and I made some very good friends with people like Sister Fuller, Sister Gill and Mrs Trivett. I couldn't really single out anyone because they were all so helpful and obliging.

Matron M. Leworthy

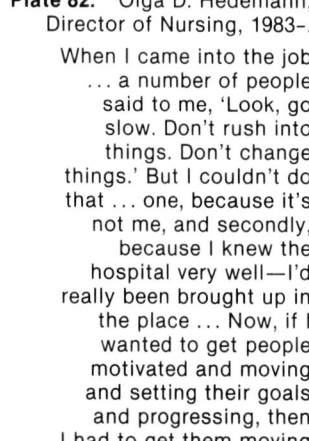

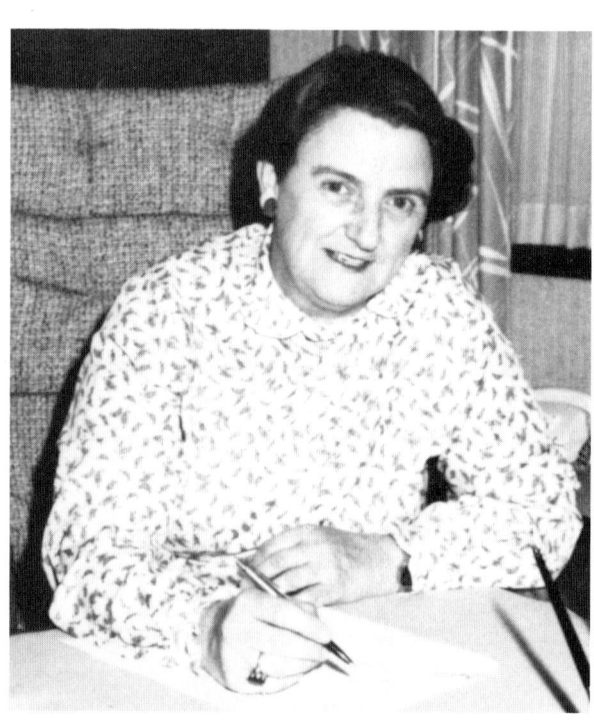

Plate 82. Olga D. Hedemann, Director of Nursing, 1983–.

When I came into the job ... a number of people said to me, 'Look, go slow. Don't rush into things. Don't change things.' But I couldn't do that ... one, because it's not me, and secondly, because I knew the hospital very well—I'd really been brought up in the place ... Now, if I wanted to get people motivated and moving and setting their goals and progressing, then I had to get them moving right from the start.

Olga D. Hedemann
Director of Nursing, 1983–

However, such a mouthful of a title was it, that the building was soon affectionately abbreviated in general conversation to 'Di's wing'. In April 1983, the Princess, with the Prince of Wales, visited the hospital named in her honour, and captivated by her grace and friendly concern, those who saw and talked with her.[155]

It was a momentous year in 1983, with the change to state Labor Government, and *Australia II* sailing to victory at Newport. Both events would have an effect at the hospital. Another event important for the hospital was the resignation of Mavis Leworthy after 21 years as matron. She was succeeded by Olga Hedemann on 4 March 1983 at a difficult time when the old system of nursing training and organisation was being reviewed and reformed. For most of its years, the board of management had leaned to the Labor party in its membership, but politics was not an issue among members. While he was chairman between 1970 and 1983, Cliff Bennett forbade discussion of a political nature at board meetings, and under William Wauhop, the board was more Fremantle and hospital oriented than politically motivated. At various times, board members contributed their wisdom gained in different areas: Greenslade had a produce business in Hamilton Hill; Douglas Gawler, who seemed to live in a trench-coat, was an ophthalmologist; Max Minchin, a representative of the honorary staff, also brought the experience of accountancy to the board; K. G. Smith, who died in 1971, was the manager of the Australian and New Zealand Bank, and Ron Christian the manager of the West Australian Newspapers in Fremantle; William Wauhop was Mayor of East Fremantle and Bill McKenzie the Mayor of Fremantle. Les Priest had connections with the Friendly Societies movement and wove beautiful cane prams and pushers for a living. Cliff Bennett was educated at Fremantle Boys' School, worked at Robbs Jetty, and became general manager of the W.A. Meat Export Works at the jetty. Lindsay Brown was a Fremantle councillor and a Fremantle person. There were Medical Department representatives, but most on the hospital board were:

> ... people who were really Fremantle people ... they were all really Fremantle people and they earned their livings and lived in the place and had an attitude towards the place—and the old ship sailed extremely well.[156]

Some distinctly felt the boat rock with the new appointments to the board under the Labor Government in 1983. Only Harry Fletcher, Ron Porter and the medical school representative, Professor R. A. Joske, were reappointed. The new members included the Hon. Mr Justice Howard Olney, a judge of the Supreme Court; Bill McKenzie; Stephen Hales, of the Commonwealth Development Bank of Australia; Dr Noel Dougan; Mr Anthony van Merwyk with Dr J. Turner as his deputy; Ms Helen Cattalini, a social worker; and Mrs Golda Alexander, a business director. When Porter died, Mrs Lorna Noonan, a retired schoolteacher, took his place in April 1984. Two months later, following the resignation of Fletcher, Olney was elected as the new chairman and Lindsay Bickford, formerly of the Fremantle Port Authority, joined the board. When McKenzie resigned, Mrs Jean Hobson, a Fremantle City Councillor, was appointed in his place in 1985. With their sympathy for

---

[155] FH Annual Report, 1983.
[156] Rowe, interview.

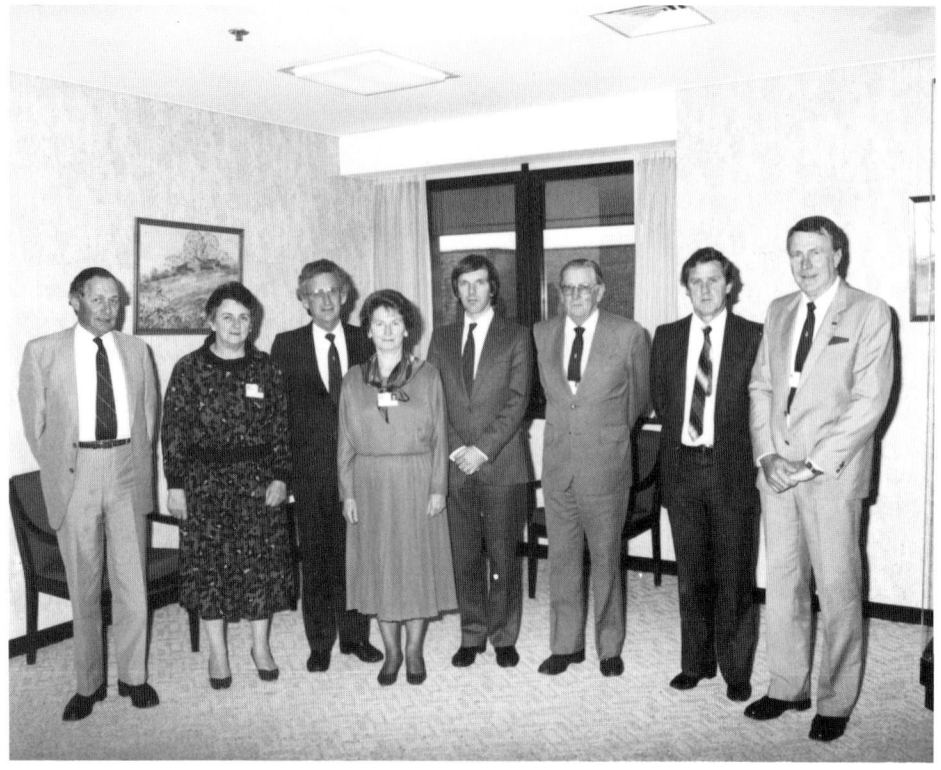

Photograph courtesy Fremantle Hospital

Plate 83.   Fremantle Hospital Board of Management, 1987.

(Left to right): Professor R. A. Joske, Miss O. D. Hedemann, Mr Justice H. W. Olney, Mrs J. Hobson, Dr J. H. Turner, Mr L. S. Bickford, Dr N. Fatin, Mr R. J. Marshall.

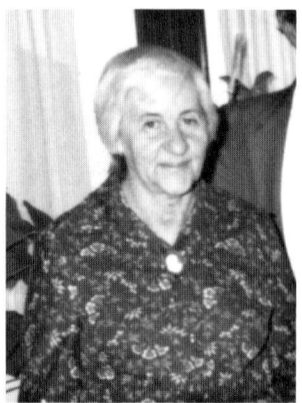
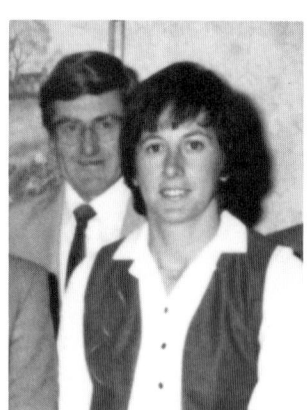
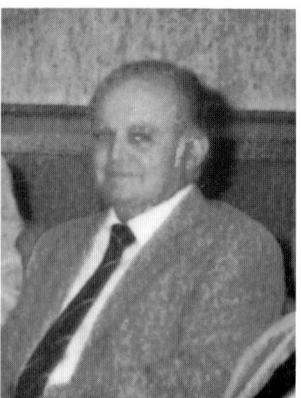

Mrs L. V. Noonan   Miss H. Cattalini   Mr S. G. Hales.
                            Mr A. J. van Merwyk

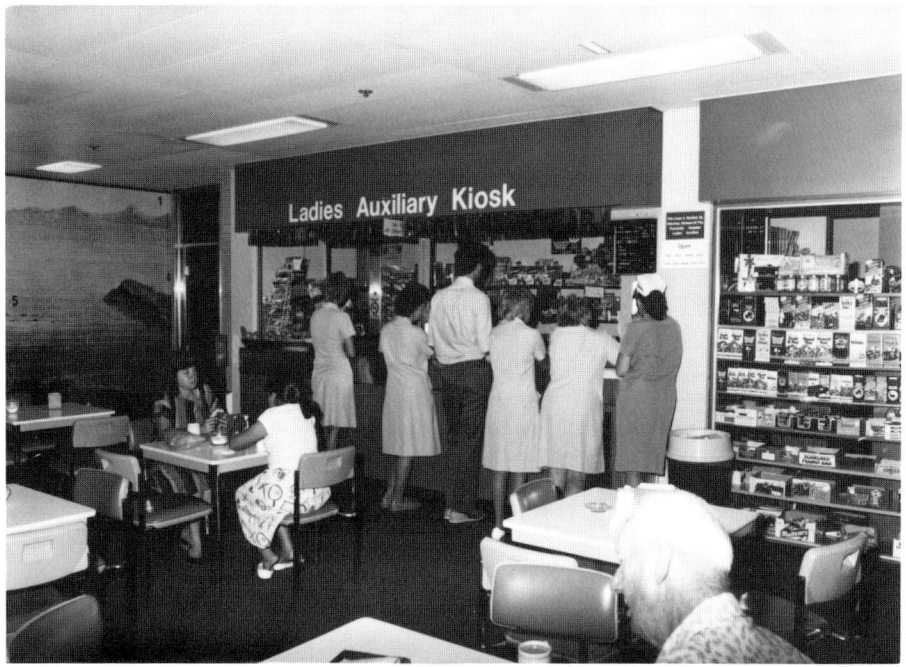

Photograph courtesy Fremantle Hospital

Plate 84.
The Fremantle Hospital Ladies' Auxiliary continues to operate two excellent kiosks at the hospital on a voluntary basis and has put to very good effect the profits from this enterprise by purchasing items of equipment for the benefit of patients in the hospital.

Fremantle Hospital Annual Report, 1984

government policies, as Chairman Olney suggests, a more welfare-oriented approach in administration has been taken by the board.[157]

When Alan Bond won the America's Cup and the right to a challenge in Fremantle waters, all the port was affected. Overseas, interstate and local visitors flocked to the Fremantle area in 1987. Patients at the hospital had an unobstructed view over the fishing harbour and out to the Indian Ocean and they watched the return of the challengers and spectator craft daily. With all the anticipated activity, hospital resources were organised to cope with an increased demand for its services, but the number it was called upon to treat was comparatively small. Nevertheless, the hospital was prepared. It was also ready when inspections for Hospital Accreditation were conducted in 1986, and the certificate and acknowledgement of the high standard of patient care by staff for diagnostic and treatment facilities at the hospital which it earned, is valid until January 1989.

There is certainly a lot of kudos associated with it when you become fully accredited . . .

[157]   H. Olney, interviewed by C. Jeffery, 9 March 1986.

and it's certainly a great thing for the hospital to achieve this at its first attempt and certainly demonstrates to everyone that it has systems, the staff and the capacity to provide first class services to its patients.[158]

Although it is a hospital of 363 beds, with another 40 at Woodside Maternity Hospital which it administers, Fremantle Hospital is still closely linked to its community. In 1986, when the Health Department released a report on suggested hospital services for the metropolitan area, recommendation was made for Perth's public hospitals to be classified primary, secondary and tertiary, treating minor complaints, general medicine and complex conditions respectively. The report suggested that Fremantle Hospital's tertiary level services would not be developed, and there was much talk of downgrading it to a secondary-care level. Fremantle citizens were not prepared to accept the move lightly. Already there were 100 patients visiting the Fremantle Hospital cardiologists, and a busy emergency department treated 70,000 people each year. The Minister for Health, Ian Taylor, denied that moves were in hand to actually downgrade the hospital, but inside and outside the hospital opposition to the suggested move swelled. Petitions organised by the nursing staff were signed by over 6,000 people in three weeks. Fremantle's Mayor John Cattalini, declared that he would fight for the hospital's status, public meetings were held, and letters of protest submitted to the press. If the hospital lost its tertiary status, a public meeting at the hospital concluded, it would mean 'death by attrition'. Not until early March, when the Minister for Health gave an assurance that Fremantle Hospital would not be downgraded and that extended care and psychiatric treatment would be improved,[159] did Fremantle people relax their protest.

Could Henry Calvert Barnett who, in 1894, stumped into the boarding house at Point Street and enthused over its potential as a casualty ward, see the improvements and changes in medical care at Fremantle, he would marvel. There are no longer open cesspits in the town. Typhoid, smallpox, cholera and even measles and pneumonia are rare. The laboratory and therapy departments conduct tests and procedures with equipment that would have Barnett shaking his head in disbelief. Computers have revolutionised many departments, from X-ray to administration. A CAT scanner supplements other X-ray equipment; there is an important medical research centre contributing greater knowledge about health and treatment of disease; a chapel with a full-time minister; a pathology department essential for diagnoses; an innovative and supportive psychiatric ward which is suggesting new directions in mental care and development. The pharmacy shelves are lined with drugs which Barnett would consider work miracles. Patients walk days after operations where once it took weeks or months. There is a fine library, staff change and rest rooms, and an operating theatre where many are restored to health. It is yet a time of great change, with financial constraints, with continuing learning which results in new methods and use of resources, and with major differences in the training of nurses. It is a time when people are questioning their rights and roles in society and the workplace.

If he looked further, Barnett would see a concerned community supporting its

[158] R. Marshall, interview.
[159] *Ibid.*

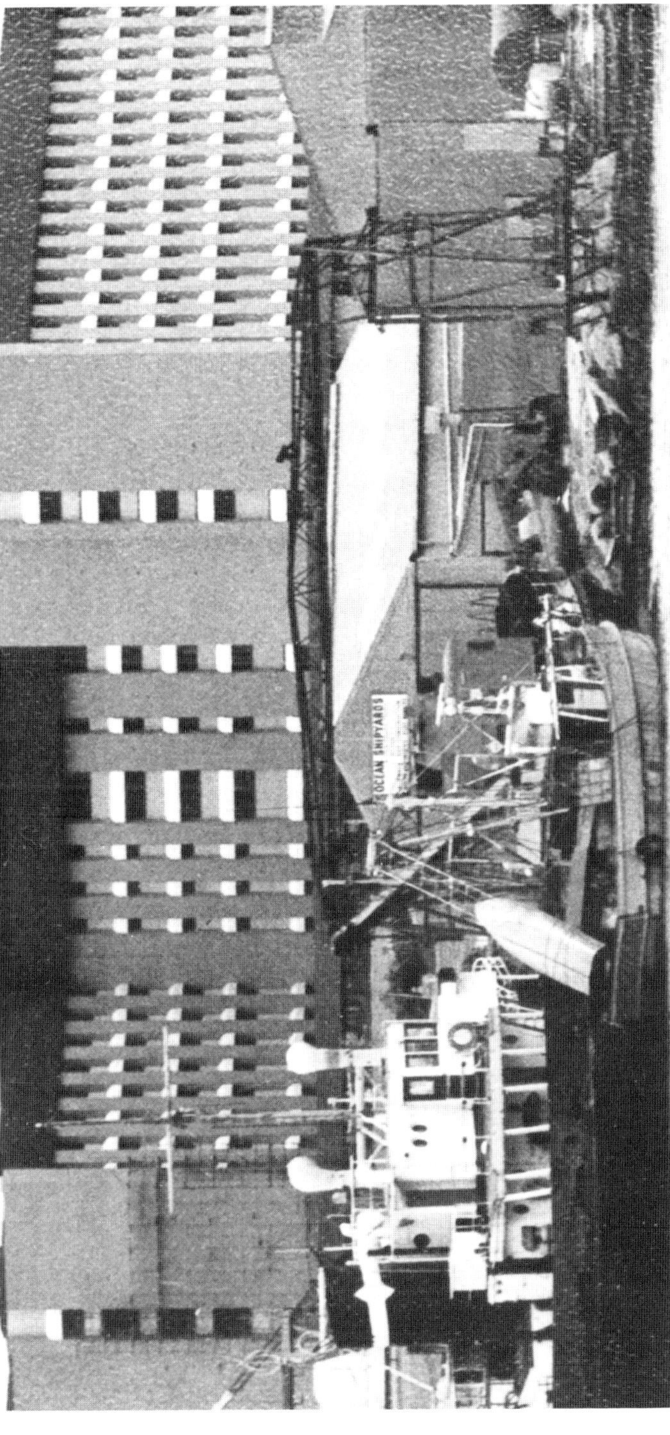

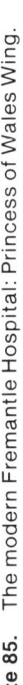

Plate 85. The modern Fremantle Hospital: Princess of Wales Wing.

Photograph courtesy Fremantle Hospital

hospital. A board of management freely gives time and expertise for the benefit of the institution, members of the ladies' auxiliary give hours and energy, keeping open two well-run canteens for staff and patients and raising thousands of dollars for the hospital. Others, including nurses, raise funds both for the hospital and outside concerns such as the asthma foundation, through walkathons, stalls and other means. Children come to sing, or they write to the elderly. Some have Brownie meetings in wards where patients can watch.

'I think that a hospital's a little bit like a church. I don't think it will ever really stop being built,'[160] observed Roy Marshall, the administrator. There are plans to build a new intensive-care unit, another coronary unit, a primary care unit, and in the more distant future, an improved psychiatric ward and a maternity wing. But a hospital is more than bricks and mortar. Care and concern, knowledge and efficiency form the foundations. Relationships between staff, patients, voluntary workers and visitors are important too. Without buttresses of compassion the walls would fall. Pain and peace, joy and laughter also have a place in this building.

One hospital administrator, speaking of the people of Fremantle, explained that Fremantle Hospital 'was *their* hospital and they were fiercely proud of it'.[161] The sentiment is not misplaced. Fremantle Hospital meets the medical needs of those who attend it, and through its motto, gives a blessing to its community: 'Vive Valeque' . . . 'live, and be well'. Barnett and those who have gone before would not be disappointed.

[160]   *Ibid.*
[161]   A. Smith, interview.

APPENDIX 1

NOSOLOGICAL REPORT FOR THE TOWN OF FREMANTLE TO DECEMBER 1833

Medico-Chirurgical Review and Journal of Practical Medicine, 1838

Gleanings during Three Years spent in the Indian Seas.
Swan River and King George's Sound.

For the following sketch, we are indebted to our friend Mr. William Barrett Marshall. Our readers will probably remember a notice of the medical establishment of the British Auxiliary Legion in Spain. This was from the same pen. Mr. Marshall, now one of the surgeons of the Kensington Union, has seen much in the Royal Navy of disease abroad, and has not only seen but observed it. We hope we shall be enabled on many occasions to introduce him to our readers.

Nosological Report, for the Town of Fremantle, in the Colony of Western Australia, from the Commencement of the Colony in 1828, to December 1833.

DISEASES	Number of Cases	Recovered	Died	REMARKS
COELIACA.				
ENTERICA. Dysphagia Mulosa	Six	Six		
PNEUMATICA.				
PNEUMONICA. Bex Convulsiva	Unknown	Unknown	Unknown	No case of this disease occurred in the Colony until after the arrival of the 21st Fusiliers. The Children belonging to the detachment were affected on their arrival. A few of the cases proved fatal at Perth, but none at Fremantle.

DISEASES	Number of Cases	Recovered	Died	REMARKS
HAEMATICA.				
PYRECTICA.				
Auctus Tertiana	Four	Four	. . .	The subjects of this complaint were all sailors, who arrived, sick, in the Colony.
PHLOGOTICA.				
Apostema Empyema				
Empresma	Six	. . .	Six	The patients were Lascars, and brought the disease with them from India.
Cephalitis	Twenty-six	Twenty-six	. . .	The attack was, in every case
Pneumonitis	Four	Four		slight; and yielded readily to the
Gastritis	Two	Two		antiphlogistic treatment.
Enteritis	Three	Two	One	In two out of the three cases,
Hepatitis	Five	Five		the sufferers had been inmates of the Penitentiary at Millbank, and, while there, were attacked with the epidemic dysentery that prevailed.
Ophthalmia.				
O. Purulenta	. . .	. . .	. . .	The number of cases was not to be obtained; every man in the Colony being said to have experienced the disease once at least. In a few instances, it has recurred a second time in the same individual—the greatest sufferers were those of intemperate habits.
Dysenteria.				
D. Acuta	1 Hundred and one	Ninety-five	Six	From Sept. 27th, 1829 to Nov. 20th, 1833—average duration of the complaint, ten days—bloodletting indicated in only four cases.
DYSTHETICA.				
Marasmus Tabes	Three	. . .	Three	One of these cases was that of an invalid from India, the others were of individuals who had the complaint before they came to the Colony.
Porphyra Simplex	Forty	Unknown	. . .	Characterized by soft, spongy bleeding gums; and aggravated by contractions of the joints. It commenced with the arrival of the first settlers, but is now a rare disease, not a case having occurred for 18 months; it proved fatal in numerous instances.

DISEASES	Number of Cases	Recovered	Died	REMARKS
NEUROTICA.				
PHRENICA.				
Ecphronia Mania	Six	Two	One	The death was suicidal. Two of the cases were removed from the Colony, and one is still afflicted.
ESTHETICA.				
Neuralgia faciei	One	. . .	. . .	
manus	One	One	. . .	This case yielded to a course of dietetic and alterative remedies.
SYSTATICA.				
Carus Apoplexia	One	. . .	One	
ECCRITICA.				
CATOTICA.				
Paruria Retentionis	Fifteen	Fifteen	. . .	Ascribed to water-drinking, and dram-drinking both—the water of the place being very brackish; and the greater number of patients, sailors, of alleged intemperate habits.

The data from which the foregoing Report has been drawn up were supplied me by the courtesy and kindness of Mr. Harrison, Assistant Colonial Surgeon. They refer almost entirely to Port Fremantle, and the district within which it is situated. Further particulars I failed to obtain from the Colonial Surgeon who resides at Perth, the capital of the territory—and this report, therefore, only conveys a partial view of the 'ills to which flesh is heir' in the new settlement of Swan River.

The cases of dysentery and scurvy had their origin in privation and want, the earlier settlers having had more than an ordinary share of difficulties to contend with, and having been peculiarly improvident, or unfortunate, or, perhaps, both.

Here, as everywhere else, among civilized men, inebriety has added its multitude of victims to the sick-list—and aggravated the diseases of others—and, in many more instances, indisposed the system to receive benefit from medicine where the disease itself has not arisen from intemperance. Many of the cases of paruria retentionis, empresma cephalitis and ophthalmia, were examples of this.

But, although the ophthalmia which so universally spread among the settlers, assumed an aggravated character when occurring in persons of intemperate habits, its universality must be accounted for in some other way—and to do this is not difficult. Port Fremantle is built on a small isthmus, the sides of which are washed by the waves of the sea on the one hand, and the waters of 'the Swan' on the other. The soil is a white sand, glistening with particles of rock-salt, and crystal, and constituting a mirror from which the glare of the sun is reflected upon the eye of every settler; the houses are, for the most part, built of lime-stone. The winds which set in, alternately, now hot from the land, and now cold from the ocean, lift up the finer grains of sand, and convey them over miles of sea and land by turns—these, touching the eye, irritate, and irritating, inflame. And these, being causes continually present, and universally applicable, will sufficiently account for the prevalence of so painful an affection, in the case of almost every settler in the Colony.

The temperature varying from the freezing point of Fahrenheit to 106°, and frequently differing more than twenty degrees in the same day—and the climate subject to sudden changes, the surprise is that there have happened so few cases of rheumatism. During H.M.S. *Alligator*'s stay at Swan River, December, 1833, the thermometer ranged from 70° to 105° in the shade; the evenings and mornings being much colder than the intermediate portions of the same day. A hot land-wind prevails during the forenoon—a refreshing sea-breeze from the cold South sets-in in the afternoon; the latter is equally conducive to the health and convenience of the inhabitants, cooling the air they breathe, and facilitating their commerce with the interior by means of the principal river.

The numerous cases inserted in the report as cases of empresma cephalitis, can hardly, I should think, deserve so bad a name. I suspect they were cases chiefly of cephalia pulsatilis—arising from exposure to the sun, and principally occurring in persons of drunken habits; the symptoms being, sudden and violent headache, flushed face, vertigo and sickness; but without delirium; continuing not longer, upon an average, than two or three days—and readily yielding to venesection, purgatives, and the application of refrigerant lotions to the head.

The above may serve to convey a tolerable estimate of the state of health in Western Australia, although a register only of diseases occurring in a single locality. Perhaps the modifications of disease in other places is slightly in favour of the inhabitants—as at Perth, the capital of the Colony, where the presence of the Government exerts a salutary influence over the habits of the settlers recommending temperance by its example, and repressing excess by its influence.

There is a colonial surgeon at Perth, A. Collie, Esq. R.N., with a salary of £200. per annum, and, of course, the private practice of the whole of the respectable families located there. There is also an assistant surgeon at Port Fremantle, Mr. Harrison, who has the responsibilities of a surgeon, and the care of the gaol; with the duties of quarantine to attend to besides. Medicines are provided at the Government expense. A room has been fitted up at Perth for the reception of patients, and is sufficiently roomy during the infancy of the settlement, and the paucity of sick poor.

At King George's Sound, Mr. Lyttleton is the Colonial Assistant-Surgeon, with the pay and allowances of an assistant-surgeon in the Army—and At Port Augusta there is a third medical officer, with an allowance of five shillings per diem.

Besides these four medical men, who are permanently attached to the Colony, there were, in December 1833, two others, assistant-surgeons in the Army, Messrs. Davidson and Milligan, who accompanied detachments of His Majesty's 21st Fusiliers, and 63rd Regiment. There was also a private practitioner at Fremantle, who divided the practice of that place with the official one. Two others are said to be living elsewhere, not so much upon their professional earnings, as by their skill in agriculture—to which they have been obliged to turn for that daily bread which the practice of medicine failed to secure to them.

At King George's Sound, I requested Mr. Lyttleton's assistance to draw up an account of the diseases of Albany—and am indebted to him for the concise yet comprehensive intelligence, that all the disease which have befallen the settlers there, had their origin in privation, or in excess. A testimony which speaks volumes for the climate.

[*Extract from the M.S. Journal of W. B. Marshall, R.N., author of* A Personal Narrative of Two Visits to New Zealand, *London, 1836, Nisbet.*]

APPENDIX 2

DR. DAVY—SOME MORE OR LESS LEGENDS

Sunday Times, 7 June 1908

Away back in the late Nineties the late Dr. Davy was a central figure in the social and professional world of the Old Camp. His vast scientific knowledge was unquestioned, and his thorough acquaintance with seven countries and their languages gave him a big pull over argumentative fellow clubmen.

One night, a coterie, including Dr. Davy, A. E. Morgans, Jack Sinclair, Larry Goodrich, and others, were walking home from the said club.

'If I had your learning,' said one of the party to Davy, 'I'd be Prime Minister of England.'

The doctor, who was always painfully hard up, struck a dramatic attitude.

'Then tell me,' he exclaimed pathetically, slapping his chest as he spoke, 'how the devil it is I'm so deucedly hard-up.'

Immediately, as he slapped his chest, there was a burst of flame and smoke from the inside pocket of his coat, wherein was a box of wax matches.

The blow had ignited them!

For a few seconds no-one knew what on earth was the matter.

Then A. E. Morgans tried to wrench the now burning coat off, but the doctor held it closely around him to smother the fire. A night porter rushed out of the adjacent hotel, darted in again, and coming out with a bucket of water, dashed it at the Doctor—and missed.

Jack Sinclair got the lot! By this time A. E. Morgans had got a firm hold on the coat tails, and by a vigorous effort ripped the coat asunder, and, in consequence, sat down violently on the footpath!

Finally the night porter, who had missed with the only available bottle of water, ran back and knocked their heads off, and poured over the burning sawbones the contents of two bottles of lager!

The fire consumed (without seriously burning the wearer), his coat, waistcoat, and braces. And then a policeman came along, and demanded to see the Doctor's visible means of support for his pants!!!

Another yarn, and a true bill.

The Doctor ran a motor, which was reckoned to be absolutely the most erratic machine on the face of the globe.

After a while the public became aware that it was the doctor's playful mechanical eccentricities that accounted for the break-downs.

One day, a week after purchasing the stormy petrol, it whirred suspiciously, gave a few spasmodic coughs, and stopped dead, but with the underneath machinery going around at a terrific rate.

The Doctor jerked and tugged at every available lever and tap, and finally descended, and rushing into the Palace Hotel rang up the agents for the motor-man to come and take the blanketty dash away, and throw it on the scrap heap.

When the Doctor came out he saw a terrific convulsion, the motor, luckily a weak horse power one, was snorting and grinding furiously along the street with half-a-dozen cabmen and as many casuals hanging on to it to keep it back.

Someone had accidentally touched the right button, and set her going.

The ensuing grateful shout cost the Doctor fifteen shillings.

Again:—

The Doctor was once careering madly along the street at fully five miles an hour, when he ran down a Chow, the off-wheels passing over the Mongolian's legs.

With the cunning of the yellow-fanged race the Chow lay quiet on the road, and pretended to be next door to mincemeat.

Seeing what he had done, the doctor gallantly circled around in a big sweep, intending to come up alongside the prostrate Chinkie, and pick him up preparatory to running him to his home, or to the hospital.

Just as he approached the Chow, something went wrong with the stopping gear, and the car kept on full speed!

Then the Doctor lost his head, and consequent control of the stearing gear, and RAN OVER THE CHOW A SECOND TIME!!!

DRYBLOWER

APPENDIX 3

FREMANTLE HOSPITAL TRAINED NURSES
KNOWN TO HAVE SERVED IN
WORLD WAR I

BAILLIE	Lavinia	KIMBER	Alice
BOTTLE	Ruth	KIRKHAM	Sarah
BUTTERLEY	Ellen	LIMPUS	Florence
CARSON	Mary	LOWRIE	Jean
CONNELLY	Annie	LYONS	Lena
EDSALL	Florence	McKAY	Ethel
McGURK	Lily	McLAREN	Lily
HAYES	Mary	WILSON	Edith
HORNSBY	Ada	WOOD	Blanche
KIERNAN	Irene		

Compiled by Victoria Hobbs

APPENDIX 4

PNEUMONIC INFLUENZA

Cases Admitted to Fremantle Hospital
1 August–14 October 1919

Report for	Admitted	Discharged	Died	Remaining In
1–19 August 1919	104	22	33	49
20 August 1919–16 September 1919	41	57	7	26
17 September 1919–14 October 1919	37	46	5	12
	182	125	45	87

Compiled by C. Jeffery from Minutes of BM, FH

APPENDIX 5

FREMANTLE HOSPITAL TRAINED NURSES
KNOWN TO HAVE SERVED IN
WORLD WAR II

[Due to the nature of ill-kept military records
this listing may be incomplete.]

BRAID	Margaret
DAVIS	Hilda
HUGHAN	Isobel Mara
JONES	Ada
KERR	Dolly
McCORMACK	Pat
McDOWELL	Matilda
McELVIE	Elsie
PEGRUM	Ursula
TOPHAM	Nellie
WHEATLEY	Jean

Compiled by Florence Welch and Marjory Thomson

APPENDIX 6

FREMANTLE PUBLIC HOSPITAL:
EX GRADUATES WHO SERVED IN THE
AUSTRALIAN ARMY NURSING SERVICE,
IN WORLD WAR II

BARNARD	Jean Burnside	JOLLEY	Thelma M.
BATES	Lavinia Mary	LEFROY	Margaret
BELL	Edith Margaret	LINDSAY	Janet
BLOWFIELD	Madge	MACKIE	Gwendolyn
BORWICK	Millicent	MALES	Violet
BRAID-YOUNGER	Margaret	MALLETT	Florence
BREARLEY	Alice	MARTIN	Gwen
BUTSON	Ruth	MATTHEWS	Phyllis
CRAIG	Hazel	NICHOLSON	Francis M.
DODD	Jessie	O'DONNELL	May
DRUMMOND	Jean	ONGE	Ella Blair
FIELDING	Edna	PERRYMAN	Dorothy Alice
FREEMAN	Adelia	PRINCE	Helen
GARDINER	Cynthia Catherine	ROBINSON	Jean
HARRIS	Alice	SMITH	Elizabeth
HAWKSLEY	Mary R.	STENT	Maud Annie F.
HEDGES	Christine	THOMSON	Marjory F.
HODGSON	Ethel	VEITCH	Ruth
HOPKINS	Maud Emily	WALTERS	Winifred
JAMIESON	Olga	WELCH	Florence

Compiled by Florence Welch

APPENDIX 7

FREMANTLE HOSPITAL
STAFF NOTICE

General directions are being reissued as hereunder for the benefit of the Staff and in order to obviate the possibility of chaos and panic should an Air raid occur.

Every member of the Staff is urged to co-operate in seeing that these instructions as far as possible are put into effect.

1. A Warning will be given by short blasts on a siren for two minutes that a raid is impending and when the raid is over, one long blast for two minutes will be given.

2. Immediately the siren is heard each member of the staff will take up his or her allotted duty as previously determined.

3. The control officer will take up duty in the Board Room from where general instructions will be issued.

4. The Secretary, as Chief Executive Officer has been appointed the Control officer and the Assistant Secretary, Deputy Control Officer. Should the raid occur at night or at any time during the absence of the control officer or his deputy then the Matron will assume this responsibility or in her absence the Assistant Matron, until such time as the Control officer takes up duty or appoints another deputy.

5. The Sisters in charge should immediately prepare for emergencies as follows:

   A. All patients in the *alcoves* to be shifted into the wards, out of danger from flying Glass.

   B. List of patients for transfer to their homes to be supplied immediately to the Control officer who will arrange for transport and evacuation by the Transport Officer appointed.

   C. All windows to be adjusted so that the bottom sash protected by wire netting covers the upper window. The Sister in charge of each ward or Department *must make certain* that this precaution is strictly carried out.

   D. Primus stoves and hurricane lamps to be placed in readiness.

   E. If the raid occurs at night time the blinds in every section of the Hospital must be *correctly* drawn to obtain a *complete* black-out.

   F. Water supplies should be conserved in Baths, sinks, kettles or any other available receptacles.

6. *Fire Fighting parties* should take up their allotted positions under the fire fighting control officer or in his absence under the direction of the Hospital control officer or one of his deputies.

7. Theatre & Minor theatre staffs to take up duty in order to be in complete readiness.

8. The following Departments will not be in operation during an Air raid and the Staff should report immediately to the Control officer for instructions:

   > Path. Laboratory.
   > X-ray Department.
   > Orthopaedic Department.
   > Out-patients' Department.
   > V.D. Clinic.

9. The rest of the Staff not under the control of the Matron immediately take up duty in their allotted posts and await instructions from the control officer.

10. The Gas main will be turned off immediately the Raid occurs.

11. The boiler will be reduced to ten (10) lbs of steam pressure.

12. Should a fire be reported in any section of the Hospital, the Control officer will issue instructions for the Electric light switch at the main to be turned off, and all duties thereafter must be carried out by the aid of any other lighting systems available.

13. If the raid occurs at night the members of the Staff off duty should see that the windows and blinds in *all sections* of the quarters are correctly adjusted according to instructions. They should also seek shelter as may be provided or stay indoors in that part of the premises offering most wall protection from flying glass.

14. If Incendiary bombs fall and no fire party is near, the matter must be immediately reported to the control officer.

15. The Telephone *must not* be used during an Air raid except in cases of extreme urgency.

16. The traffic officer appointed will take up duty to control traffic in order to avoid congestion—at our entrance and exit.

The following are general hints that it would be useful to observe.

1. Ward Sisters should appoint nurses or maids for special duties as here under:
   A. Attending to the windows and blinds as instructed.
   B. Attending to patients to be evacuated.
   C. Filling Receptacles for water supplies.
   D. Other duties for emergencies.

2. All fire escapes to be kept clear of anything that might prevent easy access to them.

3. All trade waste, paper etc. to be disposed of daily to reduce fuel for fire to a minimum.

4. Have a point of assembly on each floor for evacuation.

5. Fire fighting equipment provided to be got in readiness by Staff appointed.

6. Heads of Departments & Wards to prevent panic among patients and Staff.

7. See that all bottles containing spirits of any kind are kept correctly corked.

8. If bathing or helping to bath a patient, never touch electric equipment or appliances that are being used in a bathroom, do not stand on the floor if it is wet.

9. To prevent being overcome by smoke the best precaution is to throw yourself flat on the floor and crawl towards the fire escape, stairs or open window. Should you open the window to summon help, put your head out and then pull the window down on the neck and spread your arms out along the opening to prevent the inflow of air.

APPENDIX 8

FREMANTLE HOSPITAL
RULES FOR PATIENTS

(1) Patients, when able, are requested to help in the needful duties of the Wards, and attend upon other Patients and do such light work as requested by the Nurses.

(2) Patients are to keep their beds neat and tidy, the bed clothes properly arranged, and attend scrupulously to personal cleanliness; and are to assist in keeping the premises clean by depositing all rubbish in the receptacles provided for that purpose.

(3) Patients' valuables or money must not be held in the Ward, but be forwarded through two members of the Staff to the General Office, where a receipt will be issued for the property so received.

(4) All parcels, food or drink brought into the Ward shall be examined by the Nurse-in-charge.

(5) Patients found gambling or using profane or indecent language, or being intoxicated shall be liable to instant discharge by the Medical Superintendent.

(6) Patients are not allowed to leave the precincts of the Hospital without the special permission of the Medical Superintendent.

(7) Patients are not permitted to wander around the grounds but must remain in the vicinity of the Wards.

(8) Any breach of the above rules will render a Patient liable to instant discharge from the Hospital.

By Order,
J. M. SCRYMGEOUR,
Managing Secretary.

19th JUNE 1950

Bibliography

Official Records — Unpublished

Colonial Secretary's Office. Correspondence (W.A. State Archives).
Minutes of Fremantle Local Board of Health 1886-1902.
Minutes of Fremantle Municipal Council.
Plans of Fremantle Hospital (Building Management Authority).
Public Health Department Files (W.A. State Archives).
Registers of Deaths, Fremantle District (W.A. State Archives).
Supreme Court Records (held in Supreme Court of W.A.).

Official Records — Published

Legislative Assembly Rolls 1904.
Statutes of Western Australia.
Western Australian Blue Books.
Western Australian Government Gazette.
Western Australian Industrial Gazette.
Western Australian Parliamentary Debates.
Western Australian Votes and Proceedings of Parliament.
Western Australian Year Books.

Reports

O'Connor, S. and Thompson, R., 'Report into the Aboriginal Heritage of the Arthur Head Area, Fremantle', Fremantle City Council, 1984.
Harrison, T., 'Nosological Report, for the Town of Fremantle, in the Colony of Western Australia, from the Commencement of the Colony in 1828, to December 1833', in *Medico-Chirurgical Review and Journal of Practical Medicine*, no. 5, vol. 28, 1838.

Fremantle Hospital Records — Primary

Annual Reports, June 1940-1984 (incomplete).
Clinical Supervisor: Reports on Nurses, June 1951-May 1952.
Fremantle Hospital Collectors' Book, 1933-1944.
House Surgeons' Report Books, December 1924-July 1937.
Major Operation Theatre Books, 1908-1916; 1935-1944.
Matrons' Report Books, 2 October 1903-28 February 1911.
Minutes of the Board of Management, 1908-1987.
Minutes of the Building Committee, 13 February 1961-9 April 1974.
Minutes of the Executive Committee, August 1933-August 1949.

Minutes of the Honorary Staff, Fremantle Hospital, March 1937-March 1955.
Minutes of the House Committee—various volumes to 1933 (incomplete).
Miscellaneous correspondence Fremantle Hospital, 1939–1942.
Notebook, 'The P.T.S.', kept by Matron Olive Jones.
Nurse Mavis Fuller's Lecture Notes, 1926.
Plans of Fremantle Hospital—various.
Register, 'Male V.D. 1941', Fremantle Hospital.
Rules and Regulations of the Fremantle Hospital, 1898.
Scrap Books, Random News Clippings, 1909–1938, 1948–1962, 1962–1969.

Fremantle Hospital Records — Secondary

Lane, N. J., 'A History of the Laboratory Services 1939–1985', Fremantle Hospital, 1986.

Notes and Private Papers

Boordaak School, Notes, FH.
Buzza, R. (née Bowden), Notes, FH.
Christie, M., Notes, FH.
Cole, K., Notes: 'History of the Pathology Lab., Fremantle Hospital', FH.
Curran, J. (née Strange), Notes, FH.
Davies, E., Notes, FH.
Davis, M. (née Mawson), Notes, FH.
Edinger, P. (née Murray), Notes, FH.
Foster, N. J., Notes. FCL.
Garswell, Notes, FH.
Gaughin, L. (née Hamilton), Notes, FH.
Gray, Mrs E. H., Notes, FH.
Grimshaw, K., Notes, FH.
Hanrahan, A., Notes, FH.
Hardey, J., Diary 1830–39 (WA State Archives, Acc. No. 566A), BL.
Hatch, M. (née Borwick), Notes, FH.
Heath, H. (née Hannaford), Notes, FH.
Jeffery, C., Notes, FH.
Lancaster, J., Notes, FH.
Lane, M., Notes, FCL.
McCarthy, Doreen, Notes, FH.
McPherson, M., Notes, FH.
Moorehouse, L., Notes, FH.
Morgan, R. (née Hood), Notes, FH.
Morrisey, J. (née Bailey), Notes, FH.
Pilling, B. (née Weedon), Notes, FH.
Peek, H. (née McCall), Notes, FH.
Roper, E. (née Bell), Notes, FH.
Semmens, D. (née Clark), Notes, FH.
Toy, N. (née Gray), Notes, FH.

Newspapers

Daily News
Evening Mail
Evening Times
Fremantle Advocate
Fremantle Gazette
Fremantle Districts Sentinel
Fremantle Herald

Independent Review
Inquirer
Morning Herald
Perth Gazette
Sunday Times
Truth
West Australian
Western Mail
Westralian Worker

Books, Articles and Theses

ABEL-SMITH, B., *A History of the Nursing Profession*. London: Heinemann, 1960.

ABEL-SMITH, B., *The Hospitals 1800–1948: A Study in Social Administration in England and Wales*. London: Heinemann, 1964.

APPLEYARD, R. T. and MANFORD, T., *The Beginning: European Discovery and Early Settlement of Swan River, Western Australia*. Nedlands: UWAP, 1979.

ASHDOWN, A. M., *A Complete System of Nursing*. London: J. M. Dent and Sons Ltd, 1924.

BARBALET, Margaret, *The Adelaide Children's Hospital 1876–1976*. Netley: The Griffin Press, 1975.

BARNETT, H. C., 'Suggestions Respecting Sanitary Improvement in Western Australia' [pamphlet]. Perth: R. Pether, Government Printer, 1876.

BATTYE, J. S. (ed.), *Cyclopaedia of Western Australia*, 2 vols. Perth: Cyclopaedia Co., 1912–13.

BELL, E. M., *The Story of Hospital Almoners: The Birth of a Profession*. London: Faber and Faber, 1961.

BERNDT, Ronald M. and Catherine H., *Aborigines of the West, Their Past and Their Present*. Nedlands: UWAP, 1979.

BERRYMAN, I. (ed.), *A Colony Detailed. The First Census of Western Australia 1832*. North Perth: Creative Research, 1979.

BERSON, M., *Cockburn: The Making of a Community*. Cockburn: The Town of Cockburn, 1978.

BOLTON, G. C., *A Fine Country to Starve In*. Nedlands: UWAP, 1972.

BOLTON, G. C., 'Who Were the Pensioners?', in C. T. Stannage (ed.), *Studies in Western Australian History*, Vol. IV, December 1981.

BOLTON, G. C. and HUNT, S., 'Cleansing the Dunghill: Water Supply and Sanitation in Perth 1878–1912', *Studies in Western Australian History*, Vol. II, March 1987.

BOLTON, G. C. and JOSKE, P., *History of Royal Perth Hospital*. Nedlands: UWAP, 1982.

BROWN, M., 'Probationary Prisoner 270: Thomas Bushell', in C. T. Stannage (ed.), *Studies in Western Australian History*, Vol IV, December 1981.

BRUCE, J. W., 'West Coast Radiography', in *The Radiographer*, Vol. 21, No. 5, December 1974.

BURTON JACKSON, J. L., *Not an Idle Man: A Biography of John Septimus Roe, Western Australia's First Surveyor-General (1797–1878)*. Fremantle: FACP, 1982.

CARTER, J., *Bassendean: A Social History 1829–1979*, Bassendean Town Council, 1986.

CHAPMAN, B., *The Colonial Eye*, The Art Gallery of Western Australia, 1979.

COHEN, B. C., *A History of Medicine in Western Australia*. Perth: Paterson Brokensha, 1965.

COLEBATCH, H. (ed.), *A Story of A Hundred Years: Western Australia 1829–1929*. Perth: Fred Wm Simpson, 1929.

COTTESLOE, Lord (ed.), *Diary and Letters of Admiral C. H. Fremantle, G.C.B. Relating to the Founding of the Colony of Western Australia 1829*. Fremantle: FACP, 1979 (first published London, 1928).

COWAN, E. D., 'Letters of Early Settlers', *RWAHS*, Vol. 1, Pt 1, 1927.

COWAN, P. (ed.), *A Faithful Picture: Letters of Eliza and Thomas Brown at York in the Swan River Colony 1841-1852*. Fremantle: FACP, 1977.

CROWLEY, F. K., *Australia's Western Third: A History of Western Australia from the first settlements to modern times*. Melbourne: Heinemann, 1960.

CROWLEY, F. K. and de GARIS, B. K., *A Short History of Western Australia*. South Melbourne: Macmillan, 1969.

CUFF, H. E. and PUGH, W. T. G., *Practical Nursing including Hygiene and Diabetics*. London: William Blackwood and Sons, 1924.

CUMPSTON, J. H. L., *Influenza and Maritime Quarantine in Australia*. Melbourne: Albert J. Mullett, 1919.

CUMPSTON, J. H. L., 'The Evolution of Public Health Administration in Australia', in *The Medical Journal of Australia*, February 1932.

CUMPSTON, J. H. L., *The History of Plague in Australia 1900-1925*. Melbourne: H. J. Green, 1926.

CUMPSTON, J. H. L., *The History of Small-Pox in Australia, 1788-1908*, Commonwealth of Australia, Quarantine Service Publication No. 3, 1914.

CUMPSTON, J. H. L. and McCALLUM, F., *The History of Small-Pox in Australia 1909-1923*. Melbourne: H. J. Green, Government Printer, 1925.

DE MOUNCEY, P. E. C., 'The Historic Duel at Fremantle Between George French Johnson, a Merchant, and William Nairne Clarke, a Solicitor, in the Year 1832', *RWAHS*, Vol. 1, Part V, 1929.

Dictionary of Western Australians 1829-1914 (also known as W.A. Biographical Index), various volumes. Nedlands: UWAP, 1979.

DUNN, F., *A Speck in the Sky: A History of Airlines of Western Australia*. Australia: Airlines of Western Australia, 1984.

ELLIS, A. S., *Eloquent Testimony: The Story of the Mental Health Services in Western Australia 1830-1975*. Nedlands: UWAP, 1984.

EWERS, J. K., *The Western Gateway: A History of Fremantle*. Nedlands: UWAP, 1971 (2nd edition).

FACEY, A. B., *A Fortunate Life*. Ringwood: Penguin, 1981.

FERNIE, W. T., *Kitchen Physic: At Hand for the Doctor, and Helpful for Homely Cures*. Bristol: John Wright & Co., 1901.

FORSTER, A. L., 'Physiotherapy: A Response to a Challenge', *The Australian Journal of Physiotherapy*, Vol. 21, No. 4, December 1975.

GAULT, E. W. and LUCAS A., *A Century of Compassion: A History of the Austin Hospital*. Melbourne: Macmillan, 1882.

GROVES, E. W. and Fortescue-Brickdale, J. M., *Text Book for Nurses: Anatomy, Physiology, Surgery and Medicine*. London: Humphrey Milford, 1925 (3rd edition).

HAGGER, J., *Australian Colonial Medicine*. Adelaide: Rigby, 1979.

HAMERSLEY, H., 'Radiation Science and Australian Medicine 1886-1914', in *Historical Records of Australian Science*, Vol. 5, No. 3, 1982.

HASLUCK, A., *Thomas Peel of Swan River*. Melbourne: OUP, 1965.

HITCHCOCK, J. K., *The History of Fremantle: The Front Gate of Australia 1829-1929*. Fremantle: The S. H. Lamb Printing House, 1929.

HOBBS, V., *But Westward Look: Nursing in Western Australia 1829-1979*. Nedlands: UWAP, 1980.

HUNT, L., *Westralian Portraits*. Nedlands: UWAP, 1979.

INGLIS, K. S., *Hospital and Community: A History of the Royal Melbourne Hospital*. Carlton: MUP, 1958.

JACOBSEN, E., *Tinctures and Tact*. Perth: St George Books, 1982.

JAMES, R. M., *The Meath Story: A History of the Ministering Children's League and the Cottesloe Convalescent Home*. Perth: Meath Ministering League Anglican Home, Western Australia, Anglican Diocese of Perth, 1982.

JOSKE, E. J. P., 'Health and Hospital: A Study of Community Welfare in Western Australia 1829-55', MA thesis, UWA, 1973.

KERR, W., 'Architecture in Fremantle 1875-1915', Dissertation towards degree, Bachelor of Architecture, UWA, 1973.

KIMBERLEY, W. B., *History of West Australia: A Narrative of her Past together with Biographies of her Leading Men*. Melbourne: F. W. Niven, 1897.

LEE, Jack, *This is East Fremantle: The Story of a Town and its People*. West Perth: Publication Printers, 1979.

McWHINNEY, A., *A History of Pharmacy in Western Australia*. Perth: The Pharmaceutical Council of Western Australia, 1975.

MAGGS, C., 'Oral History and Nursing History', *Nursing Times*, 19 October 1983.

MAGGS, C., *The Origins of General Nursing*. London: Croom Helm, 1983.

MILLETT, Mrs E., *An Australian Parsonage or, the Settler and the Savage in Western Australia*. Nedlands: UWA (facsimile ed., 1980. First published 1872.)

MITCHELL, Ann M., *The Hospital South of the Yarra: A history of Alfred Hospital Melbourne from foundation to the nineteen-forties*. Netley: The Griffin Press, 1977.

MOORE, G. F., *Diary of Ten Years Eventful Life of an Early Settler in Western Australia*. Nedlands: UWAP (facsimile edition 1978. First published 1884.)

NAIRN J., *Walter Padbury: His Life and Times*. Padbury: North Stirling Press, 1985.

NIGHTINGALE, F., *Notes on Nursing: What it is and what it is not*. Glasgow and London: Blackie, 1974 (first published 1859).

OGLE, N., *The Colony of Western Australia: A Manual for Emigrants 1839*. London: James Fraser, 1839 (reprinted Sydney: J. Ferguson, 1977).

OSBORNE, G. and MANDLE, W. F., *New History: Studying Australia Today*. Sydney: George Allen and Unwin, 1982.

PASQUARELLI, G., 'The General Medical and Associated Problems of the Italian Migrant Family', *The Medical Journal of Australia*, 8 January 1966.

PEARN J. and O'CARRIGAN C., *Australia's Quest for Colonial Health: some influences on early health and medicine in Australia*, Dept of Child Health, 1983.

PERRY, W., 'Major General Sir Charles Rosenthal, Soldier Architect and Musician', *The Victorian Historical Magazine*, Vol. 40, No. 3, August 1969.

PHILLIPS, P., *To Comfort Always. A Hospital and its Community*. Adelaide: The Griffin Press, 1976.

PRESTON, F. I., *Lady Doctor Vintage Model*. Wellington: A. H. & A. W. Reed, 1974.

RAFFA, J., *The Happy Children*. Perth: Artlook Books, 1984.

REECE, R. and PASCOE, R., *A Place of Consequence: A Pictorial History of Fremantle*. Fremantle: FACP, 1983.

REID, P. D., 'A Brief History of the Influence of Friendly Societies', work as part of course at Graylands Teachers' College, 1956, BL Q334.7.

ROE, J. (ed.), *Social Policy in Australia: Some Perspectives 1901-1975*. Stanmore: Carsell Australia, 1976.

ROSNER, D., *A Once Charitable Enterprise: Hospitals and Health Care in Brooklyn and New York, 1885-1915*. Cambridge: CAP, 1982.

SHANN, E. O. G., *Cattle Chosen. The Story of the First Group Settlement in Western Australia 1829-1841*. Nedlands: UWAP, 1978 (facsimile edition. First published 1926.)

SMITH, F. B., *The People's Health 1830-1910*. Canberra: ANU, 1979.

SNOW, D., *The Progress of Public Health in Western Australia 1829-1977*, Public Health Dept, 1981.

SPILLMAN, K., *Identity Prized: A History of Subiaco*. Nedlands: UWAP, 1985.

STANLEY, N. (ed.), *The First Quarter Century (1957-1982)*. Nedlands: UWAP, 1982.

STANNAGE, C. T., *The People of Perth: A Social History of Western Australia's Capital City*. Perth: Perth City Council, 1979.

STANNAGE, C. T. (gen. ed.), *A New History of Western Australia*. Nedlands: UWAP, 1981.

STATHAM, P. (compiler and researcher), *The Tanner Letters: A Pioneer Saga of Swan River and Tasmania 1831–1845*. Nedlands: UWAP, 1981.

STUBBE, J. H., *Medical Background: Being a History of Fremantle Hospitals and Doctors*. Nedlands: UWAP, 1969.

TEMPLETON, J., *Prince Henry's: The Evolution of a Melbourne Hospital 1869–1969*. Melbourne: Robertson & Mullens, 1969.

THOMAS, J. E. and STEWART, A., *Imprisonment in Western Australia: Evolution, Theory and Practice*. Nedlands: UWAP, 1978.

TRUTHFUL Thomas (pseud.), *Through the Spy-Glass: Short Sketches of Well-known Westralians as Others See Them*. Perth: Praagh & Lloyd, 1905.

UHL, J., *Mount Royal Hospital: A Social History*. Maryborough: Hedges & Bell, 1981,

VOGEL, M., *The Invention of the Modern Hospital: Boston 1870–1930*. Chicago: University of Chicago Press, 1980.

W.A. Parent, Vol. 2, No. 1, March 1980, 'Catering for Sick Students'.

WILLIAMS, G., *The Age of Miracles: Medicine and Surgery in the Nineteenth Century*. London: Constable, 1981.

WOODWARD, J., *To Do the Sick No Harm: A Study of the British Voluntary Hospital System to 1875*. London: Routledge and Kegan Paul, 1974.

Interviews — Fremantle Hospital.

Sister L. Allen, interviewed by C. Jeffery, 28 August 1985.

Nurse L. Anderson, interviewed by C. Jeffery, 24 July 1987.

Doctor S. Barrington Knight, interviewed by C. Jeffery, 10 December 1986.

Surgeon F. Bell, interviewed by C. Jeffery, 14 March 1987.

Chairman of the Board C. C. Bennett, interviewed by C. Jeffery, 23 March, 3 April and 1 May 1985.

Chief Physiotherapist R. Black, interviewed by C. Jeffery, 10 September 1987.

Domestic A. Brain, interviewed by J. Lancaster, April 1987.

Surgeon L. Daly-Smith, interviewed by C. Jeffery, June to July 1984.

Pharmacist J. Dickson, interviewed by C. Jeffery, 27 March and 12 June 1987.

Doctor H. Ferguson, interviewed by C. Jeffery, 10 July 1987.

Sister S. Fitzgerald, interviewed by C. Jeffery, 10 September 1987.

Patient H. Fosbery, interviewed by C. Jeffery, 11 July 1987.

Secretary L. Frame, interviewed by C. Jeffery, 31 July 1987.

Deputy Matron M. Fuller, interviewed by C. Jeffery, 18 November and 13 December 1984.

Tutor Sister A. Harris, interviewed by C. Jeffery, 24 November and 1 December 1984.

Sister H. Heath, interviewed by C. Jeffery, 15 May 1984.

Director of Nursing O. Hedemann, interviewed by C. Jeffery, 11 October 1985 and 11 and 19 April 1986.

Sister V. Hobbs, interviewed by C. Jeffery, 21 January and 5 February 1985.

Pathologist J. Holme, interviewed by C. Jeffery, 5 March 1986.

Storeman G. Hunt, interviewed by C. Jeffery, 13 August 1987.

Chief Pharmacist J. Jeffery, interviewed by C. Jeffery, 1985 to 1986.

Engineer M. Jones, interviewed by C. Jeffery, 9 July 1987.

Matron O. Jones, interviewed by C. Jeffery, May to July 1984.

Chief Technologist N. Lane, interviewed by C. Jeffery, 27 July and 3 September 1987.

Medical Superintendent G. Leyland, interviewed by C. Jeffery, 25 June and 9 July 1987.

Matron M. Leworthy, interviewed by C. Jeffery, 3 and 17 April 1985.

Doctor N. Marinovich, interviewed by C. Jeffery, 24 September 1987.

Teacher B. Marshall, interviewed by C. Jeffery, 7 August 1987.

Carpenter L. Marshall, interviewed by C. Jeffery, 4 February 1986.

Administrator R. Marshall, interviewed by C. Jeffery, 20 and 28 February and 6 March 1987.

Doctor M. Mayrhofer, interviewed by C. Jeffery, 21 May and 5 June 1987.
Doctor D. McCarthy, interviewed by C. Jeffery, 3 April 1987.
Radiographer J. Millar, interviewed by C. Jeffery, 26 January 1987
Surgeon M. Minchin, interviewed by C. Jeffery, 15 August 1985.
Sister B. Needle, interviewed by C. Jeffery, 31 August 1985.
Chairman of the Board H. Olney, interviewed by C. Jeffery, 9 March 1986.
Nurse E. D. Parker, interviewed by J. Lancanster, 1986.
Sister H. Peek, interviewed by J. Lancaster, 1987.
Orderly V. Poklad, interviewed by C. Jeffery, 30 August 1985.
Radiographer J. Pugh, interviewed by C. Jeffery, 2 September 1985.
Wardsmaid J. Purdy, interviewed by C. Jeffery, 5 September 1985.
Medical Superintendent J. Rowe, interviewed by C. Jeffery, October 1984 to February 1985.
Plumber G. Schneider, interviewed by C. Jeffery, 5 April 1987.
Almoner N. Seadon, interviewed by C. Jeffery, 21, 23 and 28 August 1985.
Administrator A. Smith, interviewed by C. Jeffery, June to July 1985.
Medical Superintendent P. Smith, interviewed by C. Jeffery, October 1985 to October 1986.
Doctor E. Strahan, interviewed by C. Jeffery, 26 June and 3 July 1987.
G. Trivett (Red Cross), interviewed by C. Jeffery, 5 and 18 December 1984.
Doctor H. Uther Baker, interviewed by C. Jeffery, 27 March and 7 April 1986.
Sister D. Western, interviewed by C. Jeffery, 29 March and 4 April 1987.
Patient and Telephonist W. Wilkinson, interviewed by C. Jeffery, 2 September 1985.
Doctor C. Wilson, interviewed by C. Jeffery, 11 November 1985.
Seamstress A. Wren, interviewed by C. Jeffery, 10 September 1987.
Occupational Therapist E. Wylie, interviewed by C. Jeffery, 5 September 1987.

Interviews — Fremantle City Library.

C. Crowther, interviewed by M. Howroyd, 28 October 1983.
H. Fletcher, interviewed by L. Stevens, 17 and 24 November and 2 December 1981.
M. Foster, interviewed by G. Fowler, 27 March 1983.
S. Gore, interviewed by G. Fowler, 3 October 1980.
F. Harrison, interviewed by M. Howroyd, 8 February 1984.
A. Healy, interviewed by G. Fowler, 12 March 1983.
S. M. Kingsbury, interviewed by M. Howroyd, 12 March 1984.
F. Manns, interviewed by M. Howroyd, 9 December 1983.
E. McGuffie, interviewed by A. Reid, 8 September 1983.
M. Mundy, interviewed by L. Stevens, 12 September 1979.
E. Notley, interviewed by M. Howroyd, 13 April 1984.
A. Parry, interviewed by L. Lauder and J. Brodsgaard, 5 February 1975.
A. Prior, interviewed by D. Brooks, 16 April 1985.
N. Silich, interviewed by L. Stevens, 17 and 24 September 1983 and 14 January 1984.
H. V. Sunderland, interviewed by L. Stevens, 27 February and 13 March 1985.
F. Thacker, interviewed by M. Howroyd, 22 November and 13 December 1983.
L. Thomas, interviewed by M. Davis, 25 May 1984.
E. Ulrich, interviewed by M. Howroyd, 24 February 1984.
H. A. Watson, interviewed by M. Howroyd, 7 and 8 May 1984.
H. Wilkison, interviewed by M. Scott and K. MacGill, April 1976.
A. Williams, interviewed by M. Howroyd, 25 October 1983.
W. E. Wray, interviewed by M. Howroyd, 9 and 10 May 1984.

Interviews — Battye Library.

Doctor C. Anderson, interviewed by M. Adams, June 1981 to September 1983.
Sister R. Bottle, interviewed by V. Hobbs, 1975.
Sister M. Lund, interviewed by C. Jeffery, 2 December 1985.

Index

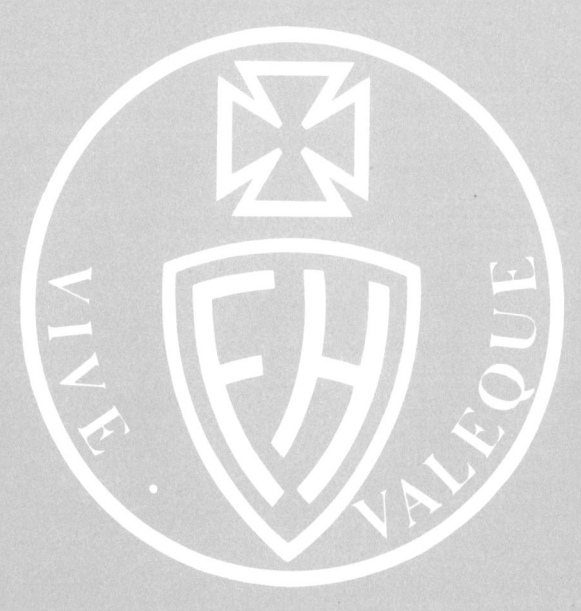